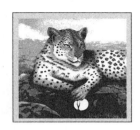

FATAL PAUSES

Getting Unstuck Through

the **Power of No** and the **Power of Go**

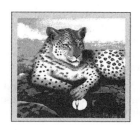

FATAL PAUSES

Getting Unstuck Through

the **Power of No** and the **Power of Go**

By

Stuart C. Yudofsky, M.D.

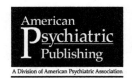

American **P**sychiatric Publishing

A Division of American Psychiatric Association

Washington, DC
London, England

If you would like to buy between 25 and 99 copies of this or any other American Psychiatric Publishing title, you are eligible for a 20% discount; please contact Customer Service at appi@psych.org or 800-368-5777. If you wish to buy 100 or more copies of the same title, please e-mail us at bulksales@psych.org for a price quote.

Copyright © 2015 American Psychiatric Association
ALL RIGHTS RESERVED

Manufactured in the United States of America on acid-free paper
18　17　16　15　14　　5　4　3　2　1
First Edition

Typeset in Trade Gothic and Janson Text.

American Psychiatric Publishing

A Division of American Psychiatric Association
1000 Wilson Boulevard
Arlington, VA 22209-3901
www.appi.org

Library of Congress Cataloging-in-Publication Data

Yudofsky, Stuart C., author.
　Fatal pauses : stuck in pause and getting unstuck through the power of no and the power of go / by Stuart C. Yudofsky. — First edition.
　　p. ; cm.
　Includes bibliographical references and index.
　ISBN 978-1-58562-500-0 (pb : alk. paper)
　I. Title.
　[DNLM: 1. Mental Disorders—therapy—Case Reports. 2. Psychotherapy, Psychodynamic—Case Reports. 3. Cognitive Therapy—Case Reports. 4. Self Care—Case Reports. WM 420.5.P75]
　RC455.4.I56
　155.9'3—dc23

2014020315

British Library Cataloguing in Publication Data
A CIP record is available from the British Library.

To Beth,

there's a lambence,

a soft luminous quality to the light,

as though it came not just from today.

—William Faulkner

Light in August

CONTENTS

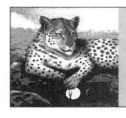

Preface: "Pause"

Simply dashing
in vertical slashings,
you pose in parallel
to pause.
"Press me to hold out!
Press me to hold over!
Press me and hold on!
Press down to hold up,"
is your
buttoned-down beckon.
Mind to muscle,
skin to plastic,
we do press down,
and we are held up.
But you press on
to distort our sense
of time
and self
to keep us down.
Conceived by engineering,
deceived by marketing,
you disguise to entice.
"I'm here to help you,"
you say.
Yes, we've all heard that before.
And yes,
we've been betrayed to believe
you're our harmless tool,
a Trojan tool
to infect us
with the virus
of your metaphor:
"Wait a while.
Process what you've experienced.

Think it through a bit
before you act."
"Take a break!"
Sounds so sound,
so reasonable,
doesn't it?
Until we ask,
"Who brakes what?"
"What breaks whom?"
And
"For how long?"
Your virus
invades our very cells
to seduce the splicings
of our DNA
with your dilatory code.
You replicate our wait.
You hold us up.
Until we ask,
"For how long
must we pause?"
And you say,
"Be patient!"
Our bodies did not evolve
to resist your fatal germ.
We weren't spawned
to stall.
Until we ask,
"Did we devolve
To need suspenders?"
To be patient patients?
"Can our chemistries
catch up
to what they've hatched?"
"Do we submit
to the stings
of your switch?"
and
For how long?
Beware, be wary
of the
Pause button.

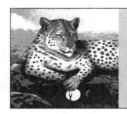# Acknowledgments

As the initial incentive to write this book came from my patients and from readers of a previous book, *Fatal Flaws*, I am deeply grateful to them all. They had requested written information about the "3-D method" that I had used to help them get "unstuck" from a wide range of psychosocial problems that had unsettled them for protracted periods of time. This book is the product of their requests.

Lynn Yudofsky, M.D., "our middle daughter," originated the concept and name of the *Power of Go*. This concept is derived from techniques that she and I use for our personal and professional improvement—especially to accomplish those tasks that we would prefer to delay or not to do at all, such as exercising or completing administrative paperwork.

I thank my dear, career-long friend and colleague, Robert E. Hales, M.D., M.B.A., Editor of American Psychiatric Publishing's Books Division. Bob provided me with encouragement and wise, practical editorial guidance throughout the three years of my writing *Fatal Pauses*. Beth Yudofsky, M.D., my beloved wife and esteemed professional partner, read and gently critiqued every word of this book, and her suggestions and input transformed the final product. She collaborated with our eldest daughter, Elisa Yudofsky Nord, to craft the menu selections for those readers who might dare to try the Fatal Pauses 3-D Diet (Chapter 6, "Stuck in My Body, Part II (Decide and Discipline)"). And to complete this "family project," our youngest daughter, Emily Yudofsky, who is employed at a high-technology firm in Silicon Valley, California, and our son-in-law, Daniel Nord, a computer sciences engineer, who also works in California in a large company that develops video games, both read and revised Chapters 12 and 13, "Stuck in Adolescence and Cyberspace," to ensure the accuracy of technical aspects of computer games and compulsive gaming. Additionally, because I am not well versed in video games, I enlisted the help of Robert T. Brockman II, a brilliant computer scientist and electrical engineer. Robert insisted that I learn to play a wide range of video games so that I could write with some authenticity about this subject. He also helped me understand subtleties and intricacies in the development and design of computer games that could lead to a person's becoming dependent on them to the point of withdrawing from real-life interpersonal relationships.

For more than a quarter of a century I have worked on many books with the gifted editorial team at American Psychiatric Publishing. From the inception of the concept of this book until the book was published, Rebecca Rinehart, Publisher, and John McDuffie, Associate Publisher, provided me with unwavering encouragement, steadfast support, and vital direction. Greg Kuny, Managing Editor, oversaw all aspects of this project, and they went swimmingly. A consummate professional and warm and gracious person, Greg is a person with whom it is an absolute pleasure to work. I thank Rick Prather for designing the beautiful cover and for the many other seminal technical and visual elements that improved the readability and aesthetics of the book. The American Psychiatric Publishing marketing team, comprising Alyson Stiffel, Christie Couture, and Patrick Hansard, have worked hard to promote the book and ensure that those who might benefit from *Fatal Pauses* know of its existence.

In writing *Fatal Pauses*, I strived to craft every sentence in a clear, grammatically correct, and scientifically accurate fashion. Carrie Farnham edited the manuscript version of the book and discovered many opportunities wherein the book could be improved. Although the revision process between an editor and an author like me has the potential to become tense, I immediately respected, admired, and appreciated her extraordinary craft and professionalism. What a great privilege and pleasure it has been for me to work so closely with a person of her expertise, work ethic, and integrity. Thank you, Carrie, for making the book so much better.

The exquisite painting on the cover of the book is the work of family practitioner and artist Christy Morgan, M.D. The subject of her oil painting is a parable found at the beginning of Chapter 2 ("Getting Stuck: Evolutionary and Neurobiological Overview"), and in her work, Dr. Morgan has magically succeeded in capturing and portraying what I believe to be the evolutionary underpinnings of how we become "stuck in pause." No surprise: Dr. Morgan is the granddaughter of a distinguished female artist and is also a dedicated, compassionate diagnostician and clinician.

Mrs. Patricia (Tricia) Hoffman, my devoted administrative assistant at Baylor College of Medicine, was of invaluable assistance to me with the manuscript preparation. Gracious, warm hearted, and generous of spirit, Tricia is beloved by my patients, students, and colleagues, and she provided me with moral support and encouragement throughout the process of my writing this book.

The primary goal of *Fatal Pauses* is to inform people about why and how they become stuck and to help them get unstuck. I asked two dear friends to help me determine whether or not I had succeeded in this goal and to help me improve the book in areas in which I had not been successful. Mrs. Maureen Hackett is one of our nation's best known, most effective, and most admired advocates for those among us with mental illnesses. She also has a keen sense for what constitutes effective communication on the subject of mental health advocacy and what does not. Maureen carefully read the entire book and provided me with candid and insightful ways to improve the content and, hopefully, to inspire the reader to make changes in his or her life. Mrs. Dorothy Kay Brockman is an experienced and successful writer of mass market books about important medical topics. Not only is she a gifted writer and editor who understands the intricacies of crafting a book that will appeal to and be readily understood by the general public but she also knows the ins and outs of publishing. Dorothy Kay spent a summer poring over every word in this book and making helpful suggestions about how the book could be made more accessible to the lay reader and how it should be marketed. The encouragement, generosity, and competence of both of these wonderful friends gave me the incentive and courage to forge forward to the finish line with *Fatal Pauses*. Thank you both.

Stuart C. Yudofsky, M.D.
Houston, Texas

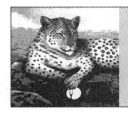

Introduction: Why This Book?

I wasted time, and now time doth waste me.
—*William Shakespeare*, Richard II, *Act V, Scene 5*

Only those who will risk going too far can possibly find out how far one can go.
—*T.S. Eliot, Preface*, Transit of Venus

Why This Book?

Fatal Pauses is an outgrowth of my 40-year practice as a neuropsychiatrist as well as of a book called *Fatal Flaws*, which was published in 2005. *Fatal Flaws* is an unconventional book about understanding, helping, and dealing with people with personality disorders. Many of the readers of *Fatal Flaws* were in important relationships with people with personality disorders. That book focused on depicting the manifestations of personality disorders as expressed in close relationships. Somewhat surprising to me, a large number of these readers called or wrote me to ask for advice and help in disentangling themselves from their intense, debilitating relationships. Most often the individuals from whom they desired to become free were unwilling to work on understanding themselves, changing their behaviors, or improving their relationships.

Movingly and vividly, these readers communicated to me their anguish and frustrations as they struggled, without success, to break free from these relationships. Invariably, they would say, "I am stuck; can you help me out?"

Quite directly, my readers were letting me know that although *Fatal Flaws* had been helpful to them in illuminating the characteristic features and treatments of people with personality disorders, it failed to offer sufficient help for *them*—the spouses, children, siblings, business partners, employees, etc., of people with personality disorders—to become unraveled from these relationships. Unwittingly, they were also asking how to get help in understanding more about themselves—particularly how and why they became ensnared in the relationships in the first place and why they were unable to let go. They felt *stuck!*

Similarly, I frequently am referred patients who have previously received extensive psychiatric treatment to which they believe that they have not responded adequately. Invariably, many of these patients also report "being stuck," but not solely in relationships with people with personality disorders. Over the years I have come to appreciate that people can become stuck in many important areas of their lives and for a multiplicity of reasons. I now accept that rarely is there a simple source of or solution for their plights and have learned to recognize characteristic patterns of dysfunction in people who are stuck. Because most people who feel stuck are failing in significant realms of their lives, it has become my responsibility to work with them to help them discover the causes of their problems and to devise and implement an effective treatment plan to "get unstuck." Plaintively and movingly, they will say to me and to other clinicians with similar practices, "*You* have to come up with something, otherwise *I* won't make it." I wrote *Fatal Pauses* to share what I have come up with to help people get unstuck.

Being Stuck

I define *being stuck* as follows:

1. Not *stopping* something that is *bad* for us and
2. Not *starting* and *staying with* something that is *good* for us

People can become stuck in many ways and for a wide variety of reasons. For example, they may have been unsuccessful in *stopping something* such as smoking, drinking too much, taking an addicting drug, overeating, remaining in an abusive relationship, wasting time, procrastinating, being dishonest, being critical of their spouses, putting themselves down, and the like. Others have been unsuccessful in *starting and staying with something:* an exercise program, a new career path, a new school, a challenging job assignment, a diet, a committed relationship, a positive attitude, writing a book, and the like. They feel frustrated and defeated, and many, wittingly or unwittingly, have given up. They tell us "I know that I must get going with my life, but I don't know how or where to begin"; "I'm just not getting anywhere"; or "In truth, I feel that it is impossible for me to change." These people feel *stuck*, and they are stuck, in what I term a *protracted pause*.

Evolutionary Disequilibrium

It might surprise you that being stuck is a relatively recent—although tragically pervasive—phenomenon. For the vast majority of the history of our species, human beings could not afford to pause—even for a brief period of time. For our ancestors to stall was to die, quite literally—by being eaten by predators, by being killed by human rivals, or by dying through starvation. Is "pausing in neutral" any less dangerous in our contemporary world? Yes and no.

As opposed to the decisions of our ancient ancestors, these days our decisions do not have *immediate*, life and death implications. Therefore, we frequently put important decisions into deep freeze—at great cost. We *take actions* with destructive consequences that are quite delayed—such as smoking cigarettes, overeating, taking drugs, or remaining in stressful relationships or dead-end jobs. We also fail to take actions that have far-reaching deleterious implications to our physical and mental health—such as not exercising, not quitting stressful dead-end jobs, or not working on relationships that are souring. Finally, we become anxious when we are stuck in pause, and chronic anxiety is erosive to our relationships and the quality of our lives.

Over the past several hundred years, the agricultural and industrial revolutions have dramatically changed our lives and how we live them, but our bodies adapt and evolve much, much more slowly. A race between a supersonic jet and an earthworm would understate the differences between the speeds of our socioeconomic advances and our genetically based, adaptive, somatic changes. This discrepancy between the technologically driven changes in the ways we live and our adaptation to these changes leads to many serious health problems. Our biological drives evolved for times of "feast and famine," not for a world of supermarkets and almost infinitely available food quantities and choices. Technological progress over the past 300 years has massively enhanced our ability to grow crops and to capture, breed, and harvest animals, which has exponentially increased the amounts of and access to food. Simultaneously, we are being plagued by an epidemic of obesity and concurrent diseases such as type 2 diabetes, coronary artery disease, hypertension, stroke, and a vast array of orthopedic disorders.

Our brains and, therefore, our mental health are also vulnerable to the vast and increasing divide between technologically driven, socioeconomic "progress" and our ability to adapt to such. For example, technology-driven agriculture and industries have also led to the broad availability of alcohol, drugs, Internet pornography, and video games, while the adaptation of our minds, bodies, and behavior to these innovations has not kept pace. We get stuck trying to resist and trying to overcome the consequences of these relatively recent "advances." Throughout this book I will offer effective strategies and useful approaches to surmount and straddle the negative consequences of this divide.

Our neurological and endocrine systems—which control our thinking, emotions, movements, and behavior—have remained essentially the same for millennia. Therefore, the neurobiology and neuroendocrinology of contemporary human beings is 99.99% identical to that of our ancient ancestors who were hunter-gatherers. We are genetically and evolutionarily wired to go or to stop. Fight or flight. But we are not wired to spend endlessly protracted amounts of time *deciding* whether to go or to stop. Even today, we have no "pause button" or neutral gear! Our biological systems must keep active at all times—even and especially during sleep states. No matter whether it is the exchange of oxygen for carbon dioxide at the cellular level or the neural stimulation of our heart muscle at the tissue level or in our deepest state of stage 4 sleep or our paying attention to the traffic when we cross a busy street, our brains must keep active for us to stay alive. To pause in neutral in any of these realms leads to the same result today as it would have for our ancient ancestors 10,000 years ago: it endangers our survival.

An exact parallel of yesteryear's fatal consequences of protracted pausing occurs today in the business world. For example, if a modern-day technological product—such as a mobile communications device—were to lag the field for even 6 months, that product is likely to be surpassed by a rival in a few months. That is precisely what is happening at the moment this book is being published to the once-dominant BlackBerry mobile device at the hands of the Apple iPhone and the Google/Android-based mobile devices. At this point many experts in the field of communications technology do not expect BlackBerry to survive, even though the company currently has tens of millions of regular users of its product. We humans are no less vulnerable when we become stuck.

The Fatal Pauses 3-D Method of Getting Unstuck

The method of *Fatal Pauses* derives from the distillation and application of pivotal, recent knowledge and evidence gleaned from the medical, behavioral, social, and anthropological sciences and, as importantly, from my clinical practice and personal life. In my method and recommendations, I have tried to be practical and nondoctrinaire. I distrust, and therefore eschew, "quick fixes." Quick fixes without insight-guided changes inevitably lead to a return to the quicksand of protracted pauses. This book embraces a wide variety of theoretical approaches in psychiatry, psychology, and the behavioral sciences and blends these in ways designed to enhance your understanding of yourself and of how you became stuck and to offer a "prescription," the 3-D Method, to help you become unstuck.

"Just say no" is the well-known slogan that was used intensively since the early 1980s by the U.S. government to discourage drug use in children, and "Just do it" is the epic, trademarked advertising catchphrase of the Nike Corporation to encourage participation in physical activities. When we become stuck in pause, it is the *just* component of these slogans that gives us problems. The word *just* is a conceptual black hole that we are supposed to vault in order to get to the action components of these phrases. The problem is that the black hole of just sucks us into a state of oblivious inaction: we can't *just* "say no," or we can't *just* "do it," without first discovering why we become stuck in the first place and, on the basis of these insights, deciding to become unstuck. Only then can we assert the discipline required for us to become unstuck.

The *D* components of the Fatal Pauses *3-D Method of Getting Unstuck are* 1) to *discover* the ways in which people become stuck; 2) to utilize this discovery, which involves identifying the underlying conflicts inherent in being stuck, to *decide* whether or not we want to become unstuck; and 3) to muster the *discipline* through wielding what I term *the Power of No and the Power of Go* to get unstuck. I will try to bring to life, through the clinical examples in the book, this approach, which has worked well over the years for many of my patients who are stuck—as it has in my personal life.

Case Examples

Although my method of getting unstuck is forthright and may even appear simple, I realize that *people* are not simple. The brains of people are also not simple, nor are the unique life experiences that affect their brains, genes, and, consequently, their thinking, emotions, choices, and behavior. Thus, I will present representative, detailed case examples derived from my patients who have been stuck. In the case examples I hope to convey the excitement, infinite variability, and mystery inherent in all human beings—and, for better and for worse, in the mental health profession. Even though I realize that these case examples reflect the unique, elegant complexity of my patients' lives, I nonetheless believe that their circumstances, challenges, frustrations, and dysfunctional behavioral patterns will parallel and are applicable to those of others—and perhaps even to you.

Interspersed with the case examples throughout the book are treatment principles that highlight special concepts of and approaches to treatment that apply to most patients in psychotherapy. These therapeutic principles are assembled in a table that appears in the Appendix. Additionally, many people who are profoundly "stuck in pause" are challenged by having two or more compounding psychiatric disorders and/or by a significant traumatic experience, which leads to their symptoms and "complicates" their treatment. These compounding factors are designated in the chapter titles.

The heart and soul of this book are in the case examples. If these examples do not communicate stirringly the inherent mystery, tension, joy, excitement, and power of my field and the heroism of human beings striving to overcome the misery of being stuck, I have failed in what I have tried to accomplish.

For purposes of maintaining the complete confidentiality of my patients, all clinical examples in this book are composites, with the specific distinguishing details absolutely disguised. Nonetheless, I have tried to render the clinical vignettes realistic, representative, and revelatory of patients who were stuck and how they became unstuck to pursue and achieve their unique potentials. If you believe that you recognize yourself or someone else whom you know in the case studies, you are wrong. What you are recognizing is a common pattern of dysfunction, not any specific person.

Possibilities and Potentials

Paradoxically, *Fatal Pauses* is an optimistic book that is all about possibilities and potentials. Why, then, the word *Fatal* (other than it works well with the title of my previous book)? For many people who are stuck in the pause mode, the corpses of their pivotal potentials and exhilarating opportunities will lie forever interred. For example, the fulfillments of meaningful marital intimacy will languish forever unconsummated for a person stuck in a loveless marriage. The satisfactions of an occupation more delightful than a holiday will be but an evanescent dream for a person who works solely to make a living and "get by." The pauses are *fatal* only if nothing is done to understand and correct their underlying problems, which need not be the case.

The goals of this book are to help people get unstuck and to get them going on positive, productive life paths. I am confident that if people learn and apply the method presented in this book, they will achieve their goals, gain control of their lives, and change their lives for the better. But first it is necessary to determine whether or not you, or someone whom you know, or a patient whom you are treating, is, in fact, stuck, which can be done by taking or administering the Am I Stuck? Scale in Chapter 1.

Hybridized Components

Like *Fatal Flaws*, this book is a hybrid, as manifested in the following three ways: *Fatal Pauses* is part casebook for mental health professionals and part self-help manual for people who, for multifarious reasons, are stuck. As a consequence, throughout the book there is a blending of writing styles that reflects whether or not a specific point is being addressed to a patient or to a clinician. Although some readers might find this unconventional approach somewhat disorienting, I believe that it also has advantages. Success in understanding and escaping being stuck *must* be a joint enterprise between patient and clinician. We are in it together: the pilot of the plane is also a passenger. By using an intimate writing style, I hope to bring to life how experienced clinicians think through, discuss therapeutically, and work through problems with our patients and their families. Many readers of *Fatal Flaws* who are not clinicians told me that they appreciated "inside" insights into how clinicians conceptualize psychiatric disorders and construct treatment approaches. They found that this technique and information helped to demystify the process of psychiatric care and was educational and respectfully inclusive.

Second, the method for getting unstuck espoused in *Fatal Pauses* comprises, for the most part, a hybrid of an insight-oriented, psychodynamically based model combined with cognitive-behavioral-based treatment approaches. The former model enlightens assessment, diagnosis, and treatment, and although the latter model informs assessment and diagnosis, it also greatly expedites the treatment process—and the results.

Third, similar to many modern technological devices—such as computers or automobiles—the foundations and "working parts" of whatever wisdom the book imparts derive from innumerable inventions and inspirations of gifted, creative thinkers, many of whom, in this case, have been and still are my teachers, patients, students, and colleagues. To all of these generous, selfless donors, I express my heartfelt gratitude.

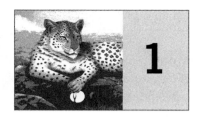

The Am I Stuck? Scale

The Am I Stuck? Scale will help determine whether you, someone with whom you have a close personal relationship, or one of your patients or clients might be stuck in pause.

Part 1: Taking Score of Yourself[1]

For each of these questions, answer yes (y) or no (n).

1. Am I stuck in making the decision to leave a destructive relationship (e.g., accepting abuse, accepting belittlement, compromising my values)?

(y) (n)

2. Am I stuck in making the decision to stop a bad habit that endangers my health (e.g., smoking, overeating, drinking excessively, taking drugs, risk taking)?

(y) (n)

3. Am I stuck in making the decision to stop compulsive behaviors or procrastinating habits that waste my time (e.g., Internet surfing, hours on Facebook, excessive TV watching, gambling, video games, sexual addictions, pornography seeking, compulsive shopping)?

(y) (n)

4. Am I stuck in making the decision not to lie, break the law, or break rules (e.g., lying, compulsive exaggerating, drinking and driving, stealing, illegal betting, taking drugs)?

(y) (n)

---

[1]This scale may be administered to others by substituting "Are you" for "Am I," "your" for "my," and "yourself" for "myself."

5. Am I stuck in making the decision to stop hurting others (e.g., being overly critical, misleading, demeaning, unfaithful, insensitive, mean, exploitative, negativistic, abusive, prejudiced)?

(y) (n)

6. Am I stuck in making the decision to stop diminishing, demeaning, hurting, and/or hating myself (e.g., being self-critical, submissive, passive, insecure, pessimistic, irritable)?

(y) (n)

7. Am I stuck in making the decision to pursue and engage an optimal life partner (e.g., looking my best, acting my best, getting out, networking, making "the effort," taking "the risk," making "the commitment")?

(y) (n)

8. Am I stuck in making the decision to use my time constructively (e.g., improving my mind, my body, my health, and the lives of others)?

(y) (n)

9. Am I stuck in making the decision to protect my body and enhance my health and safety (e.g., eating a healthful diet, exercising regularly, driving safely, getting into psychotherapy, avoiding physical and mental risks, attending Alcoholics Anonymous meetings)?

(y) (n)

10. Am I stuck in making the decision to improve my mind and advance my career (e.g., studying hard, working hard, doing my best, attending classes, completing assignments, preparing for tests, attending college or graduate school, maintaining a positive attitude, risking career changes)?

(y) (n)

11. Am I stuck in making the decision to be honest and live honestly (e.g., telling the truth, attending religious services, managing anger, assisting others, volunteering, avoiding bad influences, making new friends)?

(y) (n)

12. Am I stuck in making the decision to treat others fairly and respectfully (e.g., being thoughtful, being kind, expressing appreciation, thanking, apologizing, compensating, remediating)?

(y) (n)

13. Am I stuck in making the decision to treat myself fairly and with respect at all times (e.g., being positive, pleasing myself, ac-

knowledging my successes, acknowledging my abilities, accepting compliments, accepting gifts, forgiving myself, rewarding myself appropriately)?

(y) (n)

Part 2: Calculating Your Am I Stuck? Score

A. For each "yes" answer in Part 1, write the number (in parentheses) that most closely correlates with the length of time that you have been stuck in making the respective decision:

6 months (1)
6 months to 2 years (2)
2–5 years (3)
More than 5 years (4)

The number in parentheses constitutes your score for each item for which you replied "yes."

B. To total your Am I Stuck? score, add the numbers in parentheses.

Examples:

- If you were stuck with item 3 for 5 years (4 score) and item 9 for 3 years (3 score), your total score is 7.
- If you were stuck with item 1 for 1 year, your total score is 2.

C. Rating yourself on the basis of your total Am I Stuck? score.

0: You are not stuck in pause and would not likely have a great deal to gain personally from reading and applying the principles in this book.[2]

1–2: You are, minimally, stuck in a partial pause and most likely can benefit from reading and applying the principles in this book.

3: You are stuck in pause and will benefit from reading and applying the principles in this book.

4 or more: You are stuck in fatal pause, or a protracted pause. This means that unless you do something definitive to change your

---

[2]Nonetheless, reading this book might be helpful to you in understanding and helping others who *are* stuck—including if you are a mental health professional or have a close relationship with someone else who might be stuck in pause.

situation, you will not achieve your potential or feel fulfilled or be happy. You are also likely, unwittingly, to affect your loved ones in ways that are not positive. You owe it to yourself and to your loved ones to read and apply the principles in this book.

In Chapter 2, "Getting Stuck," we will examine how people get stuck in the first place.

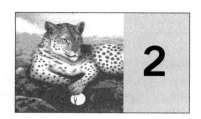

Getting Stuck

Evolutionary and Neurobiological Overview

The world is too much with us; late and soon,
Getting and spending, we lay waste our powers;
Little we see in Nature that is ours;
We have given our hearts away, a sordid boon!
—*William Wordsworth, "The World is Too Much With Us"*

In my beginning is my end…
—*T.S. Eliot, "East Coker," Four Quartets*

I will show you fear in a handful of dust.
—*T.S. Eliot, "The Waste Land"*

In this chapter I provide a highly condensed neurobiological and evolutionary overview of how contemporary humankind has become stuck in pause and the scientific and theoretical principles on which the Fatal Pauses *3-D Method of Getting Unstuck Through the Power of Go and the Power of No* are based. (Some readers may prefer to skip this chapter, which focuses on behavioral and biological science, and proceed straight to Chapter 3, which gets right to the point: how to go about getting unstuck using the Fatal Pauses 3-D Method.)

Origins

It was the dry season. A parched autumn trailed the scorching summer along the vast and ancient African savanna. The only clouds to darken the skies were smoke-like swarms of locusts that devoured the rare remnants of the desiccated grasses and the scatterings of seeds that had been spared by the relentless, consuming wildfires. Starving and emaciated, she hid her skeletal brood in the shadows of their yawning cave and, once more, braved forward on her interminable search for food.

Beyond the hushing locusts, the dry, empty air carried no sounds of life—only those of her blistered feet as they beat a grim rhythm against the baked, barren, dusting clay: *dry and empty, dry and empty, dry and empty.*

Spurred by hunger, she ventured ever deeper into the vast dryness. Suddenly, behind a massive termite mound, she saw it: a patch of green wetness stitched within the quilt of beiges and browns. And near the center of the patch was a date palm that had relinquished about its roots copious quantities of its amber treasure.

With racing heart and moistening lips she hastened toward the mound. But, just as suddenly, she paused. Blending fear and desire, a novel ache drained her brimming hope. Was a lion lurking behind the termite tower, or did it melt invisibly within the quilt's thorny fringes? Perhaps a wily leopard blended into the shadows of the palm's lofty green. Cagey carnivores, both, waiting patiently to feast on a desperate primate.

For a few unbearable seconds, as her anxiety flooded to fear, she did not move—her fathomless hunger pitted against the terrifying unknown. As this struggle stormed within her, she also understood that to pause, even briefly, on this desiccated plain was to invite certain death.

Neither betrayings of branches nor shiverings of leaves unveiled the crouching cats. Contrasting with this silent stillness was the gnawing, groaning ache that now knitted and knotted her shrunken belly. Courage waning, she abruptly turned and raced back to her ravenous offspring. The ache of uncertainty overpowered her cramping, famished belly.

On this long-forgotten day along the ancient, arid African plain, your ancestor and her wasting babies went unfed—as did the predators lying in ambush in the tree and behind the baking termite mound. That she decided and acted rapidly—and correctly—is why *you* exist today. Her genetic code that you carry is also why you know anxiety. And you feel it in your gut whenever you pause in conflict.

Getting Stuck and the High Cost of Evolutionary "Success"

Among our ancient ancestors (1.8 million to 20,000 years ago), anxiety most likely accompanied immediate, conflicting, life-and-death choices. But they couldn't be anxious for long. Survival depended on making the right choice—and making it fast! Your starving hunter-gatherer ancestor who was described above fought with herself about whether or not to gather the fallen dates and risk being devoured by a hidden leopard. Momentarily, she froze in place while contemplating "go" or "no." Accompanying her indecision was this strange, uncomfortable, unsettling emotion: anxiety, which, on that occasion, saved her life and the lives of her offspring.

Our ancient ancestors did not have the luxury of prolonged pauses, for to pause in indecision meant to be discovered and attacked by the omnipresent predators that were perennially on watch for their unwary primate prey. Additionally, to pause meant to be vulnerable to our human rivals, who competed with us for limited resources, territories, or mates. Daily survival depended directly on *fight or flight* decisions—with precious little time to choose which.

Over the last 20,000 years, our relationships with our previous predators changed dramatically. We began to live more safely in larger groups, hunt in teams, and cultivate our own vegetables and animals for food and shelter. We developed great skills at making tools, deadly weapons, and transportation machines such as boats, automobiles, and airplanes. We invented imaginative technologies for information storage, communications, and environmental monitoring that have revolutionized our individual and social behaviors and group potential to anticipate and avoid dangers. As a result, our lives are now rarely endangered by larger predatory animals and are much less immediately vulnerable to lethal forces of nature such as droughts, tornadoes, fires, hurricanes, and floods. Therefore, most of us have far less of the minute-to-minute, day-to-day survival fear from predators than was endured by our ancestors. The main exceptions, of course, are predatory behaviors within our own species. In the so-called "developed world," we now live in material abundance with an unprecedented range of options for food, shelter, defense, and early warnings of life-threatening dangers. As we will discover, however, these options and this abundance have come at a high cost to our health and equanimity.

It is true even today that our survival can depend on immediate decisions and actions—such as stopping when a traffic signal turns red, not running across a busy interstate highway, or not venturing across an international border into a war zone. But deaths from these causes usually occur from risk-taking patterns that are long-standing and multidetermined.

These days, our most important decisions related to our survival and well-being do not have immediate repercussions, but the deadly consequences come home to roost many years later. Daily, we battle with ourselves to make the right choices, but, because the reinforcements of making poor choices are immediate and deleterious consequences are so remote, we usually lose these battles. Not deceiving ourselves completely, we become conflicted, anxious, and self-loathing. We become stuck in pause.

The Human Brain: A Brief Overview

The purpose of the following summary of selected properties and functions of the human brain is to emphasize key principles that help explain how people become stuck in pause as well as the principles that underlie the Fatal Pauses 3-D Method of Getting Unstuck Through the Power of Go and the Power of No. This summary is by no means intended to offer a comprehensive, representative, or inclusive review of what is considered one of the most complex entities in the observable universe: the human brain.

Structure, Complexity, Capacity, and the Human Brain

A healthy human brain comprises approximately 100 billion nerve cells, most of which are neurons. A neuron is a specialized cell that processes and transmits information both electrically and chemically. The prototypical neuron has four components:

1. The *cell body* possesses and processes information that it receives from and sends to other neurons. It also manufactures and reprocesses specialized proteins called neurotransmitters that are used for chemical signaling to other neurons.
2. *Axons* conduct electrical signals away from the cell body to communicate with other cells at junctions called synapses. There is

usually only one axon per neuron. The electronic components of axons operate through action potentials that work like an off/on switch: there are no firings in resting (or "off") states, and electrical impulses are initiated to travel down axons to nerve endings during active (or "on") states.

3. *Dendrites* are thin structures with multiple branches that conduct electrochemical messages from other neurons toward and into the cell body of a particular neuron. A single neuron generally has many thousands of dendrites.

4. A *synapse* is a junction wherein chemical messages are carried from one neuron to another through a space called a synaptic cleft. Signals pass from the axon of one neuron to the dendrite of another via neurotransmitters.

It is estimated that there are hundreds of trillions of synapses in the human brain, and synaptical nerve endings can be formed from different combinations of at least 1,000 proteins that can be affected by at least 60 known neurotransmitters and, no doubt, many, many more that are yet to be discovered (McAllister et al. 2008). Adding further to the brain's complexity and potential, numerous protein-based enzymes are involved in the manufacture, release, and degradation of neurotransmitters. Each one of these myriad elements enables and affects information coding and processing. On the basis of these elements, the capacity of the human brain to intake, process, store, and transmit information is almost unfathomable.

Computers and the Human Brain

Comparisons of the human brain to man-made machines have been made throughout history, and these relationships reflect both the state of humankind's contemporaneous technical advancement and that era's knowledge of the workings of the brain. For example, several hundred years ago the "mechanisms" of the brain were compared to those of a clock, a comparison that would be untenable to the point of being absurd today. Manifestly, we did not know very much about our brains in that age. These days, computer-brain comparisons are common for reasons that we can all understand. Among the similarities are that both computers and our brain have analogous functions such as memory storage, information processing, and mathematical computation. Both have parallel working components and structures such as those used for electrical signaling, memory storage, and input and output processing. An important difference is that the human brain utilizes both electrical and chemical signaling mechanisms, which gives our brain a considerable current advantage over computers with regard to the "connectivity units" that underlie both memory storage capacity and information processing speed. On the other hand, computers use high-conductivity wires that can transmit far more rapid electrical signals than can axons in the brain. Another difference is that most computers can be "shut down," whereas the human brain must continue to be dynamic in both the so-called "active" and "resting" (which turn out to be highly active) states.

For the purposes of understanding how people get stuck in pause and *Fatal Pauses'* approach to becoming unstuck, I will focus only on one among the many similarities and on one among the many differences between the human brain and computers.

Important Similarity of the Human Brain and Computers: Binary Code

The electrical component of neurons (as contrasted to the chemical transmission across synapses through neurotransmitters) and the basic coding mechanism of computer software have one critical similarity: they are both what is termed *binary functions*. Binary functions can communicate in only two basic ways: on and off. The sequence of instructions that a computer can interpret and/or execute, often called the computer program, is based entirely on ones and zeroes. Correspondingly, the electrical signal that moves down the axon and dendrites of a neuron relies on action potentials that function like a switch—*on* or *off* or *fire* or *don't fire*. During an *on* stage, the signal triggers chemical messengers that can then communicate across synapses in almost infinite permutations and combinations to other brain neurons.

As will be amplified in Chapter 3, "The Fatal Pauses 3-D Method of Getting Unstuck Through the Power of No and the Power of Go," I believe that this basic, binary simplicity has behavioral parallels that can be helpful in understanding how some people become stuck in pause and how to craft and execute a plan to escape being stuck and to move forward in life.

Important Difference Between the Human Brain and Computers: Evolution

Computers and other technological tools are evolving much more rapidly than the human brain, and this has critical ramifications for our health and peace of mind. Over the last five decades computers have "evolved" at a breathtaking, breakneck speed. Many of the important functions of computers—including memory capacity and processing ability—are dependent on the number and processing speed of transistors that can be placed on an integrated circuit. In 1965, Gordon Moore predicted that, for the foreseeable future, the number of transistors that could be positioned inexpensively on an integrated circuit would double every 2 years. His prediction has proved accurate for almost 50 years, and this has enabled computers to become far more powerful, smaller, and less expensive from year to year.

On the other hand, notwithstanding the rapid pace of the *early* evolutionary advancement in the size and complexity of the primate brain, over human beings' more recent history, some scientists believe that this evolutionary change has slowed down considerably. Wang et al. (2007) concluded that the more complex the brain, it seems, the more challenging it becomes for brain genes to change. If this proves to be accurate, the implications are profound: paradoxically, our bodies' adaptive effects based on natural selection, which involve genetic changes, may not be able to keep pace with the technological advancements made possible by our brains. Many of the changes in how we live are dependent on the Industrial and Agricultural Revolutions, which are but a brief instant in the time required for significant mammalian evolution.

For example, our evolved brains have enabled us to develop tools and technologies to produce, process, and distribute food in great abundance and varieties, without the intense labor and risks to life and limb required of our ancient ancestors. Nonetheless, our bodies have not kept pace with the effects of these changes to the point that we are now jeopardizing both individual and group survival. We eat too much and exercise too little. Recent data confirm that 34.9% of American adults are obese and two-thirds of our adult population are either obese or significantly overweight (Ogden et al. 2014). Stated another way, notwithstanding the dire effects on quality of life, health, and survival, somehow, more than two-thirds of Americans, or hundreds of millions of us, can't resist ingesting unhealthful foods in excessive quantities. Nor can we get ourselves to exercise regularly. Thus, the sad truth is that most of us are stuck in pause with regard to making decisions and choices that are healthful for our bodies and minds. If we do not use our minds to intervene, over time, natural selection will have its inevitable sway through the process of disease and death—at an incalculable cost in the form of human misery.

Repetition, Consistency, and the Human Brain

Repetition

The human brain has evolved to recognize and rely on patterns—both in organizing and retaining information, as well as in interpreting and making decisions based on data. Relatedly, the brain "learns" most things through repetition. As has been reviewed in the section "The Human Brain: A Brief Overview," the brain consists of neurons that are connected at synapses. Synaptic pathways can be changed by previous activity, a process that is called *synaptic plasticity*. Changes in neural pathways and the creation of new pathways and networks enable learning and form the basis of what is conceptualized as thought, mind, and memory. The strength of the stimulus and the number of times it is repeated are all important elements in learning. And, as we all know, we can learn things that are good for us or bad for us, that either enable or endanger our survival. When we become stuck in behavioral and mental ruts—such as ruminating about our weight, about stopping drinking, about leaving a destructive relationship, or about doing our homework or exercise regimen that day—we are actually reinforcing the persistence of those pathological thoughts and behaviors. *Rumination about, without resolution of, important life problems* is a hallmark of being stuck in pause.

Consistency

On planet Earth, most living organisms—and all mammals—evolved and adapt according to cycles of the sun and the moon. As a consequence, vital human functions such as hunting, gathering, farming, eating, sleeping, reproducing, and protecting ourselves from the elements and predators have rhythms that are linked to solar and lunar cycles—so-called circadian rhythms. Each of these functions is enabled and regulated by brain biology and function that have evolved over millennia to comply with solar and lunar cycles—a phenomenon called *chronobiology*. However, recent "advances" in technology have challenged our physical and mental integration with these cycles. One among many examples of technologically induced chronobiological disequilibrium is that modern jet aircraft have enabled us to travel great distances in hours that would have, for most of humankind's existence, required from many months to many years to traverse. Today, when we fly across time zones, not only do we have difficulty regulating our sleep and ability to concentrate and think clearly, but our mood can also be affected in disabling and dangerous ways. I advise many of my patients with "brittle" bipolar illness not to travel great distances by air across longitudes at the risk of their triggering severe manic or depressive events. Another example is that the very recent (on an evolutionary calendar) invention of electric light makes it possible for many college-age students to stay up all night studying or partying and then to "fit in" whatever sleep they can manage during daylight hours. Given that we did not evolve to be nocturnal primates, this reversal of day and night inevitably leads to mental and somatic dysfunctions, many of which can have quite serious implications for our health and futures.

Our very survival depends on our ability to recognize recurring *patterns*, which encompass our visual, auditory, tactile, gustatory (taste), olfactory (smell), and proprioceptive (spatial) perceptions. Neurobiologists believe that even our sense of beauty, appreciation of music, and enjoyment of athletics relate to our recognition of consistencies and symmetries. As infants we are introduced to processing consistent social patterns through recognizing the faces and expressions of our caregivers and associating these expressions with safety and satiety. As very young children, we constantly are gazing at our parents for approval and reassurance and react with startle and alarm when our parents have fearful expressions. We learn that this change in facial pattern communicates that danger lurks. Consistency in these patterns leads to a sense of trust, whereas inconsistencies in pattern expectations are associated with anxiety, insecurity, confusion, and physical and emotional disorders.

Because we evolved to have structure and order in the key realms of our daily lives, *inconsistency in the structure and patterns of our daily lives* is another hallmark of being stuck in pause. In subsequent chapters I will reveal how pattern inconsistencies lead to fatal pauses such as eating disorders and addictions and how these disorders can be countered by limiting the variety of and introducing consistency and structure to *all* of our daily activities.

Fight or Flight and the Human Brain

Automobiles have accelerators to move forward and backward and brakes to stop all movement. We know that if we gently depress both the accelerator and the brake at the same time, nothing happens. However, if we simultaneously jam on the brakes and floor the accelerator, not only does the car not move but also its motor, brakes, and transmission will be damaged. Similarly, human beings have ancient anatomical and chemical systems that are responsible for going and stopping, for fight and flight, and these are mediated in the brain by the parasympathetic and sympathetic nervous systems. When a person is in a calm, relaxed state, the *parasympathetic nervous system* prevails in regulating the body's activities that are required for survival. In this situation, the heart beats slowly and regularly, and breathing is also slow and unlabored. Alternatively, when we are under real or perceived threat or are launching an attack, our *sympathetic nervous system* prevails: our heart races, our blood pressure elevates, our pupils dilate, and even our body hair may stiffen or stand "on edge." Accompanying both states are chemical changes in our brain and throughout the rest of our body. Cholinergic and serotonergic release prevail in restful states, and catecholamines— epinephrine, norepinephrine, and dopamine—and glutamate are most active in states of fight or flight.

Because our brain biology is still based on the ancient fight or flight patterns that prevailed when we all were on the menus of carnivores, we now react to the real or perceived threats to our social status as if we were in danger of imminently being killed and devoured. In modern times, however, in the vast majority of occasions when we feel threatened, we do not take action. Nonetheless, the chemistry of our brains and bodies responds as if we are either furiously going on the attack or running for our lives. Although we are frozen with regard to our overt behavioral responses, our internal states go on the rampage: we can feel fearful, anxious, or even panicked; we ruminate and obsess over our safety and future and those of our loved ones; we become depressed and suffer headaches, back pain, high blood pressure, and heart disease; we develop eating disorders and alcohol and other substance use disorders; and, likely as the result of compromised immunological systems, we can even become at risk for other serious medical illnesses including cancer and arthritis. And, tragically, we do not take the actions that would make things better. These biological changes occur when we are stuck as the result of the socially based and choice-based conflicts described above. And when we are stuck in these ways, over time, our pauses can actually become life threatening, or fatal. *Indecisiveness and failure to take action in fight or flight choices and conflicts* are another hallmark of being stuck in pause.

Fear, Anger, Anxiety, and the Will to Persevere

The Emotions of "Pause"

The emotions fear, anger, and anxiety are inextricably associated with being stuck in pause.

Fear is a basic, simple emotion. Evolutionary biologists explain that for millions of years humankind's principal threat came from other species of animals. We were on the regular diets of innumerable predators—including mammals such as lions, tigers, cheetahs, leopards, wolves, hyenas, and bears; reptiles such as alligators, crocodiles, and snakes; and sea animals such as killer whales and sharks. Our ancestors had good reason to be fearful because each of these animals could kill them in great numbers. And the *ways* in which our ancestors were killed by such predators—being ripped apart and devoured—were also terrifying. Our fear alerts us to keep our distance from these dangerous "beasts." In our far more complex and subtle contemporary world, we are fearful of things that are far more ephemeral than lions and leopards. Our fears of failure at work or school, of being embarrassed among colleagues, or of being rejected by people whom we deem to be important are prototypical examples. Many of us are fearful of taking the risks or making the changes that are required to optimize our potentials or escape from destructive habits or relationships. We are fearful of invoking the anger of others or losing what is familiar and regarded as safe. Fear is always involved in being stuck and must be overcome to become unstuck.

Thus, *fear (the "flight" component of the fight or flight dyad) and accompanying avoidance behaviors* are another hallmark of being stuck in pause.

Anger, manifestly, is the emotion that accompanies the *fight* factor of the *fight or flight* equation. Anger impels us to pursue and kill threatening species before they can harm us. Angry emotions are also protective and are expressed when we defend our offspring or other members of our tribe and families from survival-related threats. Both killing and kissing cousins, anger and fear are also closely related to survival *within* our species—often coupled with mating, feeding, and territorial behaviors. Among our ancient ancestors our anger was almost always externalized—whether we were fighting off predators, enemies from other tribes, or rivals within our own tribes. We screamed, threatened, hit, bit, kicked, maimed, and killed.

In modern times, however, almost all of these expressions of anger are impractical, impotent, or prohibited in the usual circumstances of our daily lives. So often, when we are frustrated and feel stuck, we don't even know at whom to be angry. For example, if our car breaks down on a busy and dangerous highway, how do we express our immediate anger toward the engineer in Detroit or Tokyo who designed the faulty mechanical part? Or to the disappearing driver of the speeding car that roars by deadly close to our stalled car? Additionally, we are usually prohibited from threatening or attacking our rivals and those with whom we disagree. For example, we are instructed to smile and appear pleasant while being cross-examined in court by a prosecutor who might wish to ruin us financially, take away our medical licenses, put us in jail for life, or even sentence us to death by an executioner—a process from which, ironically, all anger has been sanitized. Even in violent contact sports, such as football, ice hockey, or boxing—in which the victors frequently inflict concussions on their opponents—we are not permitted to express overt anger, either verbally or physically, by trying to belittle or "intentionally" injuring our opponents. In such athletic engagements, the combatants are encouraged to shake hands and embrace after battle to show that they are "good sports."

So where does our anger "go" in modern times? We suppress our anger and internalize it, often at a significant cost to our physical and mental health. Internalized anger is associated with somatic symptoms such as migraine headaches and muscle aches, stomach and esophageal ulcers, and colitis. Anger turned inward is also a classic model of and theory for the underlying causal dynamics of depression, self-destructive thoughts and behaviors, and, in extremis, suicide. *Self-directed anger, as expressed through irritability, self-deprecation, self-destructive thoughts and behaviors, depression, and somatic symptoms,* is another hallmark of being stuck in pause.

Anxiety is a more complex emotion than anger and fear, and it has been conceptualized as deriving from many disparate sources. A displeasing, unsettling, and upsetting emotional state, anxiety can actually be conceived as an adaptive emotional signal that enhances our survival. This intensely uncomfortable feeling heightens the senses, allowing our hunter-gatherer ancestor to be more vigilant, to stop in her tracks as she became paralyzed by the conflict between her desire for food and her fear of being ambushed by a deadly predator. *I conceptualize anxiety as a symptom that occurs as a result of being stuck between fight or flight or between go and no. An unsettling amalgam of anger and fear, anxiety, I believe, is a symptom of conscious and unconscious conflicts about critical choices.* Thus, *anxiety, per se,* is another hallmark of being stuck in pause.

The Will to Persevere

The will to persevere is a drive fundamental to animal survival. Why fight or try to escape danger if we don't care to live? Recently, Dr. Josepf Paravizi and other scientists at Stanford University localized components of this drive in a group of neurons in the anterior midcingulate cortex (Paravizi et al. 2013). These cells coordinate the complex behavioral and psychological states that enable a person to anticipate a challenge to survival and to mount the motivation required to overcome that challenge. Even more complex psychological and biological states influence the regulation of this system, which will be essential to motivate an individual who is stuck in pause to *want* to change. Otherwise, that person will be unable to *decide* to change or exert the motivation and *discipline* required to become unstuck.

Conflict and Being Stuck in Pause

Freud brilliantly conceptualized anxiety as being the result of unconscious conflicts between more basic and potent feelings, such as a conflict between sexual lust and fear of reprisal. His theories have been continuously revised, clarified, and updated by succeeding generations of psychoanalysts and evidence-based behavioral psychologists and psychiatrists. Many years ago, psychologist Kurt Lewin described three basic forms of conflicts that are useful in understanding how we are stuck (Lewin 1935).

1. *Approach-approach conflicts* arise when we must choose between two things we like or between two positive opportunities or outcomes. Examples include deciding between which of two preeminent universities to attend or between devouring a crème brûlée or staying thin. These conflicts can be quite subtle and confusing and frequently occur when a person is stuck in an unhealthful or dysfunctional dependency—such as on a drug or in a relationship. Thus, to resolve this conflict we must *decide* to *avoid* something that we actually like or want in order to achieve something that we finally realize we like or want more. For example, most people with alcohol use disorder actually like the way alcohol makes them feel. These people must first understand and accept that they like alcohol before they can choose between their affection for alcohol and their desire to be healthy and not destroy their jobs and relationships. A component of acceptance is the recognition that we actually like alcohol too much. Once we clarify (i.e., *discover*) that what we truly like is not good for us, we then must *decide* what we like and want more—for example, alcohol versus good health and mature relationships. Then we can finally decide to avoid what we like; this always will require *discipline*.

2. *Approach-avoidance conflicts* are common among people who are stuck in pause, and they also can be difficult to discover and confusing to comprehend. These conflicts occur when something we like or want leads to things we don't like or don't want. This commonly includes an emotion, such as anger, or a biological drive, such as the sexual drive. For example, we might justifiably *want* to express anger at someone with whom we have an important relationship but also wish to *avoid* evoking the negative response of the other person. Or we may wish to express our sexual attraction for another person but avoid acting on our desire out of fear of being rejected.

3. *Avoidance-avoidance conflicts* occur when we have to decide between or among several things or actions that we don't like. We

would prefer not to partake of *any* of the options. These conflicts occur when we must choose to do something that we don't like to do in order to avoid something else that we don't like. An example would be paying our taxes to avoid going to jail. (Note that avoidance-avoidance conflicts are different from approach-avoidance conflicts, wherein we must choose to *avoid* something that we *do like* to *avoid* something we *don't* like—for example, eating chocolate cake versus becoming overweight.)

There are many other types and permutations of conflicts that occur that are even more complex and confusing than the examples above, but, for the sake of clarity, I will not include them in this book.

Modern-Day Sources of Conflict and Getting Stuck

Anxiety

A thesis of this book (and of many other clinicians and investigators) is that in modern times, anxiety no longer *enables* survival. Rather, it *disables* survival as a result of our pausing too long in our effort to resolve conflicting *fight* or *flight* or *go* or *no* choices. It is important to understand that these *no* choices correspond to *flight* decisions that are *active states* that require catecholamine activity in the brain and throughout the body. Anxiety always occurs when we become paralyzed or stuck between *go* and *no* and has been labeled as the signature symptom of our era, the so-called *Age of Anxiety*. I believe that the Age of Anxiety is a result of our having far too many choices, about which we become conflicted, and, in turn, we become stuck in pause. A second major source of conflicts and anxiety is our increasingly complex dependencies on others.

Too Many Choices

Over the vast preponderance of our evolutionary history, we did not have access to the extraordinary variety and amounts of foods that so many of us "enjoy" today. Nor could we protect ourselves from the vicissitudes and ravages of climate and environment in the multifarious ways that we are currently able. The opportunities and options for social, vocational, and recreational choices were far more limited for our ancient ancestors than they are for us at the present time. The day-to-day survival of our ancestors was dictated by so much that was outside of their control—such as where they were born, the season of the year, the presence of predators, and the immediate availability of food and shelter.

Today, many of us can walk into a supermarket and choose from among nearly limitless types of foods that emanate from distant and disparate parts of the world. And once we bring ourselves to arrive at a choice of the type of food for our main course, the act of choosing only raises seemingly infinite other decisions that we must then make. For example, if we choose to have fish for dinner, we then must select one from among the almost innumerable species of fish that come from nearly infinite locales. They all stare back at us from a single icy reef in the supermarket, and we must choose one. We then can move on to white wines that, similarly, derive from nearly infinite varieties of grapes that were grown, mashed, and fermented in nearly innumerable regions of our planet. Our ancient ancestors could never dream of such variety and abundance, nor did they pause in indecision beneath such a crushing avalanche of choices. Unfortunately, associated with so many modern-day choices are the inevitable problems and conflicts: 1) we make the wrong decisions, such as choosing unhealthful foods that we ingest in excessive quantities, or 2) we fail to decide and take action. The former leads to our being stuck in our inability to assert "no" to choices that disable our survival, and the latter leads to our being stuck in our inability to say "yes" to taking actions that enhance our health and personal potential.

Complex Dependencies on Others

Within our current social systems, *every* person depends on other people for his or her survival. Securing food, building shelter, and protecting ourselves are no longer possible without the cooperation and consent of others. We seek to belong to tribes or to more intimate social groupings within our own tribe that will protect us from the omnipresent rival tribes and inhospitable social groupings. Although this was also somewhat true for our ancient ancestors, today, within our own tribes, our survival also depends much more on our perceiving and mastering subtle nuances involved with fitting in with and being accepted by other individuals within our respective social systems. For example, the competition of cavemen for suitable mates was based on physical size and strength and dominance/submission paradigms more than it is for so-called "modern men." Today, we rely on *mentalization*, which is our capacity to perceive and respond to what is on the minds of other people in order to maintain our social connections and status. Deficits in our capacity to mentalize, such as those that can occur with psychotic disorders, severe autism, or personality disorders, often place the individual at severe disadvantage with regard to social acceptance and advancement.

As a consequence of the survival value of our complex dependencies on others, many of us are vulnerable to becoming stuck in pause as we constantly monitor and evaluate our social status and safety within our particular systems. We must make sure that we are safe, secure, and prioritized before we take action. We spend countless hours on Facebook as we check and try to influence our social status. However, we do not take the necessary actions to resolve our fears. We ruminate about such questions as "Am I successful enough for her?" or "Am I attractive enough for him?" without doing much about our concerns. We want to be accepted and prioritized, but we don't want to make the decisions and do the work that will enable our being exceptional. Approach-avoidance conflicts like this burgeon like weeds from the fertile fields of our indecisiveness. And we become more and more anxious the longer we stay stuck while trying to figure out what we want to do. When we find ourselves in these circumstances, we usually require some professional help in understanding why we have become stuck in the first place and in discovering what to do to become unstuck

On the basis of the concepts touched on in this chapter, in Chapter 3 I will present the Fatal Pauses 3-D Method of Getting Unstuck Through the Power of No and the Power of Go.

References

Lewin K: A Dynamic Theory of Personality. New York, McGraw-Hill, 1935

McAllister AK, Usrey WM, Noctor SC, et al: Cellular and molecular biology of the neuron, in The American Psychiatric Publishing Textbook of Neuropsychiatry and Behavioral Neurosciences, 5th Edition. Edited by Yudofsky SC, Hales RE. Washington, DC, American Psychiatric Publishing, 2008, pp 3–43

Ogden CL, Carroll MD, Kit BK, et al: Prevalence of childhood and adult obesity in the United States, 2011–2012. JAMA 311(8):806–814, 2014

Paravizi J, Rangarajan V, Shirer WR, et al: The will to persevere induced by electrical stimulation of the human cingulate gyrus. Neuron 80:1359–1367, 2013

Wang HY, Chien HC, Osada N, et al: Rate of evolution in brain-expressed genes in humans and other primates. PLoS Bio 5(2):e13, 2007

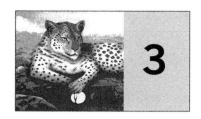

3

The Fatal Pauses 3-D Method of Getting Unstuck Through the Power of No and the Power of Go

Blessed be He who speaks and does;
Blessed be He who decrees and performs.
—*Hebrew Morning Prayer*

To make anything a habit, do it;
to not make it a habit, do not do it;
to unmake a habit, do something else in place of it.
—*Epictetus*, The Discourses of Epictetus (*as quoted in*
Life Witness *by Byram Karasau*)

Make everything as simple as possible,
But not simpler.
—*Albert Einstein*

"I knew smoking could kill them, but somehow I
didn't really realize that smoking could kill me!"

Brief Overview of the Fatal Pauses 3-D Method of Getting Unstuck

The Fatal Pauses 3-D Method of Getting Unstuck has three fundamental, interacting, and indelibly linked components: *Discover, Decide, Discipline.*

1. The D1 component is an approach process to *discover* the conflicts and causes that underlie your becoming stuck in pause. After you discover and understand why you have become stuck in the first place, you are in a position to move on to the D2 component.
2. The D2 component is where you *decide* whether you wish to choose to remain in your patterns of thought and behavior that led to being stuck or to do the necessary work to change. In order to make this decision, you must understand the *basic conflicts* that underlie your being stuck. This will help you clarify what you *most* want to do.

- Should you decide to remain stuck, treatment can help you deal with that decision, which usually means stopping the rumination and self-recrimination commonly associated with this choice.
- Should you decide to change and become unstuck, you are ready move on to the D3 component.

3. The D3 component constitutes your mustering the *discipline* that is required for you to make and sustain the changes required for becoming unstuck.

The Power of No and the Power of Go is a binary model and method of discipline that have been adapted from principles of neurobiology and evolution. In this chapter each component of the Fatal Pauses 3-D Method of Getting Unstuck will be amplified and explained. But first let's review the practical and theoretical principles on which this method has been based, as detailed in Chapter 1, "The Am I Stuck? Scale," and Chapter 2, "Getting Stuck."

Brief Overview of Chapters 1 and 2

Chapter 1 consists of a questionnaire, the *Am I Stuck? Scale*, that is designed to assess whether or not you, someone with whom you are personally involved, or your patient might be stuck in pause. The questions in this scale screen for the most common and important areas in which people become stuck, including destructive relationships; alcohol and other substance abuse; compulsive behaviors (e.g., video games, gambling, sexual excesses); eating-related problems; risk taking (both poles: being foolhardy or the other extreme, being overly cautious); engaging in illegal activities; procrastinating; abusive behaviors; self-destructive, self-diminishing, or self-incriminating thoughts, feelings, and behaviors; overpleasing others; problems with "life balance"; and problems adapting to aging.

In Chapter 2, the origins and biological implications of our becoming stuck in pause were reviewed from an evolutionary perspective. In this chapter, I offer a synopsis of the profound complexity of the human brain and a review of the basic elements of its function. I detail how our brains evolved to react to serious threats through binary *fight or flight* actions and how these actions are mediated by specific electrical and chemical changes in our brains and bodies. Like computers, the brain's method of processing information utilizes binary functions, which are "fire/don't fire" electrical transmissions in the axon component of neurons. Additionally, at the brain's neuronal synapses, complementary, biochemically based neurotransmissions are employed. Also reviewed in Chapter 2 were the ways we rely on pattern recognition to make sense of our external and internal environments and how this reliance is enabled by consistency and repetition.

In Chapter 2, I also discussed how, in today's world, we become stuck in pause through both conscious and unconscious conflicts related to complex interpersonal and social relationships and through having too many choices. Uncertain about what is the best course to take, we become conflicted between *fight* and *flight* or *stop* and *go* decisions, all of which are active states. Anxiety is conceptualized as deriving from a neurobiological amalgam of anger (fight) and fear (flight). Not being able to make decisions that lead to maximizing our potentials and happiness involves our failure to resolve approach-approach and approach-avoidance conflicts. When unresolved, these conflicts are associated with chronic anxiety, persistent rumination, and physical and mental dysfunctions. When we become stuck in pause, our fight or flight biophysiological responses lead to serious consequences for our psychological and physical health. Thus, anxiety, which once had survival value because it heightened our senses to make us vigilant about undisclosed danger, now endangers our survival.

Table 3–1 summarizes the hallmarks of being stuck in pause.

Let us now apply our understanding of these fundamental, evolutionary, and brain-based principles underlying getting stuck to present a method for getting unstuck.

TABLE 3–1. Hallmarks of being stuck in pause

Indecisiveness and failure to take action in our *fight or flight* or in *do or don't do* critical life choices and conflicts

Uncertainty and rumination about how to resolve important life problems

Inconsistency in the structure and patterns of daily life

Anger (the *fight* component of the *fight or flight* dyad) is internalized, self-directed, and expressed through irritability, self-deprecation, self-destructive thoughts and behaviors, depression, hopelessness, and psychosomatic symptoms

Fear (the *flight* component of the *fight or flight* dyad) accompanies avoidance of resolving conflicts

Anxiety (the amalgam of anger and fear) is the result of failure to take action in *fight or flight* or to choose between *no or go* conflicts

---

Fatal Pauses 3-D Method of Getting Unstuck: Discover

Introduction

In order to *discover* how a person has become stuck in pause, it is first necessary to gain a holistic understanding of the person as a unique individual—both strengths and weaknesses, both abilities and disabilities. In the clinical setting, this is accomplished through taking the standard psychiatric history, medical history, and mental status—to be followed by crafting a psychiatric treatment plan. Taking shortcuts in this realm is fraught with risk, and important underlying causes may not be identified and resolved. Shortcuts most often lead to recidivism. The D1 component of the Fatal Pauses 3-D Method of Getting Unstuck utilizes standard psychiatric and psychological approaches to understanding and treating people, in function and dysfunction.

Standard Psychiatric History and Treatment Plan

A comprehensive explication of how to elicit and organize a psychiatric history, how to make a psychodynamic formulation, how to diagnose a patient, and how to construct a treatment plan to reverse psychiatric disorders is far beyond the scope and focus of this book. Mental health professionals may acquire this information and these

skills from standard textbooks on the subject and through enlight-
ened supervision in the clinical setting. I recommend that people
who are stuck in pause seek consultation from a formally trained, licensed, and gifted mental health professional—in addition to reading
and applying the method and techniques presented in *Fatal Pauses*.
Through the presentation of case examples in this chapter and the
subsequent chapters of this book, I will endeavor to demonstrate how
standard psychiatric history taking and treatment planning meld
with the Fatal Pauses 3-D Method to enable people to get unstuck.
An excellent example of this approach can be found in Chapters 8
and 9, "Stuck in a Bottle," which describe a person with chronic alcohol use disorder who suffered many recurrences despite long stays
in residential settings and devoted attendance at Alcoholics Anonymous meetings. She accounts in her own words how insight gained
in psychotherapy about the unconscious roots and experiential
causes of her alcoholism has enabled her to remain sober.

Several critical components of the standard psychiatric evaluation and treatment planning merit emphasis. More than 25 years ago
it was my privilege to publish a book, *The Psychiatric Evaluation in
Clinical Practice*, with Roger A. MacKinnon, M.D., a professor of
psychiatry at Columbia University and a master clinician and educator (Mackinnon and Yudofsky 1986). In that book and a related book
that followed (Mackinnon and Yudofsky 1991), we made the following points that I utilize in my psychiatry practice to this very day:

> The most important technique in obtaining a psychiatric history
> is to allow the patient to tell his story in his own words and in the
> order that he chooses. (Mackinnon and Yudofsky 1986, p. 41)

> The most common error that the psychiatrist makes while ob-
> taining a psychiatric history is his interference with the patient's
> natural unfolding of the history by over-structuring the interview
> with excessive questions or by following a particular interview
> schedule. It cannot be emphasized too strongly that the organiza-
> tion of the history and the mental status examination outlined in
> this chapter is for the psychiatric written record; it is not a script to
> follow during the interview. (Mackinnon and Yudofsky 1986, p. 40)

Both the content and the order in which the patient presents his
or her history reveal valuable information concerning his or her
deeper feelings. From the instant a patient, his or her family or
friend, or a health care professional first contacts me or Mrs. Hoff-

man, my saintly administrative assistant, to request care, I begin endeavoring to understand and devise a treatment plan for that patient. Every detail and interaction—even those that occur prior to my first meeting with a patient—are important, if not essential, to my optimal assessment, understanding, and treatment of the patient. Although my clinical sessions with patients emphasize spontaneity and I almost never impose a structure or goal for the individual sessions, my approach to organizing and implementing a treatment plan is highly structured and formulated. Thus, there is an important distinction between my *gathering* of historical information and my *organization* and *implementation* of the treatment plan. All three elements are accomplished by full and respectful collaboration with the patient.

In our two books on this subject, Dr. MacKinnon and I also emphasized the great value in constructing a written formulation and treatment plan that conceptualize the biological, psychological, and social underpinnings of the patient's psychiatric disorder and our approach to treatment. The foundation for this approach is what is termed the *biopsychosocial model*. *Biological* factors and features include genetic predispositions, brain lesions and disorders, endocrine and other medical dysfunctions, and toxins (including alcohol and drugs of abuse). *Psychological* factors and features comprise both positive and traumatic life experiences and how they are represented in the individual's conscious and unconscious mind in the formation of psychiatric symptoms. *Social* features encompass cultural effects, family setting, occupation, interpersonal relationships, values, and spiritual life.

With most of my patients for whom it is safe and therapeutically indicated, I share all the elements of the psychodynamic formulation and treatment plan. In fact, we work together on arriving at a diagnosis and assembling and implementing the treatment plan. Until treatment is discontinued, our treatment is always a "work in progress." The wise old saying "A person never wades in the same river twice" applies directly to psychiatric treatment planning. Not only does the stream constantly change, but the person also changes with time. Inevitably during the course of treatment, important events and changes occur in the patient's life that affect the goals and purpose and, therefore, the focus of treatment. Similarly, as time goes by, our bodies and biology constantly change as the result of aging, health issues, external environments, and treatment. These changes also can require adjust-ments in the treatment plan (Yudofsky and Kim 2004).

Table 3–2 summarizes the sequence and structure for organizing and implementing a comprehensive psychiatric assessment and treatment plan for patients who are stuck in pause.

TABLE 3–2.	Fatal Pauses 3-D Method of Getting Unstuck: D1 (discover)

Comprehensive psychiatric assessment and treatment plan for patients who are stuck in pause

Classic psychiatric approach to *elicit* and *organize* a patient's historical information, chief complaints, presenting symptoms, and current mental status

Classic psychodynamic principles to *conceptualize* and *understand* the sources of the patient's psychological symptoms and conflicts

Evidence-based psychiatric and medical approaches to *conceptualize* and *diagnose* the biological aspects of the patient's psychological problem

Treatment plan to reverse the patient's psychiatric and medical disorders utilizing the biopsychosocial model and evidence-based treatments

Many extensive case examples of the *Discover* (D1) component of the Fatal Pauses 3-D Method of Getting Unstuck will be presented in the succeeding chapters of this book.

Fatal Pauses 3-D Method of Getting Unstuck: Decide

The D2 *(Decide)* component of the Fatal Pauses 3-D Method of Getting Unstuck uses the information and insights gained from the standard psychiatric assessment described above to determine the *conflicts* that underlie a patient's being stuck in pause. A brief discus-sion of theory and types of conflicts that lead to being stuck and the associated anxiety is found in Chapter 2, and these conflicts are sum-marized in Table 3–3.

I have chosen the following case to illustrate the D2 component of the Fatal Pauses 3-D Method of Getting Unstuck because of its pared down brevity and clarity. I also believe that I began to conceptualize this method as a result of this brief therapeutic encounter many years ago.

TABLE 3–3. Fatal Pauses 3-D Method of Getting Unstuck:
D2 (decide)

Determine the underlying conflicts

Utilize insights gained from the standard psychiatric assessment and
determine the principal conflicts leading to patient's being stuck in pause

Subdivide the conflicts into the following conflictual choices:

1. *Approach-approach conflicts* arise when we must choose between two
things we like or between two positive opportunities or outcomes.

2. *Approach-avoidance conflicts* occur when something we like or want to
express leads to things we don't like or that are not in our best interest.
Thus, we must choose to *avoid* something that we actually like or want
to do in order to avoid something that we don't like or that we don't
want to occur.

3. *Avoidance-avoidance conflicts* occur when we must select between or
among several things or actions that we don't like.

Case Presentation of Curtis Holbrook, M.D.

Case Example 1: Decide Component

In 1982, as a relatively junior faculty member of Columbia University College of Physicians and Surgeons, I cared for my patients in
the Atchley Pavilion, Columbia-Presbyterian's outpatient office
building for full-time faculty. One afternoon, I was treating an elderly woman who had developed depression following a stroke
when Dr. Curtis Holbrook burst into my office without knocking.
Professor Holbrook was a renowned and revered cardiovascular
surgeon. Not acknowledging my startled patient, he boomed,

> **Dr. Curtis Holbrook:** Sorry to disturb you, Stuart, but I
> have a job for you!
> **Dr. Y.:** Yes, sir?
> **Dr. Holbrook:** No matter how hard I try, I can't seem to
> stop smoking on my own. I heard that you do hypnosis
> for smoking, and I want to come in to see you this
> Wednesday at 6:00 A.M. You guys probably don't start
> working until noon, so you should have an opening in
> your schedule.
> **Dr. Y.:** Yes, sir!
> **Dr. Holbrook:** Good, then, let's get it done!

With that, Dr. Holbrook pivoted and exited as abruptly as he
had entered. Wordless, my patient and I stared at each other in star-

tled disbelief—as if a cheetah on stimulants had just pounced in and out of the office.

About Medical Hypnosis for Smoking

During my residency in psychiatry, I took a 2-year elective course in medical hypnosis from Dr. Herbert Spiegel. He was a brilliant clinician, educator, and innovator in medical hypnosis and had developed and tested thoughtful techniques that applied hypnosis to treat many medical conditions—from pain control to social phobia to certain substance use disorders.

Dr. Spiegel's general approach for using hypnosis to treat a medical symptom (e.g., pain) or disorder (e.g., nicotine use disorder) is summarized as follows (Spiegel and Spiegel 2004).

1. Take a full medical and psychiatric history of the patient to be treated. (The clinician does not want to use hypnosis to remove symptoms that identify a treatable condition, nor does the clinician want the patient to use hypnosis in ways that are unsafe.)
2. Take a focused history of the origin, course, and impact of the symptom to be treated.
3. Use the Spiegel Method to assess the patient's hypnotic profile. People have innately different capacities to be hypnotized. The "deeper" one can be hypnotized, the greater the therapeutic possibilities and effectiveness of the procedure.
4. Use the Spiegel Method to hypnotize the patient. This method utilizes a structured approach to relaxation, concentration, and focus.
5. When the patient is under hypnosis, use a highly structured approach for the specific symptom or problem to be treated.

Dr. Spiegel's specific approach for treating cigarette smoking is summarized as follows:

1. Place patient, who had previously undergone trial hypnosis, into a hypnotic trance state, which involves deep relaxation, removing all conflicting thoughts from his or her conscious mind, and focus on the hypnotist's suggestions.
2. In the hypnotic state, review, slowly and carefully, with the patient the following three steps or "truths" about cigarette smoking, health, and survival:
   - "Above all else I have a desire to protect my body."
   - "Smoking is a poison to my body."
   - "My desire to protect my body is greater than my desire to smoke; therefore, I will no longer smoke."

3. The medical hypnotist should use clear, convincing imagery to help elaborate on each of the three steps.
4. The patient should acknowledge whether or not he or she agrees with each step, focus on the truth of these steps, and make a decision to abide by their meaning and conclusion.
5. Remove the patient from the hypnotic state and teach him or her how to use self-hypnosis on a regular basis to reinforce the process.

As I applied Dr. Spiegel's method of hypnosis to smoking, the procedure required a *minimum* of four 1-hour-long meetings with my patients. The first meeting was for history taking and assessing the patient's hypnotic profile; the second was for administration of the specific procedure described above; the third, about a week later, was for short-term follow-up and reinforcement of the method; and a fourth meeting, after about a month, was for longer-term follow-up.

Given that most of the patients who came to see me for smoking had previously attempted to quit smoking many times without sustained success and given the extraordinary medical morbidity and mortality associated with smoking, I would often schedule many follow-up visits for purposes of monitoring compliance and reducing recidivism. During the 8 years that I practiced medical hypnosis (the time constraints of my neuropsychiatry practice and my increasing academic responsibilities necessitated that I discontinue administering the procedure), I used hypnosis to treat several hundred people for nicotine use disorder. Where possible, I maintained long-term follow-up data on this group. Approximately 65% of the patients so treated remained nicotine-free for 10 years and beyond. That said, many of these patients required other medical and psychiatric care beyond the hypnosis. In addition to their smoking, many patients received treatment using other therapeutic modalities for anxiety, depression, alcohol use disorder, and situational problems. Therefore, my treatment sample for using hypnosis to treat patients' cigarette smoking was not, in any way, a "clean study" of the efficacy of hypnosis per se for treating nicotine use disorder.

Dr. Holbrook's Second Visit

I had known of Dr. Holbrook and his extraordinary technical skills and seminal research contributions to cardiovascular surgery since I was a medical student. On completion of my residency, he had frequently consulted me to care for his patients who experienced psychiatric complications immediately following their heart surgery, including a fairly common condition known as postcardiotomy delirium. He was also widely known to have a "strong personality," which meant that he was assertive, abrupt, impatient, and, on occasions, volatile. (As one might imagine, his bedside manner with patients could be far less than ideal.) To work with Dr. Holbrook meant that you had to do things *his way*. I was certain that our interaction would be no different, which was likely to create a challenge for me.

A fundamental principle of medical hypnosis is that the patient *has to give up some control to the hypnotist in order to gain greater control over himself or herself*. Knowing Dr. Holbrook, I realized that there was no way on Earth that he would readily give up control—especially to a very young psychiatrist. Nonetheless, he was struggling with a potentially fatal problem, and he had come to me for help. I would do my best to help him, which certainly would transpire under *his* terms.

On the designated Wednesday, I arrived at my office at 5:15 A.M., which was fortunate because he appeared at 5:30 A.M. for our 6:00 A.M. appointment.

> **Dr. Curtis Holbrook:** It's getting late, so let's get going. I have three cases to do before noon, and the first patient is already being prepped for surgery. I need to get out of here by 6:15, at the very latest. Now put me under hypnosis!
>
> **Dr. Y.:** First, I would like to get some medical history about your smoking and explain to you the process of hypnosis.
>
> **Dr. Holbrook:** We don't need to waste time with questions. I'll summarize for you. First, I've been smoking about a pack and a half of cigarettes a day since my freshman year of college—that's 37 years ago. The longest I've been able to stop has been for 2 or 3 days, and then I go back to smoking. Second, I don't need to know anything about how hypnosis is supposed to work. We don't have time for that. I didn't explain to my patient this morning what I have to do to replace her mitral valve. Let's just get it done, Stuart!

After communicating to Dr. Holbrook that I would have preferred to take a thorough medical and psychiatric history before proceeding to hypnosis and that I believed that I was "shortchanging" him by their omission, I obediently took a hypnotic profile of Dr. Holbrook. His profile was a 3 on the 5-point Spiegel Scale for hypnotizability, which is about average. One component of the hypnotic process is a technique of relaxing the patient's mind and musculature, which involves his imagining himself to be in a place that is quiet, safe, and comfortable.

> **Dr. Y.:** Where is the place in your life that you feel the most relaxed and comfortable?

Dr. Curtis Holbrook: At my cabin in Maine. It is quite remote, on about 200 acres of forest on the bank of a big lake. No one can get to me when I'm there. It's the *only* place where I relax. I'm in the process of building our retirement home on the property.

With that, I placed Dr. Holbrook in what I hoped would be a hypnotic trance state. After he was relaxed, focused, and in the trance state, we reviewed, several times, the three steps for smoking cessation that were recounted above. One key element of the process was the following point that I made to him while he was in the hypnotic trance state:

Dr. Y.: Concentrate, Dr. Holbrook, on the fact that in the hypnotic state, your mind has become clear—like the water in the lake by your house in Maine—about what *you* want to do most. We did not say that you do not want to smoke, a statement that would be untrue. *Rather, you have become absolutely clear that you want to be alive more than you want to smoke.* You want to be alive to care for your patients, to love your wife and children, and to enjoy your lake retreat *far more* than you want whatever enjoyment you get from cigarettes. With this insight, you have now made the decision to control yourself and not to allow nicotine to control you.

I always mold the hypnotic suggestion to the personality dynamics and the life realities of the subject. Thus, I focused a great deal on Dr. Holbrook's achieving "true" control.

Dr. Holbrook would not agree to meet with me in the standard follow-up sessions for medical hypnosis, nor did he respond to several notes and phone messages in which I tried to inquire how he was faring with regard to smoking cessation. About 6 months after our first and only session, Dr. Holbrook again entered my office unannounced and exclaimed,

Dr. Curtis Holbrook: I thought that you might want to know that I haven't smoked one cigarette since we did the hypnosis thing. I am absolutely certain that I will never smoke again. But that's not why I came by.

Dr. Y.: That's great, Dr. Holbrook.

Dr. Holbrook: I came by to tell you *how* your so-called hypnosis works. As a heart and chest surgeon, I did not need *you* to tell *me* that smoking is bad for my body or could kill me. Having removed the lungs of countless people with lung cancer, I thought I knew that. The vast majority of these poor souls were smokers. I knew smoking could kill *them*, but somehow I didn't really realize that smoking could kill *me!* I never made the connection that smoking could kill *me* until you told me, under hypnosis, what a shame it would be if I died before I could retire to my vacation home in Maine. Somehow that got through to me. Before that, I suppose I always had at least 10 other things on my mind when I thought about the repercussions—for me—of smoking. I think that's because *I really like smoking.* As you probably figured out, I am very hardheaded. I don't like giving up what I like. Well, enough whining; I've got to get out of here now, Stuart. Think about what I just told you; I think it applies to a lot of people.

I realized two things from this brief third encounter in my office with Dr. Holbrook. First, this wise, tough clinician and educator was teaching me an important lesson about what it takes to make a decision to give up something that you like that isn't good for you. Second, it was his way to thank me for the help—by teaching me an important lesson.

Over the succeeding 30 years, I received an annual Christmas card from Dr. Holbrook with the same handwritten message: "I'm still around, Stuart. And still not smoking. Hope you're OK too." We both moved on. A mutual friend told me that he retired at age 65 and had moved to Maine. Not long ago, however, no card from Dr. Holbrook arrived at Christmas time. I was very upset. I later learned that he had died several months before. He was 91 years old, and I miss him dearly.

What I Learned From Dr. Holbrook

Over the succeeding years, I have thought deeply about Dr. Holbrook and what had enabled him to stop smoking. And about what he was teaching me. My conclusions were the following:

1. Dr. Holbrook had long known that cigarette smoking harmed many bodily organs and that it directly led to the deaths of innumerable *other* people. However, he never slowed down sufficiently to accept that smoking could kill *him!*
2. Hypnosis helped lead to his *discovery* and *acceptance* that smoking could also kill *him.*
3. In our last meeting, Dr. Holbrook made sure that I understood that he *liked* smoking and that he did *not* want to give it up.

4. Therefore, Dr. Holbrook's discovery that smoking could actually kill him led to a *conflict*. He would have to choose between two things that he wanted: 1) to smoke and 2) to have a long, healthy life. As a scientist and surgeon, he knew he couldn't have both. Although he had to accept that he liked cigarettes and wanted to smoke (*approach*) in order to prevent (*avoidance*) something that he didn't like or want (cancer and premature death), he taught me the value of reconstructing his conflict as approach-approach. That way he could avoid a power struggle with himself: Nobody tells Dr. Holbrook what to do—not even Dr. Holbrook!

5. Confronted with this conflict, Dr. Holbrook had to *decide* what he wanted most. He decided 1) although he liked to smoke, he liked being alive more than smoking and 2) to stop smoking.

6. After he had decided that he should not smoke, he then had to muster the requisite *discipline* to stop smoking.

For many people, discipline can be the most difficult component of the 3-D Method, but Dr. Holbrook's life was all about discipline. His routine was to be at work at Columbia-Presbyterian Hospital by 5:00 A.M. 6 days a week and rarely to leave the hospital before 10:00 P.M. At work, he did not waste time. He worked hard and was organized, productive, and efficient to the point of being brusque with patients and staff. I recognize that not everybody, once they decide to stop smoking, is able to override by sheer will power the powerful addictive qualities of nicotine and the psychosocial and social reinforcements of cigarette smoking. To change, most of us require much more insight about the factors that led to and sustain our being stuck, and most of us need support to get unstuck. Usually, we fail a few times before we succeed.

I believe that Dr. Holbrook was stuck primarily because he had *avoided* confronting himself with a clear decision every time he lit up a cigarette. His smoking was on "automatic pilot." When he allowed himself to become aware of what he was choosing between—immediate pleasure and future poor health—he assumed control for the first time. After he had decided, he had the discipline to act on his decision. It is not always so easy, as will be evidenced in the case presentations in the succeeding chapters of the book. For Clarke Myerson in Chapter 4, "Stuck in My Job," the D1 component (discovery) of why and how he became stuck in his job required the most focus, and for Lynda Jensen in Chapter 9, who was dependent on alcohol, the D3 component (discipline) was a key challenge to remaining off alcohol.

At the end of the day, however, only we ourselves can manifest the discipline that is necessary to get unstuck. No one can do that part for us. The next section of this chapter presents my technique to help you muster the discipline required to get unstuck using the Power of No and the Power of Go.

Fatal Pauses 3-D Method of Getting Unstuck: Discipline—Getting Unstuck Through the Power of No and the Power of Go

Introduction: Making It Simple but Not Easy

Although a multifaceted confluence and interplay of genetic, biological, experiential, psychological, social, and spiritual factors can lead to becoming stuck in pause, a straightforward intervention is required for becoming unstuck. Utilizing a similar binary approach, as exemplified by the basic information processing functions of computers and the action potentials of the electrical transmission of the brain (i.e., "all or none"), the dauntingly complex task of becoming unstuck can be rendered far less complicated. Simple does not necessarily mean easy. Success depends on the determination to succeed.

Definitions

The Power of No: *Not* doing something you *want* to do
 To achieve something that you want more
The Power of Go: *Doing* something that you *don't want* to do
 To achieve something that you want more[1]

Getting Unstuck Through the Power of No and the Power of Go

Table 3–4 summarizes the technique of getting unstuck through the Power of No and the Power of Go.

---

[1]For those readers who are using *Fatal Pauses* as a self-help book, substitute "I" for "you."

TABLE 3–4.   Techniques for getting unstuck using the Power of No and the Power of Go

---

1. *Identify areas in your life in which you are stuck:* In what critical areas of your life are you stuck in pause?

2. *Identify your goals for change:* What would you like to do or achieve if you become unstuck?

3. *Identify the central unresolved conflict(s) that underlie your problems and prevent change:* What are the specific approach-approach and approach-avoidance conflicts that have led to your becoming stuck? Where possible, reconstruct the conflicts as approach-approach to obviate your being in a power struggle with yourself.

4. *Identify and monitor the hallmarks of being stuck (Table 3–1):* Which among the symptoms commonly associated with being stuck do you have (rumination, obsessions, indecisiveness, anxiety, anger, irritability, self-deprecation, demoralization, depression, fear, and panic)? Do you have inconsistency in your life patterns and/or do you avoid important tasks and initiatives?

5. *Identify binary problem/solution:* What are the principal problem(s) that you must *stop* and *not do* and/or what must you *do* to get unstuck?

6. *Identify "critical decision point":* What are the key decision points that are required for you to get unstuck and to stay unstuck (e.g., for alcohol use disorder, "Don't drink!")?

7. *Identify the corollary factors required to achieve resolution:* What other factors require a *stop* or *go* decision to support the critical decision (technique 6)? For example, for alcohol use disorder, "Go to Alcoholics Anonymous meetings regularly" or "Stop going to bars."

8. *Resolve your problem through the Power of Go and the Power of No:* Do those things that are required to get unstuck or *don't do* those things that are required to get unstuck. Both decisions require action, corresponding to *fight or flight* behaviors.

Case Examples of Getting Unstuck Using the Power of No and the Power of Go

The technique of using the Power of No and the Power of Go to become unstuck is best illustrated by two more relatively uncomplicated case examples. Because we all become stuck in pause in various ways and at different points during our lifetimes, I will present two examples wherein I became stuck in my own life.

Case Example 2: The Power of No

About 1 month after having begun an internship in surgery, I was doing a postoperative examination of a patient who had had a mitral
valve replacement. Mrs. O'Brien was about to be released from the
hospital, and I was weighing her, which is a requirement for discharge.

> **Mrs. O'Brien:** How much do I weigh? The silver lining of
> having to undergo this surgery and to stay in the hos-
> pital for 2 weeks is that I'm sure that I lost weight on
> this horrible hospital food.
> **Dr. Y.:** You weigh 167 pounds, Mrs. O'Brien.
> **Mrs. O'Brien:** There is no *way* that I can be that heavy. It
> means that I have gained over 5 pounds since I have
> been here! I've hardly eaten anything. The scale must
> be wrong. Please check to see if it is accurate.
> **Dr. Y.:** I'll weigh myself on the scale to check it out. My
> weight never varies. I've weighed the same since I was
> in high school.

Clad in a green scrub suit, I removed my shoes and my white
laboratory coat (with its pockets stuffed with a surgical intern's bal-
last of medical instruments, note cards, laboratory reports, and a
beeper), and confidently stepped onto the platform of the Detecto
hospital balance scale.

> **Dr. Y.:** Not to worry, Mrs. O'Brien. I think you actually have
> lost a few pounds. This scale reads that I weigh 152
> pounds, which is about 12 pounds too high. We'll find
> another scale where you can get an accurate reading.

Over the course of that fateful day, I checked my weight on five
different Detecto scales—all with the same result. I was shocked to
learn that I had gained 12 pounds during my first month as an intern! With mounting horror, I rapidly calculated that I would more
than *double* my weight over the course of my 12-month internship—
unless I did something to intervene.

This incident occurred during the first week of August 1970,
about 2 months after I had received my medical degree. As a surgical
intern, I was at the bottom rung of the physician ladder. Those of us
who worked at the New York City Municipal Hospital System were
kept busy during literally all of the time that we were in the hospital.
We worked 6 days per week, and, on the days that we were "off call,"
we left the hospital after 8:00 P.M., only to return at 5:00 A.M. the
next "on call" day. We were on call every other day and stayed up
without sleep throughout the nights that we were on call.

The Vietnam War was just winding down at that time, and there was a physician shortage on the surgical services of the Bronx Municipal Hospital Center and Lincoln Hospital, where I was assigned. Assisting advanced residents and surgeons during an endless succession of emergency and scheduled operations, my fellow surgery interns and I were in operating rooms, running to emergency rooms and intensive care units, or at the bedside of a patient nearly every minute of our time in the hospital. Consequently, there was very little time available for us to sit down to eat.

To subsist, I had developed the habit of grabbing and gobbling down doughnuts while racing from one operation to another. Gleaming from their grease-stained, cardboard showcases like cored apples in a fluorescent-lit, antiseptic Garden of Eden, the doughnuts were irresistibly iced with chocolate, caramel, and vanilla. They enticed me from their omnipresent lairs in nurses' stations, patents' rooms, and surgeons' locker rooms. Not that I was complaining, for there was nothing that I enjoyed more than to consume a steaming-fresh, fragrant doughnut—or two....

The seed of my precipitous weight gain had fallen onto fertile, troubled soil. Weight had always been a big issue for me. For as long as I could remember, my mother was on a diet. Like almost everyone on her side of our family, she was perennially "heavy." A successful businesswoman and perfectionist who triumphed in just about all other areas of her life, she was continuously miserable about and ashamed of being overweight. She hated how she looked. Sensitive to her endless suffering, I had vowed never, never to let that happen to me.

Accordingly, I devised a plan whereby I would limit my doughnut intake to no more than six per day, as opposed to the several dozen that I calculated that I had previously been consuming each day. I checked my weight regularly to determine whether or not the plan was working. Despite considerable effort, however, the number of doughnuts I devoured daily and, consequently, my weight did not change. I was anxious and unsettled by my failure. To make matters worse, I found that I was becoming *preoccupied* with doughnuts. I ruminated about how many I had eaten that day. During long surgical procedures I kept obsessing about when and where I would get my next doughnut. Feeling weak and somewhat ridiculous, I was pretty sure that my preoccupation with doughnuts was rooted in other, more complex issues—such as the stresses associated with my transition from being a student to being a physician. Nonetheless, I focused on doughnuts. I tried to avoid the hospital locations where doughnuts, like land mines, were strategically placed. And I chastened myself each time that I lost my resolve—which was quite often.

I resolved that I would not let doughnuts defeat me and let myself become obese. On further scrutiny of my habit, I noticed that my hunger for a second doughnut intensified significantly after I had eaten the first. My extended periods of doughnut abstinence felt like torture, and those periods were punctuated with relapses in which I gorged on several at a time. In a flash of insight, I came to the following realizations:

1. It would be far easier for me to stop eating doughnuts altogether than to ration them, as I had been trying to do without success.
2. I would have to change other, related behaviors in order to remain abstinent from doughnuts. After all, I had to eat something at work because I was there most of the time.

I devised a doughnut-ending plan that included the following:

1. Because I was off call one weekend day per week, I would use that day to shop for, prepare, and pack healthful foods to take to the hospital for lunch and dinner every day.
2. On those times when I was not on call, I would awaken even earlier to eat healthful breakfasts at home.
3. Most importantly, I would not take a single bite of another doughnut—either at the hospital or anywhere else.
4. I would not replace eating doughnuts at the hospital with similar, high-caloric foods with little or no health value— such as the pastries, cookies, cakes, and candies that are also present in abundance in hospitals.

The plan worked. I found that it was far easier for me to stop eating doughnuts altogether than to limit their intake to a so-called reasonable amount. Within 2 weeks I had stopped ruminating about doughnuts or related types of food. There was no point in getting into debates and power struggles with myself about doughnuts because I had eaten my last one. Over the next several months, I lost the weight that I had gained during my first month of internship. I have not touched another doughnut in more than 40 years, and my weight has remained stable. More importantly, I had begun to appreciate *the Power of No!*

Discussion of Case Example 2

Although correcting a "doughnut habit" that had persisted for only 2 months hardly qualifies in life-altering relevance as a fatal pause, it nonetheless encompasses the fundamental elements of being stuck in pause. It is possible that my "doughnut abuse" could have developed into a fatal pause had it gone unchecked over a protracted period of time and damaged my health and self-esteem. Table 3–5 outlines the key elements of being stuck in pause with regard to overeating doughnuts, and Table 3–6 outlines the technique for getting unstuck through the Power of No.

TABLE 3–5. Key elements of being stuck in pause

1. *How I was stuck:* I was gaining weight because I couldn't stop eating doughnuts

2. *Goals for change:* Stop eating doughnuts; lose weight

3. *Central, unresolved conflict:* I loved doughnuts/I wanted to remain slim and healthy (approach-approach)

4. *Hallmarks of my being stuck in pause:* Ruminations, anxiety, guilt, self-deprecation

5. *Binary problem/solution:* Eat doughnuts, get fat/don't eat doughnuts, get and stay thin

6. *Critical decision point:* Don't put a doughnut in my mouth

7. *Corollary factors to achieve resolution:* Reallocation of weekend time, planning meals, packing and bringing meals to work, nonsubstitution of doughnuts with other pastries and sweets, weighing self regularly

8. *Resolution:* Stop eating doughnuts

Five key principles led to my success in getting unstuck from pause using the Power of No. First, I had to *decide to stop something that I liked doing in order to achieve something that I wanted more.* Notice how the emphasis is placed on what I wanted to do *most:* Although I wanted to eat doughnuts, I wanted to be thin and healthy much more. Thus, I wasn't saying "no" to myself, I was saying "no" to the donuts. In actuality, I was saying "yes" to my health and appearance, which was far more important to me than the pleasure of eating doughnuts. At the most fundamental levels, when you say "no" to yourself, you set up a power struggle that will usually be lost. The *decision* never to eat another doughnut was also, fundamentally, empowering. This principle came in quite handy when I treated Dr. Holbrook about 12 years later (see Case Example 1).

Second, the binary *none or all, go or don't go* choice was required to achieve success. My trying to cut down my doughnut intake to a "reasonable" amount (whatever that might be for such a high-fat, high-

---

TABLE 3–6. Key principles for getting unstuck through the Power of No

---

1. You must *stop* something that you like in order to *gain* something that you like more.

2. You are saying "Yes!" to something that you fundamentally want by saying "No!" to something that you want less.

3. A *none or all* binary choice is required to achieve success. This involves making a critical decision (such as *not* drinking *any* alcohol). Moderation does not work in this case.

4. The Power of Go is *always* required to achieve the Power of No to support your critical decision (e.g., going to daily Alcoholics Anonymous meetings for people with alcohol use disorder). "No" is a decision that requires action.

5. A reprioritization of your time and restructuring of your schedule are usually required to support the critical decision (e.g., making time in the day, every day, to attend Alcoholics Anonymous meetings for people with alcohol use disorder).

---

sugar, vitamin void food) did not work. Why? 1) I liked doughnuts too much; 2) eating one donut induced my craving/hunger for more; 3) just limiting the number of doughnuts led to my obsessing about *when* to eat doughnuts, *where* to eat doughnuts, and *how many* doughnuts to eat; and 4) I felt frustrated and defeated when I exceeded my target amount.

For many years a large food brand tellingly advertised a best-selling snack food by proclaiming, "Bet you can't eat just one!" As in Las Vegas, the food industry continues to win that bet. For tens of millions of Americans, the beverage industry wins its bet about our not being able to drink sugar-loaded soft drinks or alcohol-containing beverages in moderation. But who says we have to take that bet? We're OK if we don't eat that one potato chip, smoke that one cigarette, or drink that one drink. I had to accept that I liked doughnuts too much merely to limit my intake of them. It was necessary for me to stop eating them altogether. I found it hard to admit to myself that I was too weak to "eat just one." I did not realize at the time that, just like drugs and alcohol are for so many of us, foods like doughnuts hijack our brains. We did not evolve to resist food products with combinations of high fat, sugar, and (in the case of other processed snack foods such as potato chips) salt.

This principle was again useful to me three decades later when I was texting and talking on my cell phone while driving. Once again, I had tried, unsuccessfully, to limit cell phone use to when I had stopped at traffic lights, but I eventually went back to answering calls and texting while driving. Employing the Power of No (at first by locking my cell phone in the trunk of the car), I have been able to stop this dangerous practice.

Third, the binary—none or all, go or don't go—choice can be reduced to a single *critical decision*. In the case of my "doughnut addiction," I would achieve certain success if I did not take one bite of a doughnut. Not putting a morsel of doughnut into my mouth was my critical decision point.

There are two primary values in identifying and remaining vigilant of this critical decision point. If I were to engage in preliminary behaviors that could endanger my resolve—such as going into a bakery with some friends and even buying and taking home a dozen "irresistible" doughnuts "for my family," my sticking to the critical decision would protect me. Knowing that I am still OK as long as I don't put a doughnut in my mouth would be a last ditch effort to maintain my resolve. My successful recognition and application of this decision point would also have important *ripple effects* related to other difficult decisions and choices—such as having the confidence and determination not to put into my mouth other hard-to-resist, superfattening, empty calorie snacks, sweets, and desserts such as ice cream. Success with a daunting problem leads to further successes.

Fourth, to achieve the Power of No required the continuous application of the Power of Go, or doing something that I didn't want to do in order to gain something I wanted more. I had to get up even earlier every day of my internship and had to make myself go food shopping on my one day off during the week. Thus, the Power of Go is almost always required to enable the Power of No.

Fifth, in order to effect almost any change—even one as rudimentary as stopping eating doughnuts—a *reprioritization of my time and restructuring of my daily schedule* was required. In this case, it was necessary for me to go food shopping on the one day of the week that I was off of work, as well as to get up even earlier than usual (4:00 A.M.) the other days in order to prepare and pack meals to take to the hospital. These positively enabling activities—which weren't necessarily fun or interesting to me—came at a high cost: they cut into my highly limited time for sleep and recreation.

The following example from my personal life of utilizing the Power of Go required a more complex resolution and much more discipline than "just" stopping eating doughnuts.

Case Example 3: The Power of Go

Discovery

Sometimes we are stuck in pause but don't know it. In 1983, when I was 39 years old, a shocking tragedy involving an esteemed mentor and colleague ignited my decision to return to regular exercise after several years of physical dormancy. At that time, Dr. Edward Sachar was the brilliant, vigorous chairman of Columbia's Department of Psychiatry and the director of the New York State Psychiatric Institute (the Institute). However, at age 49, Dr. Sachar suffered a devastating stroke that paralyzed the right side of his body and left him unable to speak comprehensibly. Not long thereafter, Dr. Sachar died of complications related to the stroke. As the Institute's and the department's clinical director, it had been my privilege to work closely with Dr. Sachar on a daily basis. I witnessed firsthand the stress and unrelenting demands of his research and administrative duties and saw that he rarely took the time to exercise. I attributed both the stress of his job and the fact that he did not exercise regularly to be important factors, among several others, that led to his stroke. Dr. Sachar's loss raised my awareness that my own lifestyle and professional demands were not that dissimilar to his. I therefore determined to resume exercising on a regular basis. Because of recurrent knee injuries, I had previously been advised by my doctors to avoid running and vigorous walking, so I decided to try lap swimming—solely by default.

Decision

Three decades later, the following conversation took place during a coached swim team workout on a glittering Sunday morning in the 25-meter outdoor lap pool of Houstonian Athletic and Fitness Club in Houston, Texas:

> **Bryan Smyth:** Didn't you just love that last sprint set, Stu?
> **Dr. Y.:** You and I are from a different planet, Bryan. I don't love swimming. On Sundays I "just love" lifting the Sunday *New York Times* onto the kitchen table. I don't "just love" swimming; I love having "*just* swum" and how my body feels because of swimming. Unlike you and the people from your planet, I can't wait until this workout is over.

A similar conversation had taken place 30 years earlier on a cold, wet December night in New York City. I was shivering in an ancient swimming pool in the dark, dank, and dreary basement of Bard Hall, the student center of Columbia College of Physicians and Surgeons. Apart from myself and Ilene Anderson, no one was in the pool or within the dripping, mildewed, tile walls of its encasing room.

Ilene Anderson: What are you doing here, Dr. Y.? I didn't know you like swimming.

Dr. Y. (*self-consciously and defensively*): Hi, Ilene. I don't like swimming. I'm in this pool for only one reason: to survive.

At that time Ilene Anderson was a medical student at Columbia, where I was on the psychiatry faculty. Ilene had also been my patient for the past 4 years. I became patently uncomfortable for several reasons. Primarily, I was concerned about maintaining appropriate professional boundaries. Like most mental health professionals, I endeavor to limit personal contacts with my patients outside of formal sessions and also do my best to rein in information relating to my personal life in order to enhance objectivity and reduce bias. Being mostly naked and alone in a basement swimming pool with a patient hardly qualifies as maintaining appropriate professional boundaries. Heretofore, Ilene had never seen me when I was not safely concealed within the confining, defining, starched-white cotton armor of a dress shirt and laboratory coat. However, my circumstance didn't seem to bother her as much as it did me.

Another reason for my discomfort on that day was that I had become self-conscious about my body. That was one of the reasons that I was in the pool in the first place. I knew that I was "out of shape"—both physically and physiologically. Although I had not gained a lot of weight, I realized that I had lost muscle tone: I felt flabby. For most of my life, I had actively engaged in aerobic sports, including basketball, tennis, running, and cycling. Over the previous several years, however, the confluence of several factors had eliminated most of my aerobic physical activities. I had developed two exercise-limiting physical problems: lower back pain from a bulging lumbar disc and movement-induced pain in both knees secondary to traumatic joint inflammation. At the age of 36, I was advised by my orthopedic surgeon (whom I had consulted to get a different opinion from my neurologist) to stop running.

As a neuropsychiatrist, I had learned by treating the sequelae of patients with traumatic brain injuries that cycling safely in New York City is also a challenge. I had overreacted to my doctors' advice to stop running by not exercising at all over the ensuing 3 years. Additionally, as it is for most physicians, *time* to exercise was a perennial challenge for me. As the director of the inpatient psychiatric service at Columbia-Presbyterian Hospital, I was at work before 7:00 A.M. and rarely left the medical center before 9:00 P.M. Also, my wife and I were blessed with the birth of our first child that year. Therefore, I did not feel that I had much "free time" to exercise.

Although I had always enjoyed "playing around" in the water as a child, I had no prior experience with sustained lap swimming. My sole swimming instruction took place at summer day camp when I was 5 years old. Greg, my 16-year-old camp counselor, was far more proficient at motivation than technique: "Campers, you will not be allowed to play in the deep water or to go off the diving boards until you can swim from one side of the pool to the other." Somehow we all managed to do so—with far more thrash and splash than velocity and finesse. On returning to the water 34 years later for lap swimming, I was so out of shape and constantly winded that I was barely able to thrash and splash. Velocity, finesse, and enjoyment in the water were beyond my wildest fantasy.

For several months I tried to force myself to swim laps about four times per week. I despised all aspects of the experience: having to travel to a dreary lap pool at the end of a hard day's work; having to jump into uncomfortably cold water; feeling uncoordinated and inadequate while swimming; having to waste time getting undressed, taking a shower, and getting dressed again; and having to go back, with wet hair, into the chilling New York City night to fight the traffic on the George Washington Bridge en route to my home in New Jersey. Not surprisingly, I dreaded the days that I had scheduled for swimming. During work days when I was to swim, I was uncharacteristically negative, irritable, and resentful. I would come up with "good reasons"—patient care, academic conflicts, family priorities—that would interfere with the swim plans and quite often chose not to go. Thereafter, I would feel guilt for giving in to excuses not to swim and would deprecate myself for not being strong enough to follow through with my commitment to exercise regularly.

Thus, on that evening when I encountered Ilene in the dank and dreary Bard Hall pool, I was enormously conscious of and self-conscious about how out of place and ridiculous I appeared while swimming. On the other hand, Ilene was gliding rapidly through the water with the elegance and effortlessness of a sea goddess. Obviously, she came from the same alien planet as Bryan Smyth. Throughout the swim, I kept hoping that she wouldn't pay further attention to me or to my humiliating ineptitude. Nevertheless, after about 45 minutes of my gasping and Ilene's gliding, she surfaced, uninvited, up into my lane.

Ilene Anderson: Dr. Y., do you mind if I ask you a few
   questions?
Dr. Y. (*lying*): Of course not, Ilene.

With the same piercing deftness of her freestyle, Ilene asked several penetrating questions and learned 1) why I had recently taken up lap swimming, 2) that I had no prior technical instruction in swimming, 3) that I intended to swim 4 days per week, 4) that I was swimming in order to get and stay in shape and to maintain health, and 5) that I disliked swimming laps.

Ilene Anderson: Dr. Y., would you mind if I offered you a
   little advice about swimming?
Dr. Y. (*lying again*): Of course not.
Ilene: With your perfectionistic, somewhat compulsive
   personality, it is important for you to get some excellent instruction on swimming technique. Do this before you immortalize your bad habits. I also believe
   that since you don't like swimming, you should swim
   every day. Otherwise, you will drive yourself crazy deciding which days to swim and which days not to swim.
   Eventually, you'll just stop swimming altogether. Finally, since lap swimming is so boring, you might try
   swimming with a master's team. The group process
   will improve your stroke, help with the monotony, and
   work well with your competitive nature.

Feeling even more exposed than I did in my Speedo swimsuit, I replied,

Dr. Y.: Do you mind if I ask you a question, Ilene?
Ilene Anderson: Of course not.
Dr. Y.: Who's supposed to be analyzing whom? I hope I'm
   doing half as good a job with you in the office as you
   have just done for me in the pool.
Ilene: Don't worry about it, Dr. Y. Just work on your swimming like you do on everything else, and we'll both be
   fine. I'd like you to hang around for a while so we can
   complete my treatment.

Clearly, Ilene was also shaken up by the tragedy of Dr. Sachar.
   I dislike using clichés or being subject to clichés. Nonetheless, as those of us who are in professions that involve giving advice understand, I realized that advice is far easier to give than to receive. And I confess that it was not easy for me to follow Ilene's advice. I

also recognized that *I had to change my life in order to save my life.* As a devoted advocate in my clinical practice of preventative medicine, I comprehended full well the wisdom and challenge of Ilene's sage advice. It was clear to me that as I grew older my health and fitness required that I exercise; otherwise, I would be at high risk to develop a continuous succession of orthopedic, metabolic, and cardiovascular insults that eventually could be life changing and life threatening. I also knew that it was entirely up to me to follow her advice. To do so required that I significantly rearrange my priorities and daily activities. I am embarrassed to admit that prior to Ilene's "intervention," my professional responsibilities comprised about 90% of my time and focus.

As I had experienced with my "doughnut dilemma" 12 years previously, I kept setting goals for myself that I was not following. My indecisiveness and mental state regarding swimming regularly evidenced many of the characteristic hallmarks of my being stuck in pause: inconsistency, indecisiveness, ruminations, irritability, and self-deprecation. This time I was stuck in an approach-avoidance conflict wherein I wanted to stay healthy and in good shape *(approach)* but also wished to avoid the hassle of swimming regularly and the pain of swimming fast *(avoidance)*. I had found it to be a time-consuming hassle to travel to and from a pool, and I felt embarrassed and uncomfortable when I was in the pool. On the other hand, I knew I needed to exercise regularly to stay in good shape and to be in good health. I had to decide which I wanted more: to be comfortable on a short-term basis or to be fit and healthy on a long-term basis.

Let us now apply the eight steps involved in my coming to a *decision* (D2 component) to swim on a daily basis.

1. *How I was stuck:* I was out of shape, my body was deteriorating, and I wasn't exercising regularly
2. *Goals for change:* Swim vigorously every day; get and stay in shape
3. *Central, unresolved conflict* (approach-avoidance): I wanted to stay fit and be healthy but avoid the pain and hassle of swimming regularly and hard
4. *Hallmarks of my being stuck:* Inconsistency, indecisiveness, ruminations, irritability, and self-deprecation
5. *Binary problem/solution:* Don't exercise, be unfit/swim regularly, be in shape
6. *Critical decision points:* Get to the pool; get in the water
7. *Corollary factors required to achieve resolution:* Adjust schedule to include time every day to swim, plan ahead to secure place to swim laps, schedule regular swim instruction and

masters swim group participation, and work to sustain positive attitude regarding lap swimming

8. *Resolution:* Swim vigorously every day

Discipline

At age 30, for the first time since I had entered college at age 18, I established a firm time to leave the academic/work environment. Second, I carefully researched the availabilities of excellent lap pools in my region and carved out time from my schedule to swim for at least 1 hour, 7 days per week. Over the succeeding years, depending on my professional and personal obligations on a particular day, I have had to swim at different times in different pools on specific days: 5:00 A.M., noon, or 9:00 P.M. have been not uncommon times. When I travel for work or go on vacations, I prearrange swimming accommodations for each day. Finally, and most important, I have taken swimming seriously. I continuously work on improving my technique, maintaining maximum effort in the pool, and, most importantly, sustaining a positive attitude. It's all hard to do, but the latter is the most difficult…and most important.

Despite all of the planning and effort that is required to get myself to the pool, I almost always hesitate to jump in the water when I am on deck. Most of the good lap pools have cool to cold water (less than 78 degrees Fahrenheit) so that competitive swimmers don't get overheated when they are practicing strenuously or racing. Getting into water that is this temperature is like stepping into what we conventionally term "a cold shower," which, in actuality, is at room temperature. Every day, I am tempted to turn around and go back to the locker room or, at the very least, gradually immerse myself over a period of about 15 minutes. Rather, I exercise the Power of Go and immediately jump into the water and begin to swim the workout. That entire process—from hesitation until jumping into the water—takes less than 5 seconds and is what I term *my critical decision point.* Using the Power of Go has had a "ripple effect," and I no longer delay to undertake and "get done" the other, somewhat unpleasant but necessary tasks of my life, such as the mindless, annoying paperwork that is a responsibility of the administrative aspects of my job.

Over the past 30 years, with *very rare* exceptions, such as minor injuries or hurricanes in Houston, I have swum workouts 364 days per year, for a minimum of 1 hour per day and covering a minimum of 3,000 meters per swim. I try to swim at a good pace and time almost every lap, which is a measure of effort, progress, and decline. The motto of many people who exercise seriously is "If it can't be measured, it probably didn't happen." That maxim also applies to the Power of Go.

Although these two case examples from my personal life entailed significant adjustments in my priorities and schedule, they did not require psychiatric treatment to address a specific disorder or to effect fundamental changes in my psyche, personality, or interpersonal relationships. More frequently, getting unstuck requires changes that address significant intrapersonal and interpersonal conflicts that are far more complex and challenging than my doughnut and fitness issues. As will be illustrated in Chapter 4, such conflicts and changes require a far more comprehensive D1 *(Discovery)* component, which includes standard psychiatric evaluation and treatment in order to achieve resolution.

Warning About the Dangerous Application of the Power of No and the Power of Go

Maintaining a healthful *balance* is critical when applying the Power of No and the Power of Go. Like any other tool, this implement can also be misused as a dangerous weapon. Automobiles require both brakes and accelerators in order to function properly, but slamming on the brakes during a sharp turn or flooring the accelerator while going down a wet mountain road can be deadly dangerous. In dieting, overapplication of the Power of No by people with anorexia nervosa is dangerous and potentially lethal. Excessive application of the Power of Go with regard to exercise or working can also be harmful to a person's health, interpersonal relationships, and family responsibilities. Paradoxically, people who self-destructively misuse the Power of No and the Power of Go are almost always stuck in pause, and they must have their problems evaluated and treated by a competent mental health professional (D1, *Discovery*). Fortunately, these individuals are usually very good with the D3 *(Discipline)* component—after they *discover* the sources of their problems and *decide* (D2 component) to make the requisite changes.

References

Mackinnon RA, Yudofsky SC: The Psychiatric Evaluation in Clinical Practice. Philadelphia, PA, JB Lippincott, 1986

Mackinnon RA, Yudofsky SC: Principles of the Psychiatric Evaluation, 2nd Edition. Philadelphia, PA, JB Lippincott, 1991

Spiegel H, Spiegel D: Trance and Treatment: Clinical Uses of Hypnosis, 2nd Edition. Washington, DC, American Psychiatric Publishing, 2004

Yudofsky SC, Kim HF: Neuropsychiatric Assessment (Review of Psychiatry Series, Vol 23). Edited by Oldham JM, Riba M. Washington, DC, American Psychiatric Publishing, 2004

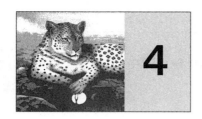

Stuck in My Job: The Case of Clarke Myerson

When Depression and Anxiety Are Complicated by Dyslexia

I sing of arms and a man…O Muse, recount to me
the causes….
—*Virgil*, The Aeneid

A tedious argument of insidious intent…
—*T.S. Eliot, "The Love Song of J. Alfred Prufrock"*

"I hate my job; I hate my life."

The Case of Clarke Myerson: D1 (Discover) Assessment Component

Precipitating Event

The menacing battle-ax who tortured his daughter was the most un-likely person imaginable to hand Clarke Myerson the pivotal piece that was missing from his life's puzzle. He had perceived Miss Brad-shaw as an akathitic grizzly bear that restlessly patrolled the bank of a frothing Alaskan stream. Ribboning and minnowing along with her schooling peers through the icy waters of that stream was Clarke's fifth-grade daughter, Brooke, whose fearful eyes locked on the ferocious, pacing pedagogue on shore. For Brooke understood that at any instant, Miss Bradshaw's clawed paw could slap her from the stream's safety to flop helplessly on the sharp rocks at the front of her classroom.

> **Miss Bradshaw:** Brooke Myerson, please come forward to the blackboard! Using the quadratic equation format that you were *supposed* to have mastered last week, demonstrate to the class how the problem that I wrote on the board should be solved.

From Brooke's pounding heart erupted a viscous anxiety that, lava-like, encased and hardened about her lungs, throat, and brain. Paralyzed of mind and tongue, Brooke once more slumped in perpetrator's silence and humiliation before her entire class. She was found out.

The following terse summons from Miss Bradshaw of Clarke Myerson and his wife was not unexpected:

> **Miss Bradshaw** (*written note to Mr. and Mrs. Clarke Myerson*): Your daughter, Brooke, has a problem that I would like to discuss with you. I have reserved this Thursday, between 3:00 P.M. and 3:30 P.M., for you to meet with me in my office. Please be on time.

Clarke understood that Miss Bradshaw held all the cards. Not performing well on the extensive admissions tests that she had taken as a 4-year-old child, Brooke was, nonetheless, accepted to New York City's elite Dulles School. The Myersons suspected that Brooke was admitted for reasons that were unrelated to her academic potential. First and foremost, as a "legacy applicant," Brooke had priority for admission. Her great-grandfather, grandmother (Jennie), two uncles, and father (Clarke) had all attended Dulles. Second, her sister, Olivia, was a sixth-grade student at Dulles and was an academic superstar. Over the ensuing years, Brooke referred to her acceptance at Dulles as "a mercy admit." Nonetheless, fueled by a combustible, albeit unstable, mix of prodigious effort and profuse anxiety, Brooke had managed to be near the top of all of her classes—until the current year. Until she found herself in the class of the terrorizing and terrifying Miss Bradshaw. Despite devoting almost all her waking hours to her school work, Brooke's grades had slipped precipitously in the fifth grade. She was pervasively anxious—both in and outside of the classroom. When called on to answer questions in class, her mind went blank while she blushed in crimson disgrace. During written examinations, almost 10 agonizing minutes crawled by before her mind could clear and her hand could stop shaking sufficiently to read the first question and record her answer. Rarely was Brooke able to complete a fifth-grade written test.

Clarke conjured and ruminated about the pending meeting with Miss Bradshaw. He envisioned Miss Bradshaw addressing his wife and him with pseudo concern and hollow laments that Brooke was judged to be not academically prepared to enter Dulles Middle School the next year. With claw and fang, she would fasten onto the tasty, comfortable loins of the Myerson family and drag them onto and over the talon-scarred terrain where she reigned supreme.

Clarke surmised that Miss Bradshaw had hit her prime a generation ago when she was a standout student at Dulles. An overweight and awkward adolescent, her sole niche and saving grace were her stellar academic performance. Thereafter, she resented those lesser scholars who had no right to pass her by on life's conventional pathways to happiness, fulfillment, and social superiority. He speculated that she was contemptuous of those prominent and protected families who posed and beamed mendaciously from the glossed Christmas cards that they sent her—but only for a while. Clarke was well aware that these cards came only during the years that the children of Dulles' elite were in Miss Bradshaw's class. Thereafter, like the inexpensive, impersonal Christmas cards that she had sent them in return, Miss Bradshaw would be tossed into some stainless steel oblivion. As used, useless, and forgotten as a discarded paper towel in a designer trash can.

Clarke suspected that Miss Bradshaw regarded the advancement and ultimate happiness of Dulles' less academically gifted children as more than just a betrayal of the ideals of meritocracy but as a form of *cheating*. And she took their swindle personally. They had cheated *her!* These inferiors had stolen from Miss Bradshaw what should have been her enduring lifetime payoff for excelling in middle school and high school. Teaching became her opportunity to avenge the successes of her fraudulent peers through exposing the weaknesses of their children—question after question, assignment after assignment, test after test, report card after report card, parents' meeting after parents' meeting. And Miss Bradshaw's revenge was never a meal consumed cold—but reheated and savored every fall with each new fifth-grade class and devoured with gusto at each grading period. And today they would be the dessert: Miss Bradshaw would cleanse her betrayed, bloodied palate with the sweet sorbet of both Brooke *and* her parents. Yum, yum! At least, that was what Clarke expected. He resented having to listen to a single savored syllable of sadistic teacher-speak hiss through the fangs of this frustrated monster. In his ruminations prior to their meeting, he even imagined the exact words that Miss Bradshaw would say to him and his wife:

> **Miss Bradshaw** (*in Clarke's imagination*): Thank you for being on time. I invited you to my office today to communicate my concern that I would be doing Brooke a grave disservice if I recommended her advancement to the Middle School at Dulles. I have minimal confidence that she could contend with the academic rigor of our middle school. Even students who are faring quite well in my fifth grade, which I deliberately make challenging in order to prepare them for the next year, find Dulles Middle School difficult…. And Brooke is perennially behind the class as a *fifth grader!* Grievously, I have come to accept that it is not in *her* best interest for me to recommend that Brooke be advanced to the Dulles Middle School.

On the day of their meeting, like salmon stiffening in the piercing clench of a bear's claws, Clarke braced himself for the inevitability of the innards-rending interchange with Miss Bradshaw.

> **Miss Bradshaw** (*in actuality*): We are all busy people, so I think that it is best to get to the point. I do not know for certain, but I believe that your daughter, Brooke, has a learning problem.
>
> **Clarke Myerson:** I *will* get to the point, Ms. Bradshaw. Are you saying that she isn't smart enough to succeed at the Dulles School?
>
> **Miss Bradshaw:** Are you listening, Mr. Myerson? I said nothing of the sort. I *know* that Brooke is highly intelligent. And I meant exactly what I said: I believe that your daughter has a learning disorder.
>
> **Clarke:** I am not following you.
>
> **Miss Bradshaw:** Differences and difficulties with processing written language, which are called dyslexia, may occur in people with all ranges of intelligence. So much of academic success in middle school and high school depends on reading with com-

prehension and the complementary processing of mathematical symbols. If students cannot do this efficiently, they cannot succeed in school because they cannot complete their assignments or finish tests on time.

As I said, in my opinion, Brooke happens to be highly intelligent. I have strong reason to believe that her current academic problems are directly related to her inability to decode efficiently written language and align numbers. I called you to my office today to recommend that she be tested by a professional— whom I will recommend—to determine if she has dyslexia.

Diagnostic testing confirmed that Miss Bradshaw's suspicions were on target on both counts: Brooke had significant dyslexia and superior intelligence. A tripartite treatment approach that included tutoring from a specialist in alternative reading techniques, extended time on assignments and tests, and supportive psychological counseling to help repair her damaged self-esteem and performance anxiety enabled Brooke to soar academically and socially—but that's another story. This case example is not about Brooke but concerns her father, Clarke.

Clarke Myerson's Referral to Treatment

Clarke Myerson is not an immodest man. Just the opposite: for most of his life he had considered himself "pretty much a failure and a phony." Clarke's father was self-made, having achieved legendary success in investment banking. For the past decade, Clarke worked in his father's large Wall Street firm as the company's fixed-asset manager. He both was grateful for and despised his job: "My bottom line is that it pays the rent, puts bread on the table for my family, and gives me something impressive to say when the parents of my children's friends ask me what I do for a living. I have no interest in the job beyond that," Clarke maintained. Forty-four other asset analysts reported to him "and most had attended an Ivy League College; everyone is much smarter than I am," he attested. Clarke believed that he never could have attained this position without being the son of the boss. Additionally, he was certain that he was accepted at the University of Pennsylvania for college and, later, the Wharton School of Finance because of his father's power and influence—and targeted philanthropy.

The one "fixed personal asset" about which Clarke took great pride and self-definition was his ability to judge people on the basis of their personalities and behavior patterns. This time, however, he believed that he had never been so wrong about anyone as he had been about Miss Bradshaw. For reasons that he did not understand, he became intensely anxious, began to ruminate about the incident with Miss Bradshaw, and was having problems concentrating and focusing on his work. He was particularly anxious at night and began to lose sleep. It took him more than an hour to fall asleep, and he would awaken several hours later and not be able to go back to sleep. So distraught was Clarke that he scheduled a meeting with his father, to whom he reported at work. Clarke filled him in on how he was feeling and asked for a leave of absence "to try to get a hold of myself." To Clarke's surprise, his father suggested that he see a psychiatrist and volunteered to help him get an appointment. As he had done his entire life, Clarke acceded to his father's suggestion.

Chief Complaint: "I'm Lost!"

Very much like the epic story presented in Virgil's poetic masterpiece, *The Aeneid*, every psychiatric treatment always and in all ways begins *in medias res*, or "in the middle of things." *The Aeneid* recounts the founding of Rome, which occurred much later than the place where the book begins. The epic also describes the events leading up to the destruction of Troy, which occurred much earlier than when the narrative commences. *The Aeneid* begins with the hero, Aeneas, fleeing, with his father, Anchises, on his back, from flaming Troy, which had been destroyed through the deceptions and hostilities of the ancient Greeks. My treatment of Clarke Myerson also began *in medias res*, with the following dialogue that came from my first session with him. Again, as with all psychiatric treatments, the events and dialogues that comprise the "precipitating event," as detailed above, were derived from many pieces of history. These pieces were revealed in many treatment sessions and discussions and were woven together by both of us into a coherent and elegant tapestry. And, as we discovered, like Aeneas, Clarke had been carrying the burden of his father on his back for a long, long time.

> **Clarke Myerson:** I came to see you because I pulled the rug out from under myself. A better analogy is of a suicide bombing,

and both the terrorist and the target were the same person: *me!* I feel like I have caused myself to come apart in a million pieces—which now seem to be flying in all different directions in space. I'm lost; I don't know who I am anymore; I don't have a clue about what is going on now or where I am going to end up. Associated with all of this is that I have been anxious beyond my ability to convey to you. And I am not even certain why. That is where you come in, Dr. Yudofsky: Figure me out and help me out! Please give me a drug or something for my anxiety! Fix me!

Dr. Y.: I want to understand you and the nature of your problem before I shoot blindly with any treatment, Mr. Myerson. You have all the clues, and I believe that you have already conveyed a few very good ones.

Clarke: I have? Like what?

Dr. Y.: One clue is your recognition of the intensity of your feelings about Miss Bradshaw. A second clue is your high level of anxiety: symptoms point to the problems. A third clue is your fabulous facility with metaphor. These clues will have far-reaching meaning and yet-to-be-discovered importance to our understanding and helping you. I say "our" because we can be successful only if we work together. Let's get busy and work together to discover why and how you became lost. It is only after we find out those two things that we can, as you say, begin "to figure you out and to fix you."

TREATMENT PRINCIPLE 1

Patients frequently seek psychiatric treatment for symptoms such as anxiety and depression that they do not directly connect to their being stuck in pause. Often they are unaware of being stuck in pause. In the course of assessment and treatment, patients become aware of where they are and how they became stuck. At that point patients have the opportunity to decide to become unstuck and exercise the discipline and behaviors necessary to bring that about.

Psychiatric History of Clarke Myerson

My treatment of Clarke began with my taking a detailed personal history with him. The very process of discussing one's problems with a caring and disciplined professional is usually therapeutic. Throughout his treatment I emphasized to Clarke that the most meaningful revelations germinate from the seeds of what might seem to be the most minor details of his life: relevant revelations from the so-called irrelevant, minor details.

Clarke Myerson's Father, Nathan Myerson
(All Roads Lead to Nathan)

The youngest among three brothers, Clarke Myerson was born with a silver shoe up his ass. This shoe encased the foot of his father, Nathan, who deposited it there with the intention, precision, and force of a National Football League all-star place kicker. And one day, young Clarke was expected to fill this silver slipper and to follow in the radiant footsteps of his dad.

Growing up poor in Brooklyn, Nathan Myerson never had new shoes, much less silver ones. Rather, like the rest of his clothing, his shoes were all secondhand, mainly from his extended family of first-generation Jewish cousins. Nathan was born just after his parents immigrated to the United States from Lithuania in 1933; they subsequently lost most of their European relatives between the monstrous pincers of unrelenting Russian pogroms and the subsequent Nazi onslaught. Yiddish was the only language that Nathan had ever heard spoken in his home. Nathan's father worked as messenger for a diamond broker in Manhattan, and his mother, who had tuberculosis as a child, mostly stayed in bed amidst the cluttered, shabby gloom of their three-room tenement apartment. In elementary school, Nathan was discovered to be a mathematical prodigy. His exceptionalism was later confirmed by his being a standout in science and mathematics at Brooklyn's Stuyvesant High School, a teeming estuary for future science professors and Nobel Prize winners in science, medicine, and mathematics. Although captain of Stuyvesant High School's national championship mathematics team, he was far more interested in the strategy, probability, and competition of chess and card games.

Attending Harvard on a full scholarship, Nathan majored in economics while earning a steady and significant income in nightly poker games by trimming the trust funds of his prep-schooled peers. Not that Nathan resented or disassociated himself from his classmates from prominent New England families and financially advantaged backgrounds. Just the opposite: he reinvented himself to become one of them. After puncturing, with his piercing brilliance, the Ivy League's unwritten 5% quota for Jews, he embraced aristocracy while epitomizing meritocracy. Nathan's rare references to his family were blemished by embellishments that broached—but never crossed—the line of lying. Nathan told his classmates that he was "raised in New York City," not that he grew up in Brooklyn; that his father was "in the international minerals trade," not a messenger for a small-time diamond broker; that he attended "a special high school for science and math," not a Brooklyn public school populated mainly by the children of immigrants.

Nathan spent most of his midterm breaks with the families of his wealthy friends and worked during the summers as an intern in their businesses. He rarely returned home after he began college. His parents were never invited to visit him in Cambridge. Although they had saved up their meager funds to attend his graduation, he discouraged them from doing so. Nathan did not dislike his parents, but he was ashamed of the drabness of their existence and detested the permanence of their impoverishment. Most of all he resented his parents' passivity: their submissive acceptance of the immutability of their immobility. But he did not blame them. He had long understood that, without education, money, or social position, they were pinned to their lowly existences—like paper patterns of cheap dresses on the cutting boards in the sweat shops on 34th Street. In response, Nathan was determined to succeed at the highest levels of education, finance, and social position, the pursuit of which was fueled by his fevered ambition and accelerated by his unyielding competiveness and blinding brilliance.

By the completion of his first semester as a freshman at Harvard, Nathan realized that he would, with ease, graduate at the very top of his class. At that moment, *summa cum laude* from Harvard no longer remained his primary goal. *That* was inevitable! Rather, Nathan believed that *reputation*, ultimately, would be of highest value to him. He wanted to be respected and feared for dominating his competition, for having a superior genius, and for being a fierce competitor. He abandoned wanting to be liked or popular, which he realized would be casualties of his brilliance, ambition, and Jewishness—the cost of doing business in that era in Cambridge. He reasoned that lots of people would obtain a Harvard degree and that several would be awarded *summa cum laude*—primarily overachievers. But only one person each year would be, by class consensus, the best of the best. And Nathan was far from subtle in establishing his reputation. For example, in the early 1950s, when he attended Harvard, organic chemistry was one of the most demanding and difficult courses in the entire curriculum. This course was taken only by students majoring in the biological sciences, primarily premedical students. It was a "sentinel course," meaning that medical schools and graduate schools in science judged applicants' qualifications and performance potential on the basis of their grades in that class. Additionally, in an era before grade inflation, students who earned one of the two or three A's awarded annually to the approximately 300 enrollees in organic chemistry had almost automatic admission to and special status in Harvard Medical School.

When it became known among the third-year Harvard premed students that Nathan Myerson was enrolled in organic chemistry, most assumed, with considerable trepidation, that he was turning premed. Why else would anyone subject himself to that torture? They were dismayed because he was an economics major who had told his friends that he was going to business school following graduation. And his classmates also knew that he had effortlessly excelled in the most challenging mathematics and economics courses that Harvard offered to undergraduates. They all recognized that if Nathan wished to apply to medical school, he would be a competitive force with whom they would have to contend. When asked by classmates why he was taking the course if he were going into business, he replied, "To learn something new. I have always been interested in science, and, besides, I am getting bored in the econ and math classes." Nathan not only received an A in organic chemistry for both semesters but his grade was sufficiently higher than the next highest grade to have "killed the curve" in the course. In other words, he was the *only* student to earn an A in organic chemistry during both semesters of that year, and his reputation was enduringly secured among the circle of intellectual elites at Harvard. The fact that he had no intention of becoming a doctor or scientist transformed "reputation into legend." Mission number 1 accomplished for Nathan Myerson.

Actively recruited by all the elite graduate schools in business, Nathan chose to attend the Wharton School of Finance of the University of Pennsylvania, from which he received both a master's degree in business administration (MBA) and a doctorate degree in economics (Ph.D.). Thereafter, Nathan worked as a securities analyst in an international investment bank, established and directed what Nathan termed "our absurdly profitable mergers and acquisition division," and departed after 15 years as a multimillionaire to found his own investment firm. His prodigious work ethic and tactical genius never faltering, Nathan spurred and guided the soaring growth of his firm to the point that it rivaled in size, income, and profits the staid investment houses that had presided prominently over Wall Street since the early twentieth century. A perennial economic advisor to U.S. presidents and a member of the Federal Reserve, he was also a fixture on the boards of trustees of important museums, universities, and charitable causes.

Clarke Myerson's "Other" Family Members

Through the lens of detachment, one could understand the near-universal admiration of—though not affection for—Nathan Myerson. With energy and talent, he played within the rules of the educational establishment, business, and society and had won his battle for the American Dream. And few among his rivals were both self-invented and self-made, as was he. But families play, fight, and, most importantly, keep score by rules that are different from those of universities or successful businesses. Nathan was as assertive, demanding, and ambitious in his family life as he was in college, graduate school, and business. During graduate school, he married Jennie, the sister of one of his Harvard suitemates. While signing the prenuptial agreement on the insistence of Jennie's wealthy, Brahmin father, Nathan stared their attorney in the eye and, with dry irritation, asked him, "Do you realize what a joke this is? In 20 years Jennie's father's estate will be chump change to me. I should be protecting my estate from his daughter!" At that point in time, however, Nathan had considerably more ambition and confidence than cash. Nonetheless, his marital prediction proved to be somewhat of an understatement. Seventeen years later and two years after founding his investment firm, he was earning twice the net worth of his father-in-law on an annual basis.

Clarke's mother, Jennie, was a quiet, compliant, and gentle Gentile, to whose Protestant religion Nathan converted. Jennie gave birth to their two older sons when Nathan was in graduate school, and Clarke was born 6 years thereafter. No different from his business, Nathan's focus in the family was on performance—the setting and achieving of lofty goals. His automatic greeting of both wife and children was "How are you doing?" never "How are you?" He never complimented his sons for their achievements but focused like a laser in identifying and demanding that they remediate their deficiencies. Jennie admired her husband and adored her sons—especially Clarke, whom she regarded as more sensitive and vulnerable than his brothers and father. She felt that he was temperamentally similar to her and that his brothers were more like their father. As did their maternal grandfather and their mother, both of Clarke's brothers attended the Dulles School, from which each was graduated valedictorian. Like their father, both of Clarke's brothers were brilliant, assertive, energetic, and independent, and, like their father, neither was particularly nurturing or involved with Clarke during the few years that they lived at home together. The headstrong brothers clashed continuously with their father over such issues as household rules and responsibilities as well as choices of courses, colleges, and career. Neither acquiesced to their father's insistence that they attend Harvard and become financiers. Instead, Nathan's oldest son attended the California Institute of Technology for undergraduate work and Stanford for graduate school, where he majored in physics and computer science. He went on to become a legendary professor at Stanford and a pioneer in the field of artificial intelligence. Nathan's middle son went to the Massachusetts Institute of Technology (MIT) and then Harvard Medical School for his medical degree and Ph.D. in molecular biology. Eschewing an internship and the traditional practice of medicine, he returned to MIT, where he focused solely on research and teaching while making important discoveries in the molecular and cellular biology of pancreatic cancer.

Clarke Myerson's Academic Career

During one of our initial sessions, I asked Clarke to tell me a bit about his earliest memories from grade school, and he responded as follows:

> **Clarke Myerson:** Two words come to mind, Dr. Y. The first word is *disappointment*. My father and all my teachers were deeply disappointed that I was not as smart as my brothers. Do you know what the word *bathos* means, Dr. Y.? That's the second word.

Dr. Y.: I believe it means "the decline from the sublime to the ridiculous." One of my friends who attended Yale had a banner on his wall that read "God, Man, and Yale," and I teased him that it was a good example of the word bathos.

Clarke: Exactly, Dr. Y., but I have a better example: my father, my brothers, and me!

Dr. Y.: Doesn't that depend on *who* is measuring and *what* is being measured?

Clarke: My teachers were doing the measuring, and they were measuring *me!* And I always come up deficient.

Dr. Y.: An example?

Clarke: Let's start with school—as far back as I can remember. What comes immediately to mind is my entire Dulles School debacle. At the beginning of every school year—that is, until I became infamous among the faculty for my idiocy—my teachers invariably would say to me, "I taught both of your brothers, and I am so delighted to have another Myerson boy in my class." As you know, Dr. Y., both of my brothers are geniuses, and I'm an idiot.

Dr. Y.: I know nothing of the sort. As I said, it depends on who's measuring and what's being measured.

Clarke: Measurement of my work began with a vengeance in kindergarten when the teacher handed out the very first graded test that I had ever taken at Dulles. The test was to reproduce, from memory, the alphabet in both upper and lower cases. All of my classmates could have done it perfectly when they were 3 years old, but for me it was like reproducing the Code of Hammurabi in the original cuneiform. The next day the teacher hands back all of the graded test papers to the class except one—that one looked like it had lined the bottom of a parrot cage for about 3 months. She holds up a tortured paper by its corner as if she's holding up a piece of soiled toilet paper and says, "We had a lot of people absent for our test yesterday, and I was not able to read the name on this test paper. Does anyone in the class today recognize it?" The entire class broke out in laughter as I raised my hand to reclaim my trophy.

Dr. Y.: Do you recall the problems that you were having with the assignment? Specifically, did you have a problem remembering the letters—and their correct sequence—or reproducing the letters per se?

Clarke: I'm not sure exactly what you are getting at, Dr. Y. It was a long time ago, but I think that I had problems with the actual writing of the letters. I am pretty sure that I knew the alphabet in my head, because I can remember singing it to my mother. But I was too stupid to remember how to construct the letters.

Dr. Y.: Please see if you can locate some of your earliest written work from school. Bring in everything that you can find, and we'll go over it together.

Clarke's mother, Jennie, was intimately involved with the lives of all of her children. She often said, "Their lives are my life." Fortunately, she had saved most of Clarke's papers from as far back as pre-kindergarten (Pre-K), and he brought them to his next session. I reserved the departmental conference room for this meeting, and we arranged the stacks of written material on the elongated table according to grade year. We started with written exercises from Pre-K. I drew Clarke's focus to a particular lesson in a workbook in which he was supposed to copy letters from adjacent examples.

Dr. Y.: What do you notice, Clarke?

Clarke Myerson: Apart from all the eraser smudges and general mess, it is clear that this assignment was way over my head. Obviously, I couldn't do it. What do *you* see, Dr. Y.?

Dr. Y.: Let's look at the lowercase letters, *b*, *d*, *p*, *q*, and *h*. What do *you* see?

Clarke: They're mostly backward.

Dr. Y.: Yes, and notice that several of the *d*'s and *p*'s are upside down as well. And when we check several lessons later when you were copying capital letters, note that many of the same mirror-image reversals occur with the same letters except for the *H*, which is symmetrical. Now let's skip to the kindergarten lessons. Note that when you tried to copy the word *bird*, you wrote the word *drib*. Same problem. However, also note that you are now reversing sequences of letters in words. Look at the word *girl*, which you wrote repeatedly as *gril*.

Over the course of the session, many examples of Clarke's problems with copying and reproducing words and letters were pointed out. In advanced grades, his written tests and themes were marred with innumerable misspelled words, which invariably reduced his grade by at least one level. In the mathematics and science courses, symbol reversal resulted in mistakes in such fundamentals as adding and subtracting columns of numbers and placing decimal points in the correct places. Additionally, Clarke recalled being unable to sound out written words, being told he was "a slow reader," and being placed in remedial reading classes throughout grade school. In middle school and high school he performed especially poorly on standardized tests, even though he had taken test preparation courses and used private tutors.

> **Dr. Y.:** Clarke, it is clear that you have a significant dyslexia—far more severe than that of your daughter, Brooke. You exhibit what we term *dyseidetic* symptoms. People with dysphonetic symptoms have auditory processing challenges, with specific difficulties translating sounds to symbols. That is not your problem. You understand verbal instructions and are fairly adept at converting oral communications to written language and symbols—albeit with your usual letter reversals and misspelling of words. As you advanced in school, your main problem was with recognizing whole words and with spelling—particularly with words that do not sound exactly the way they are spelled. You also have problems spelling words that sound the same but mean different things and are spelled differently—such as *board* and *bored*. Learning to speak and translate a foreign language from its written form would also be a formidable challenge for you.
>
> **Clarke Myerson:** This is all true. I almost failed every foreign language that I have ever taken—they were all "Greek to me." In retrospect this is all so obvious. How come I never heard the word *dyslexia* until Miss Bradshaw brought it up about Brooke?
>
> **Dr. Y.:** In the 1960s and early 1970s when you were in elementary through high school, teachers did not know much about dyslexia. Children with this condition were often regarded as "slow learners," accused of being lazy, and reprimanded for making "careless mistakes." Usually, none of this was true.
>
> **Clarke:** Aren't you just making excuses for people like me who are fundamentally dumb and just can't cut it?
>
> **Dr. Y.:** We don't think so. Those who manage to escape the phenomena of their manifest dyslectic conditions and the epiphenomena of their psychological reactions to having dyslexia can be extraordinarily creative and successful in their personal lives and careers. They also tend to be prodigiously hard workers.
>
> **Clarke:** Explain, please.
>
> **Dr. Y.:** Success in school is highly dependent—perhaps overly dependent—on reading skills. Access to most professions and many jobs also depends on doing well in school and college. Those are the phenomena of dyslexia. Over the course of your treatment, we will identify and discuss the destructive implications of the epiphenomena of dyslexia, Clarke.

Among the many sources of Clarke's low self-esteem were the "lessons" that he learned as the result of his dyslexia. Casualties of our school systems, many people with dyslexia like Clarke are "taught" such corrosive messages as "I'm dumb," "I'm careless," "I'm lazy," "I'm inattentive," "I'm irresponsible," "I'm deficient," or "I'm a bad person." Unfortunately, after achieving success—whether academically or in their careers—they often believe that they are undeserving. Not uncommonly, they also believe their successes are somehow achieved unfairly, by luck, by deception, or by some fluke. They worry constantly that they will be exposed for being unworthy of their accomplishments and that they will be humiliated and punished for their deceptions. To mitigate this dreaded event, often they will not acknowledge their achievements to themselves or others and will deflect all compliments because these make them feel uncomfortable. At every opportunity in Clarke's treatment when examples of these feelings and this behavior emerged (he put himself down mercilessly and repeatedly), I called his attention to them and interpreted their psychological sources, which were compounded by key psychodynamics—the principal one stemming from Oedipal issues related to his relationship with his father that will be addressed more fully in the next section.

Clarke Myerson's Oedipal Psychodynamics

In the ancient Greek play *Oedipus Rex*, Oedipus competed with his father, was seduced by and engaged in sexual intercourse with his mother, and was punished by being blinded. Classic psychoanalytical theory equates Oedipus' blindness with his being castrated as a punishment for challenging the authority of his father and for sexual transgressions with his mother.

In my practice of psychiatry, I interpret both the *Oedipus Rex* and Freud's brilliant psychodynamic insights somewhat differently from classical psychoanalytical theory. I believe that both the transgression and the tragedy of Oedipal violations stem from the defiance of the "natural course of things" and that the true transgressor is rarely, as conventionally conceived, the perpetrator and object of the punishment. It is only "natural" for children to become, over time, more attractive and powerful than their parents and for the parents to devote themselves to protecting and preparing their offspring to survive and prevail without them. For parents to do otherwise is to transgress nature (or, as the Greeks would conceptualize this, transgress the gods), which leads to both tragedy and punishment. Just as there is a tragic quality when a 75 year old tries to dress and act like a 25 year old, consequences of tragic proportions ensue when parents are competitive with their children. Nonetheless, as with Oedipus, it is the children who most often suffer the painful consequences of the transgressions and related punishments.

Clarke Myerson's maladaptive response to his father's over-the-top competiveness with all males—including his sons—was to diminish his prowess and pleasure in the realms that were the most important to his father—intelligence, academic success, career achievement, and career satisfaction. On the basis of their temperaments, his brothers chose to "take on" their father frontally with continuous confrontations. Of a far more sensitive and delicate disposition, Clarke "took on" himself by blunting his prowess. Success in those areas that were the most important to Nathan would make Clarke particularly anxious, so he countered any sense of accomplishment by feeling a failure. Accordingly, he was conflicted about being a superstar in finance—the same field of play in which his father excelled. This conflict was manifested in how he comported himself with all authority figures, including his psychiatrist. In treatment, patients like Clarke who have profound Oedipal issues will *initially* feel safer if they can lure their psychiatrists—as they do other authority figures—into joining them in their ubiquitous self-deprecations. My therapeutic strategy with Clarke was to facilitate his insight into the consequences of this conflict (paradoxically, feeling endangered by success), which would not be possible if I accepted his innumerable invitations to put him down and became complicit with him in this deleterious behavioral pattern. How could he trust me to help him change (and become powerful and happy) if I, in *any* way, were threatened by his power and, thus, wanted him to fail? How could he trust me if I acquiesced to his requests to reify his failures by even *suggesting* that he were not intelligent, especially when I did not believe it to be true?

Clarke Myerson's Dyslexia Combined With His Oedipal Psychodynamics

The following dialogue occurred in an early psychotherapy session when Clarke was reviewing with me problems that he was having with reading in front of his fourth-grade class. I was endeavoring to determine what types of words were challenges for him to read at the time (e.g., proper names, polysyllabic words, words that he had never before come across), and he became angry with me as the result of having to relive the experience. Clarke did not want to recall the specific details from these experiences because they unearthed deep-seated feelings of shame, humiliation, and rage.

> **Clarke Myerson:** Look, Dr. Y., we don't have to dig all of this up to come to the conclusion that I am an idiot. You and I both know that. Anyway, I thought that your job was to ask me about my feelings. Can't you make a damn good living by just asking "How did you *feel* when that happened?"
>
> **Dr. Y.:** My psychiatrists' union card was revoked many years ago, Clarke. Besides, you can hardly stop telling me how badly you feel about yourself for your putative deficiencies.
>
> **Clarke:** What are you talking about?
>
> **Dr. Y.:** Like buckshot, you pepper yourself with put-downs almost every time you speak about yourself. Most refer to your intelligence.
>
> **Clarke:** You mean my *lack* of intelligence, don't you, Dr. Y.?
>
> **Dr. Y.:** Nice try, Clarke. But I will try never to RSVP affirmatively to your innumerable invitations to join you in your self-castration party.
>
> **Clarke:** I don't follow you at all, Dr. Y.
>
> **Dr. Y.:** We will have plenty of time to discuss that in the future. At the risk of not being conventional or a psychiatric stereotype by asking you "How did you feel about that?" I believe that it is even more important to determine precisely what was causing you problems with your first test.

Clarke reluctantly devoted the next several meetings to recalling the responses of his parents, teachers, brothers, and peers to his poor performance in school—and how he reacted to their reactions. All roads led to his father, Nathan.

> **Clarke Myerson:** It seemed to me that everyone whom I knew was in awe of my father. I can't count the number of times that I saw his picture in the newspaper, in magazines, or discussing some important topic on TV. And it was clear to me that my father, whom I respected and feared more than anyone in the world, was deeply disappointed in me. And *I* was deeply disappointed in me. No matter how hard I worked, I couldn't succeed in school. I felt like I was in a no-win situation. It's bad enough to fail in school because you are goofing off; however,

when you work hard and still fail, you have proved yourself to be an even bigger dummy! Bottom line: I hated myself.

Dr. Y.: How did your mother react to your struggles in school?

Clarke: My brothers and I referred to our mother as "the blinking green light." She was consistently supportive, loved us unconditionally, and almost never said "no" to us when we asked her for something. However, Mom's acceptance seemed to mean so much less to me than Dad's disapproval. Probably because I knew that Mom's view was so biased because she loved me so much, while Dad's view was fair and objective.

Dr. Y.: How did you know that?

Clarke: Let's face it. I was not nearly as smart or successful as my brothers or most of my classmates. Somebody has to be at the bottom of the heap.

Dr. Y.: I suppose so, Clarke. But, as I said previously, it depends on who's measuring and what's being measured.

Clarke (*with some irritation*): You keep saying that, Dr. Y. Frankly, I don't know what you're talking about. I was measuring what my teachers were measuring, what my friends were measuring, what *my father* was measuring, what the college admissions people were measuring, and what everybody else—except you and my mother—were measuring.

Dr. Y.: It is clear that what everybody was measuring was conventional academic success, which is so dependent on reading with facility—which you were not able to achieve because of dyslexia. I am also interested in what they *weren't measuring*, which also can be important.

Clarke: As my kids would say, "Tru' dat, Doc." They weren't measuring good looks or great athletic or musical ability—in which I also fall short. But one area that I *would* measure at the *very* top of the heap, however, would be in the "phony-faker-fraud" category. If you can fix *that*, Dr. Y., everyone, including me, will be astonished.

Dr. Y.: I don't automatically accept that just because you happen to *feel* that you're a fraud necessarily *makes* it "true." Before we start to "fix" anything, let's start by your telling me what leads you to this conclusion.

Clarke Myerson's Experience at the University of Pennsylvania

Clarke Myerson: I have always been a fraud, so I hardly know where to start. OK, let's begin with how I got accepted to college. I was in the bottom quarter of my class at the Dulles

School. Despite going to several SAT prep courses and spending countless hours with expensive private tutors, my SAT scores were in the 600s. That is pretty low for Dulles.

One of the most humiliating hours in my entire life was in my junior year of high school when my parents joined me for my college counseling review. The counselor had prepared a list of colleges that she thought would match my abilities. Dad interrupted her as she presented her recommendations. I recall him saying something like this: "I have never heard of any of the schools you are recommending. The best school for my son is the University of Pennsylvania, which is the only school to which he is going to apply."

The counselor countered that even if my record were within the range of Penn's norms—which it was not—it was foolhardy for me to apply only to one college. Dad said, "We'll see. We're wasting each other's time. Jennie, Clarke, it's time to go."

When March came around, I was so ashamed to tell my friends that I had been accepted to Penn that I didn't tell anyone where I was going for several weeks. Most of my friends thought that I didn't get in anywhere. When I finally revealed I was going to Penn, everyone knew two things: 1) I didn't deserve to get in on my academic record, and 2) my father's power and pull got me accepted. As you can see, Dr. Y., things like that make me a total phony and a fraud.

Dr. Y.: I see nothing of the sort. It is not your prerogative, my prerogative, or your father's prerogative—even if he is a member of Penn's Board of Trustees—to decide whom UPenn accepts or whom they reject. The professionals who work in Penn's admission office are the sole arbiters of these decisions—or should be. Did you misrepresent yourself in your application, Clarke? If so, that would be fraudulent. My conjecture is that you did not. Actually, I venture to guess that you understated your abilities and accomplishments, as you have consistently done in our meetings.

Clarke: I filled out the application and wrote the essays myself.

Dr. Y.: Do you recall the subject of any of your essays?

Clarke: Strange that you should ask. My father wanted me to write my essay on a summer experience that I had working at the Philadelphia Federal Reserve—a job that he, of course, had arranged for me. That essay would have been four words: "I hated every minute." Instead, I wrote an essay on Jerry, an adult with Down syndrome, whom I helped to coach for the Special Olympics tennis competition.

Dr. Y.: I bet your mother has a copy of that essay. Would you ask her to look for it? If she can find it, please bring it in for us to read. So far, Clarke, you have not presented any evidence that you are a phony and a fraud. How did you find Penn?

Clarke: I loved Penn, but Penn didn't exactly love me. Since my brothers had absolutely no interest in going into Dad's financial firm, by default, my father designated me as the "family *heir*" to the finance business. The only problem was and is that when it comes to an *aptitude* for finance, I am "the family *air* brain." And unlike my brothers, I didn't and don't have the personal strength or the realistic alternatives to resist the onslaught of my father's will. Therefore, it was predetermined that I would be a business and finance major at Penn, an academic focus in which I had no interest or aptitude. I detested every business- and finance-related course that I took.

Dr. Y.: Why did you say that you loved Penn but Penn did not love you?

Clarke: I worked my ass off at Penn to keep up in class and to pass. I mean *every* day from early morning until late at night. Do you realize that you're talking to a guy who did not have *one* drink or one date during college in order to survive? I used to joke that if I dropped my pencil, I would be irrevocably behind. But I don't blame Penn at all. It's a terrific place and not their fault that I wasn't smart enough to benefit from all they have to offer.

Dr. Y.: But why do you say that they didn't love you? Did you get into any trouble— academically or otherwise?

Clarke: I didn't get into any trouble. I didn't let Penn down for what I *did do* but for what I *didn't* do. Penn likes its students to be involved with cultural, athletic, and community activities. I was involved with *me*.

Repeated and direct questioning was required to coax from Clarke that he had actually done quite well in college and had participated in several extracurricular activities. During a subsequent family session with his parents, I was surprised to learn from his father that Clarke was actually awarded Phi Beta Kappa. Characteristically, Clarke immediately pointed out that his father and brothers received the distinction in their junior years, "and they didn't have to study every single minute like I did."

Clarke Myerson's Strengths as a Gateway to Treatment and Change

Many individuals with dyslexia do well after they enter college. There are several reasons for their academic success: 1) the acquisition of unconventional reading skills that help them compensate for their dyslexia (such as recognizing whole words as opposed to sounding out the individual syllables); 2) creativity engendered by the necessity of approaching learning and problem solving in unconventional ways; 3) the development of the ability for sustained, intensive work; and 4) the modesty to recognize what they don't know or understand. Clarke Myerson developed all of these qualities, which facilitated his academic success at Penn. A component of our treatment was to point out, repeatedly, examples of these attributes as they occurred in his current life experiences.

> **Dr. Y.:** Thank you, Clarke, for bringing in your college admission essays. They are original, creative, beautifully written, and moving. I am not entirely surprised, because it has long been evident to me that you have a gift for metaphor and verbal expression. Did you take any creative writing courses in college?
> **Clarke Myerson:** No, but my minor was in English literature.

On my persistent questioning, Clarke eventually admitted that he not only had received A's in his English courses but that he also had enjoyed them. Paradoxically, although reading had originally been difficult for him, he nonetheless appreciated the imagery and creative use of language in poetry and prose. *Characteristic of people with both dyslexia and Oedipal psychodynamics, Clarke devalued realms in which he had talents and overvalued those areas that were much more challenging and difficult for him.* His subjective experience in his English courses was in stark contrast to his finance and business courses—both in college and graduate school at the Wharton School of Finance, where he received his MBA. Additionally, he described his work in his father's firm as "grueling and demoralizing."

> **Clarke Myerson:** I hate working in finance. I absolutely dread going in to work every day. I count the seconds, the minutes, and the hours until I can go home. I live for those weekends that I don't have to go in to work. I have been working in finance at my father's firm for 15 years—not counting the 6 years of torture in college and graduate school. It is almost as if I were serving a life sentence in prison, except that most other people think that I am the most fortunate person on Earth to have a rich family and high-paying job. The truth is that I am in a golden cage and miserable.

Dr. Y.: Ever thought about breaking out?

Clarke: Unless you are talking about acne, you must be kidding. First of all, I need the income, and second, there is nothing else that I know how to do in order to make a living. Third, even if I had the backing of the entire U.S. Marine Corps, I wouldn't have the guts to tell my father that I was checking out on him.

Dr. Y.: I'll do some counting too, Clarke. First, let's discuss *what* you would truly be passionate about doing. Second, let's figure out *how* to get there. Third, fourth, and fifth, when those two elements are determined, we can decide *when*, *where*, and *what* to tell your father. I'm no Marine, but I would be happy to join you in a family session for that discussion.

The Case of Clarke Myerson: D1 (Discover) Treatment Component

Laying the Foundation

Clarke Myerson had been stuck in pause for most of his adult life. Prior to his *deciding* (D2 component) to become unstuck using the techniques of the Power of Go (D3, *discipline* component), a treatment plan had to be formulated and executed. The following three elements were required:

1. *Information:* taking an extensive psychiatric history in order that both Clarke and I could identify, understand, and agree on the many facts and factors that led to his being stuck
2. *Insight:* identifying, understanding, and respecting the many conscious and unconscious dynamics and psychological defenses that sustained Clarke's being stuck in pause
3. *Motivation:* establishing a therapeutic alliance with Clarke that would support and facilitate his hope, courage, and willingness to change his life in fundamental ways

As emphasized in Chapter 2, "Getting Stuck," moving forward without accomplishing these three elements most often leads to false starts, frustration, recidivism, discouragement, and, ultimately, failure. The vast majority of self-help programs and quick-fix treatment fads fail our patients. There are few shortcuts that do not lead to pitfalls. As reflected in treatment principle 2, the integration of time and attention and the integration of diagnosis and treatment are essential to achieving successful outcomes.

TREATMENT PRINCIPLE 2

Effective treatment is a two-step dance: learn and do. Insight and understanding about the problem and its causes are important but insufficient. The application of this knowledge in life to effect change is essential. To do the former without the latter is more an intellectual exercise than anything that is useful, practical, or, at the end of the day, meaningful. To do the latter without the former is to shoot in the dark: one might get lucky with a "ready-fire-aim" approach, but don't count on it.

Diagnosis and Treatment

Medical/Psychiatric Diagnoses

I diagnosed Clarke with major depressive disorder comorbid with panic disorder and dyslexia (specific learning disorder with impairment in reading (315.00) and written expression (315.3) in DSM-5 [American Psychiatric Association 2013]).

Treatment of Medical/Psychiatric Disorders

As has been discussed, the experiential consequences of Clarke's dyslexia interacted with Oedipal issues to affect his self-esteem and capacity to view himself as a potent and effective adult. These factors, in turn, influenced critical life decisions and vocational choices. Finally, the biological predisposition for Clarke's depressive (major depressive) and anxiety (panic) disorders combined with his life experiences and psychosocial dynamics to lead to the severe symptoms that caused him to seek psychiatric treatment. Thus, all three of Clarke's psychiatric diagnoses are indelibly interrelated—both in causality and in symptom presentation—which necessitated that each of these problems be addressed both individually and simultaneously, as summarized in treatment principle 3.

TREATMENT PRINCIPLE 3

People rarely become stuck in pause in a single area or for a single reason. Usually, being stuck is the result of the interaction of a multiplicity of biological predispositions, prior and current experiential issues and stresses, and psychosocial dynamics. In addition, patients often have two different but related psychological and medical disorders. Examples include major depressive disorder and alcohol use disorder or antisocial personality disorder and traumatic brain injury. In treatment, the individual contributing issues of each condition must be identified and their sources must be discovered. The role of each causal factor as well as the interplay of the individual factors must be understood and addressed in the process of becoming unstuck.

Treatment of Clarke Myerson's Major Depressive Disorder

As is commonly the case for people with depression who are stuck in a protracted pause, treatment of Clarke's major depressive disorder assumed priority. Although Clarke's official DSM-IV-TR (American Psychiatric Association 2000) diagnosis at the time he presented for treatment was major depressive disorder, single episode (296.2), I became aware that for many years he had had a milder, more insidious form of depression termed dysthymic disorder (DSM-5 persistent depressive disorder [American Psychiatric Association 2013]). The conflicts, feelings, and thoughts evoked by his interchange with Miss Bradshaw intensified his chronic dysthymia into an acute depression. The severe depression from which Clarke suffered and with which he struggled rendered it nearly impossible for him to take on vigorously other treatment challenges. Among the symptoms engendered by depression were pervasive negativity, pessimism, guilt, and hopelessness; low energy, reduced motivation, little enthusiasm; diminished ability to concentrate, to set goals, and to complete tasks; and bottomless self-esteem. How could he set goals and work toward their achievement in this state of mind and mood? He couldn't. Additionally, because depression distorts perceptions and clouds judgment, I could not be certain about the degree to which Clarke's low self-esteem and hatred for his job were influenced by the general negativity associated with major depression.

Treatment must be absolutely a collaborative enterprise between patient and therapist. Gaining insights into how the patient became stuck must also be a shared adventure, and that includes frank discussions of how the unconscious elements play a vital role—as these invariably do. Over several months, Clarke and I worked at isolating and understanding the critical elements that led him to get stuck. This included illuminating the elements involving his unique temperament, biology, psychology, and life experience and how they interacted among one another. This stepwise approach is highlighted in treatment principle 4.

TREATMENT PRINCIPLE 4

Psychiatric disorders such as depressive disorders and bipolar disorders distort perceptions and cloud judgment, so major life decisions such as changing jobs, leaving a spouse, quitting school, moving to a different state, and the like must be deferred until the condition is successfully treated. Because these disorders are, in large measure, brain disorders, one cannot count on making rational decisions using a "broken brain."

For a variety of historical, genetic, and technical reasons, I placed Clarke on two antidepressants—one that modulated the neurotransmitters epinephrine, norepinephrine, and serotonin and another that primarily affected the dopamine system. Just as importantly, history taking and psychotherapy were pursued concurrently. I simultaneously encouraged ("challenged" is the better word) Clarke to address the authenticity of many of the negative conclusions that he had drawn about himself. Many studies of the treatment of severe depression confirm that medications combined with psychotherapy are superior to utilizing either alone (Keller et al. 2000). As with most antidepressants, several weeks were required for the medications to be increased to therapeutic levels, and several more weeks were required before their actions could take effect. During this time, I continued to take Clarke's personal and psychiatric history as well as to conduct insight-oriented psychotherapy. Within 7 weeks his major depression had been mitigated to the degree that his energy and motivation improved significantly, he had excellent capacities to concentrate and focus, and he no longer was hopeless, sad, and pessimistic in most areas of his life. Nonetheless, he remained self-deprecatory and continued to detest his job "and the financial world in general." At that point, both he and I agreed that his negative feelings about his work situation were the result not of a depressive disorder but of the confluence of his aptitudes, proclivities, and preferences.

Treatment of Clarke Myerson's Panic Disorder

At the time that I first evaluated Clarke, he met DSM-IV-TR diagnostic criteria for panic disorder. During the week following his fateful meeting with Miss Bradshaw, he experienced two discrete periods (lasting for several hours) in which he felt intense anxiety and the fear that he was losing control of his life and sanity. Additionally, he also endured sudden and severe somatic symptoms that included heart palpitations, shortness of breath, excessive sweating, manual trembling, and lightheadedness. Clarke was fearful that unless he received immediate psychiatric treatment, he was going to have "a nervous breakdown." Through careful history taking I learned that he had had quite a few similar episodes over the course of his life—usually coinciding with times of high stress. On those occasions he did not seek psychiatric treatment but went to the emergency room of a New York City hospital to be evaluated for a heart attack. After a thorough cardiovascular workup, he was told "nothing is wrong with you" and was discharged from the emergency department without follow-up.

After conducting a careful medical workup wherein other possible causes of Clarke's panic-like symptoms and signs were ruled out, I communicated to Clarke that he had panic disorder. He was greatly relieved that he did not have what he termed "a potentially fatal medical condition" or did not "have to be locked up forever in a mental institution." He was not being humorous or dramatic; he was truly fearful of these eventualities. Although panic disorder is categorized as an anxiety disorder, it is a close neurobiological relative of major depression, which is classified as a depressive disorder. Therefore, treatment of panic and depression are quite similar: psychotherapy is combined with pharmacotherapy with medications classified as antidepressants.

Although educating patients about their psychiatric disorders and treatment is critical to the success of all psychiatric treatment (treatment principle 5), it is especially important in the treatment of panic disorder. In a significant percentage of patients with panic disorder, panic attacks can be elicited ("detonated" is the more appropriate verb) with the initial doses of antidepressant. When this occurs without prior warning of such a possibility, patients characteristically do not return to treatment or will not thereafter consider or permit the use of another psychiatric medication. People who have experienced a panic attack often say that it is the most terrifying experience of their lives. When suspecting the possibility of panic disorder, I routinely combine the following: 1) patient education about panic disorder; 2) beginning antidepressants in minuscule doses; 3) the simultaneous initiation of benzodiazepine antianxiety medications to "cover over" any incipient panic symptoms; 4) scheduled daily communications with patients (in person if necessary); 5) inviting and encouraging 24-hour patient access to me, as needed, through my cell phone; and 6) close monitoring of blood levels of the antidepressant. I raise the antidepressant dosages slowly and work up to the standard treatment dosages for depression. At the appropriate dosages and blood levels, antidepressants are usually highly effective in the prophylaxis of future panic attacks. This procedure worked well with Clarke, who has not experienced another panic attack.

TREATMENT PRINCIPLE 5

Educating patients about what is known scientifically and what is unknown about their psychiatric disorder and psychiatric treatment *prior to the initiation of treatment* is respectful and humane and enhances treatment compliance and response.

Psychotherapy of Clarke Myerson: The First Session

Working with a patient in psychotherapy can be likened to being an art instructor assisting an artist with his or her self-portrait. Inspiring and inspired art teachers must always and in all ways, themselves, be gifted artists. Thus, they assist their student-colleagues not only in technical aspects of art creation but, most importantly, in the elucidation of the subject. From the infinite quanta of the patient's life experiences, which are shaped and shaded by the patient's unique temperament and perceptions, arise the colors, varieties, and textures that will capture the subject. The teacher collaborates with the artist in the choices of brushes, hues, and strokes and with the decisions regarding how and where the paint is to be applied to the unblemished canvas in order to achieve a pure and honest image. The new portrait is destined to replace a former work with a less distorted, more authentic self-representation. The instructor/therapist can only guide the project by his or her questions, theoretical frameworks, and artistic talent. The therapist's art lies in helping to draw out those distortions and distractions that have led to pain and dysfunction and, more importantly, to draw on nascent strengths and resources that can lead to self-actualization and peace of mind. But let us not deceive ourselves: at the end of the day, the quality and integrity of the work depend entirely on the ultimate *decisions* and *actions* of the artist/patient. The instructor/therapist must never, never apply paint to canvas. The patient/artist is the ultimate arbiter about what is true and what is right for him or her and when, how, and where to apply the paint. And it was clear to me from our first meeting that Clarke, like so many patients, was capable of discarding the crude caricature of himself and creating a masterpiece.

As stated previously, my treatment with Clarke began in the first session by my careful listening to Clarke's chief complaints and to the beginnings of his telling of his life history. I sensed immediately that Clarke took enormous solace *in being listened to* by someone whom he assumed to be "an authority." However, there also was abundant evidence by the end of our first 2 hours (the amount of time I routinely allot to an initial meeting) that a powerful authority in his life was not a good listener. This presented a conflict for him and a challenge for treatment. I sensed that a prevailing theme of treatment would be that someone influential in his life purported to know more about what was best for Clarke than Clarke knew for himself. By the end of our first meeting I realized that if I permitted Clarke to raise me too high on the pedestal of authority, our collaboration on Clarke's masterpiece was destined to be shattered by my calamitous fall.

> **Clarke Myerson:** I must confess, Dr. Y., that although I was absolutely desperate when I decided to come to see you, I had almost no confidence that any psychiatrist would have a clue

about what was wrong with me, much less be able to help me. I now find it absolutely remarkable that, in just one session, you have been able to diagnose panic disorder and depression.

Dr. Y.: You give me far too much credit, Mr. Myerson. Your signs and symptoms of panic and depression are quite characteristic of these two highly prevalent and disabling conditions. Any trained mental health professional should be able to recognize and craft a treatment plan for that component of your care. But it is only one facet of a far more complex and intriguing picture.

Clarke: Please call me Clarke.

Dr. Y.: What would you like to call me?

Clarke: I feel that it is only appropriate for me to call you Dr. Yudofsky, unless you prefer to be called Professor Yudofsky.

Dr. Y.: And you are a highly respected financier, so it would be only respectful for me to call you Mr. Myerson if you call me Dr. Yudofsky. Unless you would prefer to call me Stuart.

Clarke: First of all, no sane person in the world of finance would ever respect me. Secondly, I could never be comfortable calling you by your first name. It would be disrespectful, and I can assure you that that will never happen.

I understand that certain readers might conclude that the preceding discussion between Clarke and me was irrelevant and typical of how time is wasted in psychotherapy. They might inquire, "Why in the world would you make such a big deal about what the two of you should call each other? Who the hell cares, and what difference could it possibly make in the long run? Is that what psychiatrists do: make a big deal out of nothing?" The answers are that I cared a great deal about how we addressed one another because it is a big deal. If we did not get the power balance between us right, as reflected in some measure by what we called one another, Clarke would not be able to benefit from therapy. That means that he would continue to suffer from panic and depression and continue to be stuck in a job and life in which he was miserable. That *is* a big deal.

My being "the all-knowing professor" and Clarke's being "the passive, vulnerable, weak, and clueless patient" would represent an unequal balance of power between us that touched on a central theme in Clarke's psychological status. In the first session, as confirmed many times in our subsequent meetings, there was abundant evidence that Clarke distrusted and disliked powerful authority figures. He therefore would not permit himself to become a potent authority in his own profession or in other areas of his life and would resist following the advice of such people. So intense was his distrust of and disaffection for authority figures that he would go to the point of defeating himself in order to defeat them and to work hard to be liked by people whom he detested. Manifestly, this dynamic could be traced to his relationship with his father, whose love and approval he craved but whose approval and unconditional love he believed he could *never* attain. Additionally, Clarke, unconsciously, was fearful that his father would consider him a rival—and crush him—if Clarke ever became a powerful man. Clarke's dysfunctional response was repeatedly to diminish and demean himself in order to feel safe from the competitive wrath of his father while, at the same time, to punish his father by his having a son who was a failure in business and in life in general. This dynamic was certain to be played out in the therapeutic setting.

With an unequal balance of power, Clarke would never "permit" the medications that I prescribed to treat effectively his depression or panic. He could assure both of our defeats by being noncompliant or "developing" side effects that prevented him from taking the medications in the first place. The pills do not work well in the bottle. Additionally, there is scientific evidence demonstrating that if patients (or their doctors) do not believe that the medication will be effective, it rarely will be so—no matter how potent it is (Bingel et al. 2011). I term this phenomenon a *reverse placebo response*. If, in our treatment, I became cast as the authority and permitted Clarke to become the passive recipient of "my wisdom," he would not allow himself to accept or act on my interpretations and our insights, regardless of whether or not they were correct and could be helpful to him.

Revealingly, Clarke adamantly refused to permit me to call him by his last name and also persisted that he was "intensely uncomfortable" calling me by my first name as I had recommended. Eventually, we struck a compromise wherein I would call him "Clarke," as he strongly preferred, and he would call me "Dr. Y." Over the course of treatment, Clarke and I often referred to this interchange when discussing his issues with and responses to real and perceived authority figures. The discussion above illustrates treatment principle 6.

TREATMENT PRINCIPLE 6

In the initial stages of treatment, beware of entering into patterns and pacts with patients that replicate their central unconscious conflicts and dynamics that perpetuate their symptoms and dysfunctions. Early in treatment, such pacts and patterns appear to enhance the therapeutic alliance, but they will disable your relationship with your patient over time.

The First 6 Months of Treatment

Within 2 months, Clarke's signs and symptoms of major depressive disorder and panic disorder responded to the combination of medications and twice-per-week psychotherapy. We both became progressively more convinced that his aversion for his job and the industry in which he worked was longstanding and not solely related to his panic and depression. It was not a revelation of his treatment that his decisions to attend business school and enter a career in finance were neither his independent choice nor his personal proclivity but his acquiescence to the will of his father. Clarke had long been quite clear and resentful about why he had made that choice and blamed himself for the deleterious repercussions thereof.

> **Clarke Myerson:** What's the point of my knowing that I have made a mess of my life, when we both know that there is nothing at this point that I can do about it?
> **Dr. Y.:** I know nothing of the sort, Clarke.
> **Clarke:** I am 40 years old, married, have two children, live in an outrageously expensive apartment on the Upper East Side of New York, and spend a ton of money on myself and my family each month. I'm trapped in the proverbial "golden cage."
> **Dr. Y.:** What makes you so sure that you are trapped? Let's carefully go over your financial and personal situations so that we truly know what we are dealing with.

The following is an old "truism" among psychiatrists: "Sex is not the most delicate and difficult subject to discuss with our patients; money is." What I learned from my discussion of money with Clarke was immensely revealing, with far-reaching implications. Although throughout his treatment Clarke had presented himself as nearly destitute, it turned out that he really was quite wealthy. Clarke was not being disingenuous; rather, he did not consider as "his" the ample trust fund that he had received from his father or the staggering sums of money that he had earned and saved while working for 15 years in his father's firm.

> **Clarke Myerson:** I do not consider that I did anything of worth to earn that money. Dad just gave it to me because I am his son— like he has done almost everything else of material value in my life. So it's really not mine, unless I use it to do something that he wants me to do.
>
> **Dr. Y.:** I don't mean to alarm you or upset you, Clarke, but I surmise that you are a very wealthy man. My supposition is that, according to the laws of New York State and the United States, the money is entirely yours. I understand fully that you become anxious if you feel powerful in almost any way and that you are especially conflicted about what you regard as the source of your wealth. Nonetheless, you can do anything with your money that you want to that is legal, if you will let yourself.

With Clarke's permission (but not at his initiation), we invited his wife, Karen, to join us for a session. I learned from Karen that she had, for many years, been encouraging him to change his employment. With great empathy, she understood that he truly hated his job and just could not understand why or accept that he would continue being miserable. She welcomed his making what she termed "a big change in his life," even if it meant the family's leaving New York City. Karen looked on such a change "as an adventure and an opportunity for all of us."

After 6 months of psychiatric treatment twice per week, Clarke was no longer clinically depressed and had gained insight about the roles of his dyslexia and his parental dynamics in his low self-esteem. He disclosed in treatment that he had "long fantasized about leaving my job and going to graduate school in English literature." He also revealed, "I would love to become an English teacher and try my hand at writing." Nonetheless, other than his psychotherapy, he did not take definitive steps to undertake meaningful change in his life. Clarke Myerson was stuck in pause, and he had been so for almost 20 years.

> **Dr. Y.:** What frightens you the most about acting on what you term your fantasy to change your career?
>
> **Clarke Myerson:** I believe that you already know the two-word answer to that question, Dr. Y.: My father!
>
> **Dr. Y.:** Am I correct in my understanding that if it were not for your fear of your father, you would have the courage to leave your current job and apply to graduate school?

Clarke: Now that we have stripped away my excuses about being poor and not disappointing my wife and children, I must confess that, as you once said, "all roads lead to Nathan." And that road, my dear Doctor, is a dead end.

Dr. Y.: What exactly are you saying?

Clarke: Two things, Dr. Y.: 1) No one takes on my father and wins, and 2) I do believe that if my father were no longer alive, I would quit my job in a New York minute and apply to graduate school in English.

Dr. Y.: Who said anything about "taking on" your father or your father having to die for you to pursue your own life? Why not just talk with him about how you feel about your job and what you would like to try doing? No one has to die from this.

Clarke: With all due respect, Doctor, you have lost your mind!

The Case of Clarke Myerson: D-2 (Decision) Component

Key Conflict

After approximately 6 months of treatment, Clarke and I agreed that he was stuck in pause regarding his job and agreed on the underlying conflict that had led to and sustained that unsettling, painful state. He believed that a prime source of the conflict was his relationship with his father and his reticence to communicate to him his desire and intention to change course vocationally. Specifically, he wanted to quit his job and enroll in graduate school in English (approach) but could not face the disappointment and anger of his father (avoidance). Thus, the basic conflict was approach-avoidance. Although leaving a job that you dislike may, at first blush, seem avoidant, in actuality, it requires *making a decision and taking action* to do something that you want to do (approach). *Not* taking action on something that causes pain and dysfunction is avoidance.

Key Features of Clarke Myerson's Being Stuck in Pause

1. *How Clarke was stuck:* He hated his job, in specific, and the field of finance, in general
2. *Goals for change:* He wished to attend graduate school in either English literature or creative writing, in preparation for and pursuit of a career in teaching and writing

3. *Central, unresolved conflict* (approach-avoidance): Attend graduate school in English versus avoid his father's anger and disappointment

4. *Hallmarks of Clarke's being stuck*: Anxiety, depression, demoralization, self-deprecation, indecisiveness, rumination

5. *Binary problem/solution*: Clarke won't speak with his father about changing careers/speak with his father

6. *Critical decision point*: Meet with his father to tell him he plans to change careers

7. *Corollary factors required to achieve resolution:* Discuss implications of such a change with wife and children; make and implement plans for transition from job; research requirements for graduate school in English literature; prepare to take graduate school entrance examinations; apply to graduate schools

Clarke Myerson: This is all for naught. I don't have the guts to confront my father.

Dr. Y.: Why does it have to be a confrontation? Why can't it be a well-intentioned discussion?

Clarke: He wants one of his sons to run the business when he gives out. Since neither of my brothers is interested, he expects me to do it—by default. And my dad always gets what he wants.

Dr. Y.: Don't you think that you owe it to him, to Karen, who hates to see you suffer, and most of all to yourself to tell him how you feel?

Clarke: For what purpose, Dr. Y.? Nothing will change his iron-clad mind.

Dr. Y.: We can never know that for certain unless and until you speak your mind.

Clarke: Did you say "we," Dr. Y.?

Dr. Y.: If you would invite me. Why would my meeting with you and your father be any different from my meeting with you and Karen?

Clarke: Oh, you'll find out. There's all the difference in the world.

TREATMENT PRINCIPLE 7

People who are stuck in pause are often unaware of precisely where they are stuck. Determining the central conflict and the critical decision points that must be addressed through the Power of Go will clarify this confusion.

The Case of Clarke Myerson: D-3 (Discipline) Component

The Power of Go

Solving approach-avoidance conflicts requires the Power of Go. In the case of Clarke Myerson, he not only had to communicate to his father his intention to leave his job and begin a new career but had to deal with his idealized image of his father. By almost every objective measure, Nathan Myerson is formidable: in his abilities, accomplishments, and bearing. To his son, Clarke, who by nature has a moderate, reserved temperament and who since his infancy had been in awe of his father (and who had a lifetime of experiencing *others* in awe of his father), approaching his father was like approaching a superhuman, preternatural force. Additionally, he was going to express his intention to go against what he knew to be his father's will. His action would take courage and conviction.

In the sessions that led up to this disclosure to his father, we discussed the many pros and cons of my joining him for this meeting. From my perspective, there were more cons than pros. For many reasons that I reviewed with Clarke, I strongly preferred Clarke to address his father without my being present at the time. Primarily, I wanted him to "own" the power that he would gain from overcoming his fears and resistances to be strong and true to himself in the presence of his father. After listening to the reasons for my concerns and reservations, Clarke made the decision that I join him when he addressed his father:

> **Clarke Myerson:** From the beginning of our work together, Dr. Y., you have been consistent with two points: 1) that "we are in this together," and 2) that, ultimately, I call the shots with regard to my own feelings, decisions, and choices. I have made the decision to confront my father and have also made the decision for you to join me when I tell him. You have told me why you don't believe that it is best for you to be there, and I understand your logic. Nonetheless, I want you there. Unless you believe that it is unethical, I want you to join me.
>
> **Dr. Y.:** You have made your decision, and I am honored and privileged to join you, Clarke.

"Confrontation"

Confrontation is not a word that I like to use in or I hope would *ever* apply to my practice of psychiatry. Additionally, I regard terms such as *tough love, encounter,* and even *intervention* (which literally means "coming between") equally unacceptable. At its roots, medicine, and therefore psychiatry (and I would also include all the other mental health disciplines), is an advocational specialty. To me that means that the patient and I must be, at *all* times, on the same side. Certainly, we may not always agree about what constitutes a problem or what are the best ways to solve a problem, but we must always be "on the same side." I understand full well that the demarcation that I have drawn may become blurred at times when a patient has impaired reality testing and wishes to kill himself or herself, but these are understandable exceptions to an important rule.

In my practice of academic medicine, I almost daily have the privilege to meet with new patients (patients whom I have not "seen" before) either in a consultative setting or through interviewing patients in my role as an educator of medical students and psychiatry residents. Under these circumstances, *before* I inquire about what might be wrong or might be the problem that led them to seek help, I do my best to get to know them as a functional human being.

What I look to discover and accomplish when I *first* meet a patient or the family member of a patient are the following:

1. What that person loves and respects about himself or herself
2. Whether or not I also admire and respect what that individual loves and respects about himself or herself
3. How best to communicate to that person my understanding of his or her exceptional qualities and my *true* admiration of that person for these qualities and gifts

I have found that when these three goals are accomplished, patients invariably will begin to trust me and almost always share with me what is troubling them and permit me to try to be of help to them. There are two important caveats: 1) Not *one* molecule of this approach can be disingenuous or feigned. If I do not readily discover an area of common ground for admiration, I keep searching. 2) It is almost always unwise to point out inconsistencies in what a patient communicates to you or to use "treatment ploys" (such as sugar pills) even if you believe that it is for the patient's benefit. Such practices create distance and distrust between you and your patients, and they respond by shutting you out "so you can't catch them." These caveats comprise treatment principle 8.

Because this process is all about the patient or his or her family and *not at all* about me, I have absolutely no anxiety or fearfulness when meeting with any patient for the first time or at any point thereafter. We are on the same team.

TREATMENT PRINCIPLE 8

"Catching" patients with inconsistencies in their communications to you or using "treatment ploys" (such as sugar pills) creates distance and distrust between you and your patients, and patients will respond by shutting you out.

Meeting Nathan Myerson

Nathan Myerson: It's good to meet you, Stuart. Most of the Board of Trustees of your medical school are my close friends or business associates. I also know your Dean quite well. You should be pleased to know that he thinks highly of you.

Dr. Y.: It's my privilege and pleasure to meet you, Dr. Myerson. I admire your extraordinary business accomplishments and exemplary public service. And it's always a relief to know that my boss isn't planning to fire me—at least not today.

Nathan Myerson: The day is young, Stuart. And thank you for calling me "Doctor." Most people seem to forget that I have a Ph.D. in economics from the University of Pennsylvania. My guess is that you are here to blame me for being a terrible father to Clarke—like I heard from my oldest son's child psychiatrist many years ago. That was the first and last time I talked to a shrink.

Dr. Y.: Clarke can speak for himself. From what Clarke has told me, I believe that you have done everything in your considerable power to prepare him to succeed and thrive in a highly competitive world. A world that is not always fair.

Nathan Myerson: Fair? What's that have to do with anything, Stuart?

Dr. Y.: Do you think you were treated fairly at Harvard?

Nathan Myerson: I still don't get what you're driving at. Harvard gave me a full scholarship, a first-rate education, graduated me with honors, and invited me to be on their Board of Directors. Does that answer your question, Stuart?

Dr. Y.: Not entirely, Dr. Myerson. I never questioned that the university per se treated you fairly. But Harvard College writes in their catalogues that a significant part of their students' education derives from their interactions with one another. How did that go for you?

Nathan Myerson: You're the doctor; what would you guess?

Dr. Y.: From the composition of the Harvard student body at the time that you attended, I would guess that you felt like a member of the ball *team* but not the ball *club*.

Nathan Myerson: And how do you arrive at this inference?

Dr. Y.: From what Clarke told me about you and his relationship with you. To understand Clarke, I needed to try to gain some understanding of you, albeit through the lens of Clarke's perceptions.

Nathan Myerson: And, in a nutshell, what did you learn?

Dr. Y.: That you wanted to do more than *to succeed;* you wanted *to belong*. But, in your era at Harvard College, "to belong" meant giving away your power to others, who closely guarded their gates and kept score in ways that frustrated you.

Nathan Myerson: Kept score? How so?

Dr. Y.: Such as by when your ancestors came to the United States, by where your family takes its summer vacations, by whose parents know theirs, by what college your parents and their parents went to, by which prep school you and they attended, by which Harvard clubs they were tapped for, and the like. And I realize full well that you have been driven to make sure your children and grandchildren have "good answers" to most of those questions.

Nathan Myerson: As you might have guessed, Stuart, my all-time favorite movie is *Chariots of Fire*, in which the Jewish protagonist tried to gain acceptance at Cambridge University by winning an Olympic gold medal in sprinting.

Although I am on many boards of directors, Stuart, and I raise and give lots of money to many university programs, I *declined* Harvard's generous offer to be on their Board of Directors. Clarke, your doctor is not a fool, and he has guts. I am now prepared to address the matter at hand. And please call me "Nathan."

Dr. Y.: Like Harold Abrahams, you ran them off their feet, Nathan. And you did it "fair and square." I, for one, respect that, Nathan. The ball's in your court, Clarke.

Clarke Myerson: Please know, Dad, that I appreciate everything that you have ever done for me, and I feel terrible that I am always disappointing you. I hate myself for embarrassing you by being such a terrible student, when you and my brothers are so exceptionally brilliant. Most of all, I hate myself for letting you down at work. So I am going to ask that you do everybody and me a favor by firing me.

Nathan: Is that the kind of crap that you brought me here to listen to, Stuart?

Dr. Y.: No. But before we try to clarify, Nathan, I would like to hear your response to what Clarke just said.

Nathan: Clarke, I know that I overreacted to your performance in school—which wasn't all that bad. But it just wasn't as good as your brothers' records. But as Stuart somehow figured out, I only wanted to help prepare you to be at the very top of the pack—in the only way I knew how at the time. I would do it differently now.

As for your work performance, Clarke, you couldn't be more wrong. You are doing a fine job at our firm. It's not easy to be the owner's son, but your modesty, work ethic, and ability to get along with our other partners are superior.

Clarke: But you have to know, Dad, that I don't have the intellectual and analytical assets of the people who report to me. I feel like a fraud.

Nathan: I'll tell you what I do know: You get to work earlier than anyone else in your division, and you leave later; your division is the number two profit center among our eight divisions—only being beaten out by mergers and acquisitions, which I run. I also know that you have never had any problems with the goddamn government regulators.

Dr. Y.: Going back to the *Chariots of Fire* film, Nathan, you also have much in common with Eric Liddell, the Scottish runner.

Nathan: How so?

Dr. Y.: Eric Liddell was a natural runner. When his sister asked him to stop training for the Olympic Games and focus entirely on his missionary work in China, he replied, "I believe God made me for a purpose, but He also made me fast. And when I run, I feel His pleasure." You are a natural in finance, Nathan, and it's your passion. Unfortunately, that is not true for Clarke.

Clarke: As you said, Dad, it's not all that easy to walk in your shadow, to be a great, successful man's son—let alone to work for him. In terms of my so-called accomplishments, I *never* know what is yours or what is mine. More important and, believe it or not, much harder for me to say, is that I think that I might have a gift—and know I have a passion. But I will never know for sure if I stay in my job.

Nathan: What are you thinking about doing?

Clarke: Applying to graduate school in English literature or creative writing and then going on to teach in college. I know that I won't make a lot of money, but it's what I believe that I will be good at and enjoy doing.

Nathan: And what's your take on all of this, Stuart?

Dr. Y.: I share everyone's concerns about the practicality and timing of such a move for Clarke. Also, I don't believe that it makes sense for Clarke to change careers at this point in his life just to prove something to himself or to you, Nathan. However, I do believe that Clarke deserves a shot at doing something in which he excels and takes pleasure. And I believe he does have talent in writing.

Nathan: I had my staff write me a summary of your career, Stuart. You've been on the faculty of two pretty good universities: Columbia and the University of Chicago. What does a full professor of English get paid at those places?

Dr. Y.: I don't know for certain, but I would speculate under $100,000 a year.

Nathan: With his bonuses and options, Clarke's salary is at least that much each month. I think that you both have lost your minds.

Dr. Y.: If I may so presume, Nathan, I'd like to ask you a personal question: do any of your grandchildren have the interest and abilities to contribute to your business?

Nathan: Three of Clarke's nephews got the goods and may even be interested. And I also believe that Clarke's older daughter, Olivia, could hit the ball out of the park, if she were interested.

Dr. Y.: It might be time for you to have some talks with your grandchildren about their future plans. After all, Nathan, it's a family business.

Corollary Features

After Clarke *discovered* that he was stuck in a job that he hated, and after he *decided* to communicate to his father that he planned to change careers—and did so in several joint meetings with his father and me—the *discipline* required to effect his decision to move forward with graduate school was not that difficult for him. After all, he was pursuing what he wanted and learning what he loved.

Clarke Myerson completed the Writers' Workshop of the University of Iowa, where he received an M.A. in creative writing. Thereafter, he pursued a Ph.D. in American literature from the University of California, Berkeley, where he remained on the faculty. Currently, he is an associate professor. Clarke has become a leading scholar on American Jewish fiction writers, including Saul Bellow, Bernard Malamud, Joseph Heller, and Philip Roth. He has written several well-received books on this subject, as well as a novel of his own.

Epilogue: Ten Years Later

Several months ago, Clarke scheduled a meeting with me in Houston for what he termed "a wrap-up session."

Dr. Y.: How are you, Clarke?

Clarke Myerson: My tendency is still to say "better than I deserve to be," but I don't want to get into any more struggles with you about my Oedipal conflicts. My best answer is I am who I am, and I spend my time doing what I love.

Dr. Y.: So you *are* well, and you seem to be *doing* very well.

Clarke: So just how would you know that?

Dr. Y.: I read your books.

Clarke: I came to thank you for recognizing at our very first meeting that I have a gift for metaphor. Did you know at the time just how much that compliment meant to me? I didn't like myself very much then, and I didn't have very much else to hold on to, about which to be proud of myself. I now understand that nothing said in treatment is random. When I was falling apart, of all things, what made you focus on my ability with metaphor?

Dr. Y.: Because of the metaphoric quality of the event with Miss Bradshaw that brought you into treatment. And because of your elegant use of language and metaphor as you talked about your symptoms. And because I admire you and your gift of metaphor.

Clarke: Are you saying that *my symptoms* showed creative talent?

Dr. Y.: Indeed.

Clarke: So it turns out that my talents and problems seem to blend together. You and I may be in the same business, Dr. Y.

Dr. Y.: Perhaps....

References

American Psychiatric Association: Diagnostic and Statistical Manual of Mental Disorders, 4th Edition, Text Revision. Washington, DC, American Psychiatric Association, 2000

American Psychiatric Association: Diagnostic and Statistical Manual of Mental Disorders, 5th Edition. Washington, DC, American Psychiatric Association, 2013

Bingel U, Wanigasekera V, Wiech K, et al: The effect of treatment expectation on drug efficacy: imaging the analgesic benefit of the opioid remifentanil. Sci Transl Med 3:70–73, 2011

Keller MB, McCullough JP, Klein DN, et al: A comparison of nefazodone, the cognitive behavioral-analysis of psychotherapy, and their combination in the treatment of chronic depression. N Engl J Med 342:1462–1470, 2000

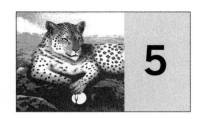

Stuck in My Body, Part I (Discover): The Case of Ms. Anita Anthony

When an Eating Disorder Is Complicated by Sexual Abuse

He jests at scars that never felt a wound.
—*William Shakespeare*, Romeo and Juliet, *Act II, Scene 2*

"I'm eating myself to death."

The Case of Ms. Anita Anthony: D1 (Discover) Assessment Component

Skin Deep: Presentation to Treatment

At 5:30 A.M. on a Monday morning, I received a call on my cell phone from Norman Campbell, M.D., the chief of orthopedics of the county hospital associated with the medical school where I work. A man of few words, Dr. Campbell is a legendary surgeon who rarely makes referrals to psychiatry.

> **Dr. Norman Campbell:** Good morning, Stuart. I hope I am not interrupting you, but I need you to see a patient as soon as possible. It's Ms. Anita Anthony, one of the best surgery nurses we have here. We got to the point that our place can't run without her, and she's been missing a lot of work lately. Although she has plenty of troubles with her body, I think most of her problems are in her head. She vehemently disagrees.

Try to fit her in today, if you can. I gotta run now. You're going to love Anita.

Following what was to have been my last appointment of that day, I met with Ms. Anthony. Sturdy of frame, lofty of stature, and tightly buttoned into a voluminous white laboratory coat, she resembled a mogul—a mountain of swollen snow that strained to burst free in an avalanche of adipose. Ms. Anthony sullenly accompanied me to my office, sat down, and, for several silent minutes, stared sourly into her glacial lap. Finally, she looked up unhurriedly, glowered directly into my eyes, and declared resolutely,

Ms. Anita Anthony: This will never work.

Dr. Y.: Why?

Ms. Anthony: Well, just look at your sad, shriveled self, and look at me. We have absolutely nothing in common.

Dr. Y.: What do *you* see?

Ms. Anthony: I see a skinny little white man in a fancy office that is set up to do a lot of talking.

Dr. Y.: And what do you think that *I* see?

Ms. Anthony: Unless you are blind, you see a big—a too big—black woman.

Dr. Y.: That's *not* what I see, Ms. Anthony. I see a person about whom I have a great deal to learn. On the surface you may be big and black and I may be little and white, but that's just the surface.

Ms. Anthony: I don't have the slightest idea what you're talking about.

Dr. Y.: On the surface, surgery, where you work, cuts and sews, and psychiatry, where I work, talks and talks. But that's just the surface. The fact is that the two specialties have a lot in common.

Ms. Anthony: Let's get this straight: In my opinion, surgery and psychiatry have absolutely nothing in common, and you and I have even less in common. Like I said, this will never work.

Dr. Y.: And like I said, that may appear to be true on the surface, but I have learned not to trust the surface. All too often, "surfaces" lead to misunderstandings. One thing in common with both surgeons and psychiatrists is that our fields are greatly misunderstood.

Ms. Anthony: Oh, here we go. According to you psychiatrists, *everybody* is misunderstood. Next thing you'll be telling me is that the reason I am 100 pounds overweight is because my mother misunderstood me when I was in diapers.

Dr. Y.: Most people think that surgeons work with their hands and psychiatrists work with their mouths. It couldn't be further from the truth. We both work with our minds, and we both do our work deep, deep beneath the surface. As you undoubtedly know, Ms. Anthony, one should never judge the quality of a heart transplant by how the skin incision looks. Nor would I ever presume to know anything about you from the color of your skin or how much you weigh. Let's start by your telling me why you came by to see me this evening. That being said, I would love to know more about your mother—and more about you.

Ms. Anthony: I'm not here to talk about my mother, and I don't want to talk about myself. The only reason I came here is because my doctor told me that I *had* to come. I'm eating myself to death. I have "high blood" everything: high blood sugar, high blood cholesterol, and high blood pressure. On top of that I have arthritis in both my knees that's so bad that I can barely walk. It all started when I had a terrible fall about 10 years ago and fractured both of my kneecaps. These days I can't even stand on my feet long enough to scrub in on an appendectomy. And I *don't* need you to tell me that my weight doesn't help anything. What I *do* need is to get two knee replacements, but Dr. Campbell won't touch me unless he gets the green light from you. That's all I need from you. I know he's worried about my weight. I've tried every diet ever invented, and none of them worked. You're looking at the only person who has ever gained 10 pounds in 2 months from eating only pink grapefruit. But please get this straight, Doctor: I don't want to see you or any other psychiatrist. Dr. Campbell told me that I *had* to come here before he will operate on my knees.

A ballet dancer could not have done a more graceful job than Ms. Anthony in tiptoeing the fine thread between recounting so much about her medical conditions and so little about herself. Nonetheless, I was able to learn a great deal—more from what she would not reveal than from what she would. The key issues of her medical status were the following:

1. She was taking two oral medications for her type II diabetes, without adequate control of her blood glucose, and her endocrinologist indicated that she would very likely place her on insulin unless she could lose weight.

2. She was being treated for essential hypertension (high blood

pressure) that was not responding consistently to a cocktail of three powerful medications, which placed her at great risk for a stroke and cardiovascular disease.

3. She was afflicted with a host of other medical problems directly related to her obesity—including sleep apnea and insomnia, arthritis of her knees and lower spine, swelling and recurrent infections of her feet, and symptoms of gallbladder disease.

In summary, although Ms. Anthony was taking 12 different medications a day to mitigate medical disorders directly or indirectly related to her obesity, her health was declining rapidly. Like so many other Americans, Ms. Anthony was, indeed, "eating herself to death."

Evolution and Diet, Part 1: Survival

Survival of the Fit: Supply Side

For most of mankind's history, food sources—whether animal or vegetable—were characteristically accessible only intermittently and required the considerable expenditure of effort to secure. As has been touched on in Chapter 2, "Getting Stuck," and Chapter 3, "The Fatal Pauses 3-D Method of Getting Unstuck Through the Power of No and the Power of Go," the relatively recent ability of human beings to work productively in groups to invent and craft tools; to raise, process, preserve, and distribute crops; and to breed and harvest animals has far outpaced the evolution of our bodies. As a result, in technologically advanced nations such as the United States, an unprecedented quantity and variety of food are ubiquitously available for contemporary men and women.

Survival of the Fit: Demand Side

In all mammals, whether rodents, canines, or primates, there are two unfortunate and inevitable consequences of abundant availability of food: obesity and overpopulation. As if nature were applying a brake, the results of unbridled increases in obesity in all mammalian species are metabolic diseases, plagues, and dramatically reduced lifespans. As the data summarized below demonstrate, human beings are currently experiencing an epidemic of obesity that is accelerating at an alarming pace, and it is killing us.

Epidemiology of Obesity

In 2012, a report of the American Heart Association (Roger et al. 2012) and a report from the National Center for Health Statistics of the Centers for Disease Control and Prevention (Ogden et al. 2012) offered the following statistics and information regarding the prevalence of obesity and overweight among American children and adults:

- Among American children and adolescents ages 2–19, almost one in three, or 32.1% of all boys and 31.3% of all girls, are overweight or obese, and of those, one in six (17.8% of all boys and 15.9% of all girls) are obese.
- In comparison with 1973–1974, the proportion of children 5–17 years old who were obese was five times higher in the year 2008–2009.
- Among American adults (age 20 and older), 149.3 million are overweight or obese, and of those, more than one-third, or 34.9 million men and 40.1 million women, are obese.
- The annual cost related to the current prevalence of adolescent overweight and obesity is $254 billion.
- Overweight adolescents have a 70% chance of becoming overweight adults.
- If current trends continue, annual health care costs attributable to obesity will reach $861–$957 billion by 2030, which would account for 16%–18% of U.S. health care expenditures.

The body mass index (BMI) is a standard measurement of obesity, and it is calculated as weight in kilograms divided by height in meters squared. *Obesity* in adults is defined as a BMI equal to or greater than 30. For example, an adult who is 5 feet 4 inches tall is calculated by this formula as being obese if he or she weighs 174 pounds or more (79 kilograms). An adult who is 5 feet 9 inches tall is determined to be obese if he or she weighs more than 203 pounds (92 kilograms). The calculations of being *overweight* are far less specific and more subjective because they relate to body type and cultural factors. In the next section, I present evidence that being overweight has important consequences for health and longevity. From the most subjective perspective, I am almost 5 feet 10 inches tall and consider myself overweight if I exceed 143 pounds.

Health-Related Consequences of Obesity

- *Cardiovascular:* coronary artery/ischemic heart disease, leading to myocardial infarctions (heart attacks) and congestive heart failure (in which the lungs fill with fluid); deep vein blood clots that can travel from legs to lungs; high blood pressure
- *Neurological:* stroke, vascular dementias (formerly called *senility*), migraine headaches
- *Cancer:* breast cancer, ovarian cancer, uterine cancers (endometrial, cervical), colon cancer, prostate cancer, kidney cancer, gallbladder cancer, stomach cancer, liver cancer, pancreatic cancer
- *Endocrine:* type II diabetes; ovarian cysts; menstrual disorders; infertility; pregnancy complications; early puberty in girls and, most likely, boys
- *Rheumatological:* gout, osteoarthritis
- *Neuropsychiatric:* depression in women; social stigmatization of men, women, and children; early onset dementia; Alzheimer's disease

Although the current epidemic of obesity has far-reaching and dire consequences for our health, we seem to have no natural resistance to this epidemic. I firmly believe that only the human mind that helped to create the epidemic can stop it: one mind, one hand, and one mouth at a time. However, like the joke about the light bulb, first, the mind must want to change itself. However, as exemplified by the case of Ms. Anthony and the incalculable number of other Americans who have tried, without success, many diets, a mind is not an easy thing to change.

Engagement in Treatment, Part 1: Don't Count on It

Notwithstanding the essential information that Ms. Anthony imparted about her dire health status, the most important information that I learned during my first hour of meeting with her was *what I didn't learn.* She would reveal nothing substantial about her personal life, family, relationships, or feelings. From every vantage she was trying to keep me at a distance from knowing her as a person, and she did so by trying to set up power struggles that I was doing my very best to elude. At the same time, I understood that if I were to engage her in any type of meaningful psychotherapy, I must respect the defensive barriers that she had erected around herself. Otherwise, she would disengage fully by leaving treatment and not returning.

After reviewing her litany of medical problems, Ms. Anthony looked at her watch and said,

> **Ms. Anita Anthony:** It's almost 9:00 P.M. That should just about do it. Now you can call Dr. Campbell and tell him that you think I'm good to go for my knee replacement.
>
> **Dr. Y.:** If I thought that would help you, Ms. Anthony, I would call him right now and advise that he proceed with the surgery. Our trouble is that I don't know you sufficiently well to come to that conclusion or to make that recommendation.
>
> **Ms. Anthony:** What else could you possibly need to know about me? I'm perfectly sane, and I can barely walk.
>
> **Dr. Y.:** I don't believe that Dr. Campbell asked you to come see me in order to determine your sanity. I think that he wanted me to work with you to solve a mystery.
>
> **Ms. Anthony:** Oh please save me, Lord. There *is* no mystery. If your knees hurt *you* the way my knees hurt *me*, you wouldn't be talking about any mystery. I don't need a detective to tell me that my knees are killing me.
>
> **Dr. Y.:** Dr. Campbell and I both know that it's not your knees that are killing you. Therefore, a knee replacement, alone, will not fix that problem or save your life. The mystery is why you—a superintelligent, highly trained medical professional—do not understand that.
>
> Dr. Campbell and I both know that you not only have pain in your knees, but you are also hurting somewhere else. I believe that if we have the chance to work together, we can solve that mystery, discover and address that pain, as well.
>
> **Ms. Anthony:** You've worn me out with all of your talk about "surfaces," "solving mysteries," and only the dear Lord knows what else. This is even worse than I expected, and I wasn't expecting a damn thing. I want to go home now. It has been a long day. You probably don't know it, but we start working very early on the surgery service.
>
> Now, I don't give you my permission to talk to Dr. Campbell or to anybody else about me. I'm sure that you know the HIPAA [Health Insurance Portability and Accountability Act] laws— I signed your forms about them.
>
> **Dr. Y.:** Thank you for meeting with me, Ms. Anthony. I both invite

and encourage you to come back to see me whenever you like. As you instruct, I will not speak with Dr. Campbell about you. Too bad, because I was going to tell him that he was absolutely right about you...and me.

Ms. Anthony: And just what *did* he say about you and me?

Dr. Y.: Now is not the best time to discuss that. Permit me to have at least one mystery, myself. I hope to see you soon.

Ms. Anthony: Don't count on it.

The Impossible Profession

Sigmund Freud is famously purported to have said that there are three impossible professions, in which one can be certain, beforehand, of unsuccessful results. The impossible professions are *teaching*, *running government*, and *psychoanalysis* (which I am confident today would have included contemporary psychiatry and the related mental health professions). Freud believed these professions are impossible because of their interminability. Why interminable? Because the work of these professions is never done: one must never stop learning, governments must continuously provide and revise services to their constituents, and there is no end to an individual's need for personal growth and self-discovery. I am certain Freud also realized that for positive outcomes, each of these impossible professions also requires the *willing* participation of those who partake of the services—and in each profession, enlisting meaningful participation can be a high hurdle to surmount.

In several ways, Ms. Anthony made it quite clear to me that she did not want or value the services that I was offering. She was both verbally assaultive and well armored. She outright told me that she did not come to see me of her own volition but was coerced to do so by Dr. Campbell as a prerequisite for her surgery. Thus, I had something that she needed, as well as the power to withhold it from her. As a result, she perceived inequity of power in our relationship, which engendered a therapeutic dynamic wherein she felt diminished. Recognizing this problem immediately, I did my best to level the playing field on all fronts, particularly by acknowledging her as a valued colleague in a potent medical discipline. She countered by trying to provoke me by demeaning me personally and my profession. She threw hard and experienced punches, and they all landed.

I tried not to counter her unremitting attack but worked to understand and feel her pain and humiliation. After all, Ms. Anthony was a proud woman needing and refusing help. Despite her denials and refusals, she bore with her the tangible burdens of her pain at all times for the entire world to see.

The therapeutic "impossibility" was that if I were more assertive and potent in my interpretations of her provocations, she would have felt even less powerful. Even worse, I could have re-created in the treatment a struggle and source of hurt that paralleled a previous, seminal root of hurt in her life—such as if she had been made to feel vulnerable and powerless to protect herself from a boundary violation as a child. Alternatively, if I held back and did not respond to or counter her provocations, I would reify her relentless contentions that psychiatry is weak, useless, and ridiculous. While vainly searching everywhere for an opening in her defensive armor, I chose the latter approach—to absorb her punches with the hope that she would eventually open up. She left without doing so, and I could only hope that I did not burn any bridges leading back to my office or to psychiatric treatment from someone else.

The public relations of psychiatry and the mental health professions is abysmally poor. My initial encounter with Ms. Anthony sheds light on one among many reasons for our poor image. I imagined how Ms. Anthony would describe her visit with me to Dr. Campbell and to all others who would listen.

> **Ms. Anita Anthony** (*as imagined by Dr. Y.*): Everybody knows that all psychiatrists are crazy, but this Yudofsky plants the flag at the top of nut mountain. These guys are supposed to have gone to medical school, but he probably was much too stupid or too crazy to learn one damn thing about medicine. He had the audacity to tell me that I didn't feel any pain in my knees, that it's all in my head. He also said that the arthritis in my knees is my mother's fault. My mother was all he wanted to talk about. I can only guess that he thought that my mother messed up my toilet training when I was a baby, or did something like that to me. I wouldn't give him the satisfaction of getting into it. No way am I blaming my sainted mother for anything. And this you will not believe—he thought surgery and psychiatry are sister professions. Maybe an evil stepsister! I did learn one important thing from him, however: Don't dare go near one of those guys. They're dangerous.

Evolution and Diet, Part 2: Of Size and Stigma

Buried among the highly abbreviated, devastating health consequences of being overweight or obese as summarized in the section
"Epidemiology of Obesity" (p. 101) is *social stigmatization of men,
women, and children.* We all recognize that many people who are
overweight or obese are subject to ridicule, rejection, and social os-
tracism by others as well as to self-imposed shame, guilt, and self-
deprecation. Untold numbers of men and women of all shapes, sizes,
and weights devote disproportionate amounts of their lives to obsessive preoccupation with what they eat and how much they weigh.
Many of the most empathic and high-minded among us reluctantly
acknowledge that they are not physically attracted to people who are
even moderately overweight—no matter how much they admire the
personal qualities of these individuals.

Why do we care so much about what we ourselves and others
weigh? There are two correct answers to this question—one short
and one long. The short answer is that we care so much because of
the *survival* implications of excessive weight. Attraction has everything to do with survival. Strong physiques; symmetrical, proportioned features and limbs; blemishless skin; and coordination and
athleticism superficially reflect our abilities to acquire food, to escape or overcome predators and competitors, to attract and retain
mates, and to reproduce and nourish offspring. These visible attributes are superficially indicative of intact genetics that have been
honed by millennia of natural selection, in which the rarest of rare
mutations that enhance our adaptation to our environments are preserved through the generations by our species. The vast majority of
mutations, however, endangers survival and, when detectable by
peers, leads to stigmatization and persecution. Wittingly—as in the
case of the German Nazi Party—or unwittingly—as in the cases of
seemingly all societies—we seem to want to eliminate nonadaptive,
survival-endangering genes from our populations. For all human
history overt manifestation of genetic differences, including facial
disfigurements, physical disabilities, and behavioral and mental disorders have led to stigmatization and persecution.

The second and more complex reason that we so deeply are
aware and care about our weight is based on our uniquely diverse life

experiences and social, psychological, and biological influences. The result is we all have distinctly divergent ideas and feelings about our own weight and that of others. Because all of these elements relate to how we become overweight and obese in the first place as well as how these complex elements affect our decision to lose weight, each significant factor must be understood and addressed for diets and weight loss treatments to be effective over the long haul. As with the myriad other ways we can become stuck in pause, I do not believe that there are any quick fixes or "one size fits all" diets for significant and lasting weight loss.

Engagement in Treatment, Part 2: Tempus Fugit

More than a year had passed since my initial (and only) meeting with Ms. Anthony. Because she had prohibited me from discussing our session with anyone, I had not heard a word in the interim from Dr. Campbell or from anyone else about how she was faring. While acknowledging to myself the fundamental impotence of any practitioner to make the decision for a patient to engage in treatment, I was nonetheless quite upset that engagement had not occurred. In my mind, I had reviewed and deliberated about what had and had not transpired in our session, about what I did, did not do, and should have done to facilitate Ms. Anthony's engagement in treatment, and I groped for what I had missed. Over the dilutions of time and distance and with new challenges and crises, I inevitably thought about her less and less. At 3:00 A.M. on a Saturday morning, I answered a page from an emergency medicine resident of the private, not-for-profit teaching hospital in which I am a staff psychiatrist and chief of service.

> **Dr. Seema Patel:** Sorry to disturb you so early in the morning, sir, but one of your patients is in the Emergency Center. She has made a pretty serious suicide attempt. At first she refused to give us any information about herself whatsoever. I told her that if she did not agree to be admitted to the psych service, we would have to commit her. At that point, she told us that she is your patient. Her name is Anita Anthony.
> **Dr. Y.:** I'll be right in.

A Wish For My Readers

As I drove to the hospital, for reasons that were not immediately clear to me, I became acutely aware of my advancing age. So many early morning calls over so many years, so many tense meetings with patients and their families, so many critical decisions made and to be made that affect prominently the lives of so many others and my own life. So much uncertainty.

Given our first meeting and the high degree of stigma associated with being admitted to an inpatient psychiatry service, I was fairly confident that Ms. Anthony would decline a voluntary admission, notwithstanding the immediacy of her suicidal potential. If she remained actively suicidal, it would be my responsibility to arrange an involuntary commitment procedure. Committing her to a hospital-based psychiatry service would, doubtlessly, intensify and, most likely, immortalize the adversarial nature of our relationship—an advent that I had tried assiduously to avoid during our first meeting. The probability was that her suicidal status would lurk in the "gray zone," where neither she nor I could be certain of her safety after she was alone again. So little would be changed with regard to the life stresses and deep-seated feelings and conflicts that had contributed to her suicide attempt. The only positive resolution would be if something were to change in her "internal world" in our impending brief meeting. Of course, that change would provide a glimmer of hope. A lot to ask of us both. Her life and my personal and professional integrity would depend on mutable intangibles such as her mood and desire to stay alive at any given point in time and my "hunches" in the emergency room about what would work best for her future—which is not always what would be the *safest* course for her at that precise moment. So much uncertainty.

On that early morning drive to the hospital, I realized once more what a blessed man I am and have been in my professional life. How much I cherish the privilege and opportunity to be an important part of the lives of so many people at such critical phases in their lives. How much my chosen profession has to offer to those whom we serve. I was confident that the sliver of an opening to help Ms. Anthony—for which I had futilely searched during our initial meeting—had arrived. Simultaneously, I recognized that I cannot go on forever practicing the profession in which I believe and that I adore with all my heart. And with all my heart, I wish these blessed opportunities and moments for all of my readers—both patients and professionals.

Getting Started

Prior to my meeting with Ms. Anthony, I met briefly with Dr. Patel.

> **Dr. Seema Patel:** Ms. Anthony was brought here by ambulance. No one came with her. The EMS [emergency medical service] said she had dialed 911 soon after cutting her wrist quite severely. When EMS arrived, she refused to be helped. However, her left wrist had a deep laceration, and she was bleeding profusely. EMS told her that they had no choice but to take her to the hospital. They insisted that if she continued to resist going to the hospital ER, they would involve the police to do so forcefully. So she chose to come here.
>
> She wouldn't say a word to me about why she tried to kill herself, even though I asked her many times and in many different ways. All she said was that she is no longer suicidal. She signed the permission form for me to clean and close the laceration, but she didn't speak to me during the entire procedure. She had hit a small vein but narrowly missed her ulnar artery, which I think was what she was going for. She made a vertical incision up the ventral part of her wrist, which, as you know is atypical of the usual horizontal slashes of most suicide attempters. It showed me that she knows a little bit about anatomy and that she was serious about killing herself. However, if you ever tried to stick a needle into someone's ulnar artery to get blood gases, you know how hard this artery is to hit— especially if there's too much adipose around the wrist. Being so fat probably saved her life. I'll pass the baton over to you, sir. Good luck on getting her to talk. At times like this, I'm so glad that I didn't go into psychiatry.

Tented in the standard cotton hospital dressing gown and compressed into the spindly confines of a small armchair in the treatment room, Ms. Anthony looked far less imposing than when I first saw her, about to erupt, in the waiting area of my office. Her mass and a large hospital stretcher dictated that I roll up too close to her on the squat, round, stainless steel surgeons' stool that was the third piece of furniture in our tiny rectangular space. Both of us were oblivious to the saddening symphony of wails, to the chorus of commands of doctors and nurses, and to the crescendos of sirens that herald the swelling stream of misery that floods endlessly into this metropolitan general hospital emergency department. We sat in silent, uncomfortable closeness for quite a long time. A cramped confessional in a chaotic cathedral is a difficult place for an angry, lost woman to gather her dignity about herself—much less to find mercy, hope, and salvation.

> **Dr. Y.:** It's been a long while since we have spoken. I have thought about you quite a bit. I'm pleased to hear from Dr. Patel that you have designated me as your psychiatrist.
>
> **Ms. Anita Anthony:** Did I have a choice? Either I deal with you or get committed to a nut house.
>
> **Dr. Y.:** When we last met, your knees were hurting you badly. Are they any better?
>
> **Ms. Anthony:** You told me that it wasn't my knees that were the problem. That it was me. I didn't believe you at the time, but it looks like you get the last laugh.
>
> **Dr. Y.:** I don't find any humor in your trying to kill yourself. Nor did I doubt for a moment how much pain you were experiencing in your knees. You and I just differed about the approach to their treatment. And between well-intended people there can be honest differences of opinion.
>
> **Ms. Anthony:** Good. Now what's your honest opinion about how I can get my bad knees and the rest of my bad self out of this damn hospital?
>
> **Dr. Y.:** The best way is for you to tell me how you became so desperate that you tried to kill yourself.
>
> **Ms. Anthony:** It's 4:00 A.M. on a Sunday morning. You've got a lot more important things to do than to listen to me complain.
>
> **Dr. Y.:** At this very moment, I have nothing more important to do than to listen to you and to learn about you. Where would you like to start?

Ms. Anthony's Scars

Ms. Anthony began by showing me the surgical scars from her knee replacements. On her right knee was a single, thin, completely healed scar that encircled the faint upper protrusion of her knee cap. By contrast, her left knee resembled a Civil War battleground—a disfigured field of bitterly contested advances and retreats.

> **Dr. Y.:** What happened to your left knee?
>
> **Ms. Anita Anthony:** The prosthesis got infected. You shouldn't

look surprised. When you wouldn't sign off on my surgeries, Dr. Campbell refused to do the procedures. So I got another surgeon, and you can see the results for yourself. He had to operate on my knee five more times to clean out the infection. I have spent much of the past year in the hospital on IVs, antibiotics, and painkillers. At one point I also had to be treated for a pulmonary embolus because of my bad circulation. I haven't been back to work in 7 months.

Dr. Y.: Are you out of the woods from a medical perspective?

Ms. Anthony: The surgeon and my other doctors seem to think so. Supposedly, the infections are long gone, but my left knee hurts me more now than it did before the surgery. I can't walk well or get off of the painkillers—despite all kinds of rehab and tapering regimens.

Dr. Y.: Are you depressed, as well?

Ms. Anthony: Anyone who has been through what I have gone through would be crazy if they *weren't* depressed.

Paradoxically, depression provided a minuscule patch of neutral ground for Ms. Anthony to answer my somewhat personal questions about her frame of mind at the time she attempted suicide and about her current living arrangements. Nonetheless, similar to the way her surgeon must have felt when he was operating on her left knee for the sixth time, I sensed that the battlefield of our incipient relationship was bristling with land mines, and one false step on my part would blow our embryonic therapeutic alliance to kingdom come.

The essence of what I had learned was that Ms. Anthony was 36 years old and had never been married. She could not identify what had precipitated her suicide attempt other than that to disclose, "I was feeling super sad, hopeless, and useless. I couldn't see any point in going on anymore." As a result of my probing, however, she also revealed that it was her deceased father's birthday and that she had two large glasses of wine in his honor and memory prior to her suicide attempt. She also confided that he was a corporal in the Army and had been killed in duty during the Desert Storm conflict when she was 16 years old. She stated that she rarely drinks alcohol and that she had the bottle of wine for more than a year before having opened it that night. The wine was a gift from a grateful patient for whom she had cared on the surgical service where she worked. She also stated that immediately after cutting herself, she regretted doing so and called 911. As predicted, she claimed that she no longer wanted to take her own life. Ms. Anthony fully met official DSM-5 criteria for major depressive disorder (American Psychiatric Association 2013).

> **Ms. Anita Anthony:** OK, we have been at this for almost 2 hours. You know everything about me that there is to know. Now tell me how I can check out of this hospital and go home to try to get some sleep.
>
> **Dr. Y.:** My preferred option is for you to sign in voluntarily to the hospital psychiatric unit where you can be safely treated for depression and tapered from the analgesics.
>
> **Ms. Anthony:** You can trust me on these two things. Number one: I will *never* voluntarily sign myself into any psych ward, and number two: if I tell you that I won't kill myself, I won't do it.
>
> **Dr. Y.:** My professional and legal responsibilities are to protect you. I also care about you. Before I make any decision about your going home, I need to be as certain as possible about two things: number one, that you won't try to kill yourself once you're alone, and number two, that you will follow, explicitly, the treatment plan that I will set up for you.
>
> **Ms. Anthony:** Although not a damn thing has changed, I give you my word I won't try to kill myself again without letting you know first. There is no way that I can prove that. You'll just have to trust me. Now before *I* agree to follow your so-called treatment plan, clue me in on what that's about. Talking forever about my mother?
>
> **Dr. Y.:** Instead of admitting you to an inpatient psychiatric facility, I must see you every day in my office to assess your suicidal potential and to treat your depression. Additionally, even if you agree to meeting with me daily, you must also agree that you will sign into a psychiatric service if, in the future, I believe you have become suicidal again. Finally, you must try to do your best to be open with me about what you are thinking and feeling. I promise to do my best to do the same.

After a long discussion/negotiation, Ms. Anthony accepted the conditions that I had posed, and we arranged specific times to meet during the next 14 days.

> **Dr. Y.:** How do you plan to get back to your home?
>
> **Ms. Anita Anthony:** I've been here for nearly 5 hours. I think my ambulance ride to the hospital has left. I'd like to take a cab, but I left my purse at home.
>
> **Dr. Y.:** I'd be happy to drop you off on my way back to my house. After all, isn't it my fault that you can't walk home?

Over my 40 years of practicing medicine, I have made countless house calls. However, I had never before—nor have I since—driven a patient home from the hospital. My careful and brilliant teachers of yesteryear certainly would *not* have approved. They would have been concerned about my blurring the boundaries between my professional and personal lives, about my giving the patient the destructive message that I was her "savior riding in on a white horse" to rescue her from all of her problems, etc. These were wise and careful mentors, and their concerns would have been altogether valid. But somehow, on this particular night of her life, it just did not seem right for Ms. Anthony to have to try to find her own way back home. She had done that too many times and had never seemed to find it. She could use a helping hand, and, if she would permit it, a guide. And besides, I was feeling a bit ancient, and maybe my time had finally come to tender and follow a therapeutic rule or two of my own.

The Case of Ms. Anita Anthony: D1 (Discover) Treatment Component

Keeping Our Bargain

Ms. Anthony kept our bargain. She was on time for each of the 14 consecutive daily sessions and felt progressively safer and more comfortable in discussing her personal history and feelings. Thereafter, we agreed to meet twice per week for 1-hour sessions. I placed her on an antidepressant medication for her suicidal depression and, simultaneously, tapered and discontinued *all* of her pain medications. Each of these analgesics had highly deleterious side effects—many of them involving her mood and mental status—and her pain nonetheless remained disabling. Within 8 weeks, she was no longer depressed and her physical pain was also markedly reduced. Most of our meeting time was devoted to my securing her personal and psychiatric history. Progressively, she became more comfortable with the process and me.

Corporal Dwight Anthony

Ms. Anthony had carefully researched the college and military background of her beloved father. Although he was away in service for much of their lives, Dwight Anthony cared deeply for and about his two children. The first in his family to attend college, Dwight Anthony was recruited to Texas A&M University on a full scholarship as a member of their Naval Reserve Officer Training Corps of Cadets. As a college junior, he became one of the first African American cadets to be chosen as a member of the Ross Volunteer Company, a highly selective honorary organization based on "honor, humility, and character." He was selected as their commanding officer as a senior in college. He was graduated with a degree in chemical engineering and with highest honors from Texas A&M, which he loved and where he was beloved by his professors and peers. Thereafter, he became an officer in the U.S. Marines. Two years later, he married Lorraine, his high school sweetheart from the small East Texas town where they had both grown up. Lorraine attended nursing school and later worked as a nurse in the pediatric intensive care unit of a large children's hospital in Houston, where she and Dwight settled and bought a small home.

After a year of marriage, Dwight and Lorraine had a son, Kyle, who was named after Edwin Jackson Kyle, an illustrious alumnus and faculty member of Texas A&M. Anita was born about 2 years thereafter. Lorraine had stopped working after the birth of Kyle.

Ms. Anthony described her mother as "a physically beautiful woman, who was passive, distant, and, for the most part, incompetent." On the other hand, she adored her father, who was actively involved in her life and that of her brother. She recalled "missing him terribly" when he was deployed overseas.

> **Ms. Anita Anthony:** The worst night of my life was on January 31, 1991. Daddy had been away for a long time. He had called about a month earlier to wish us a Merry Christmas, and that was the very last time that I heard his beautiful voice.
> I recall that three soldiers came to our little house to tell our mother that Daddy had been killed. I learned much later that he was killed during the Battle of Khafji, an early battle in the Desert Storm war. The battle wasn't even in Iraq; it took place in Saudi Arabia. He was killed by what they called *friendly fire*. I hate every single thing about that abominable term *friendly fire*. It certainly wasn't "friendly" to my Daddy or to me and Kyle. We lost our one true hero and the most important person in our lives. And what's worse, he was killed in a so-called accident. After Daddy died, my life has never been the same.

Over the next several sessions, Ms. Anthony disclosed that her mother, Lorraine, suffered a "nervous breakdown" soon after her husband was killed. Lorraine was hospitalized on a psychiatric unit of the county general hospital for about a week. After Lorraine's return home, she seemingly was either no longer able or not willing to care for her children.

> **Ms. Anita Anthony:** All she did was lie around in bed most of the day or go to church for endless hours. We did everything for ourselves. Kyle and I did all the shopping, made our own meals—and mother's meals—bought our clothes and school supplies. After Daddy died, we essentially raised ourselves.
>
> One day, about 3 months after Daddy died, Mother introduced us to a Mr. Neil Evans, whom she knew from church. The next thing you know he was living with us, and, a few months after that, they told us that they had gotten married. We were shocked and enraged. Neil insisted that we call him "Daddy," but we only called him that to his face. Neil was *not* our Daddy. In fact, he was just the opposite of our *real* Daddy. Neil was a disgusting, stupid boor who sponged off Daddy's military benefits.
>
> Neil said he was a retired policeman who was on some sort of disability. Someone in church told Kyle that Neil had been thrown out of the police force as the result of some scandal. We both believed that. We never found out what Neil did during the day, but he usually wasn't around. He said that he had a job, but Kyle and I didn't believe him. He would usually come home smelling of alcohol and spend the rest of the time watching sports or stupid sitcoms on TV. At night, I rarely saw him without a beer in his hand.
>
> One of Neil's worst traits was that he acted like he knew everything. He had an opinion about everything, and, according to him, he was never wrong. He was the total opposite of our father. I can't tell you how much I hate him.

Blind Spots

To begin to address Ms. Anthony's stony resistance to the process of psychotherapy and self-discovery, I compared the discipline of surgery, to which she was devoted, to psychiatry, which she demeaned and eschewed. In our first meeting, I primarily emphasized that a fundamental similarity is the *what:* each specialty pursues hidden mysteries that can have far-reaching implications for the survival and quality of the lives of its patients.

Although there are many important parallels in the *how*, there is also a key difference between the two specialties. In subsequent sessions, I posited that practitioners of both professions actively wield nearly all of their senses to discover hidden pathology. For example, the sense of sight is critical to both surgery and psychiatry during diagnostic assessment and treatment. Whether a surgeon notes a subtle color change in a section of the small bowel or a psychiatrist perceives a minuscule gaze aversion when a patient is discussing her grandfather, the sense of vision is critical to both specialists. In the former case, the color change could denote compromised vascularization that jeopardizes the viability of the bowel, and in the latter case, the shifting gaze might be associated with the shame surrounding a boundary violation of the patient's grandfather's.

When searching "blind spots" for pathology, there is a fundamental difference between the two professions in the *how:* surgeons rely on touch and psychiatrists depend on hearing to probe where other senses cannot reach. Both senses, of course, send messages to the memory banks and information processing centers of the brain, so *touch* becomes *palpation* and *hearing* becomes *listening*.

Listening

Because it involves a trained, experienced, and disciplined mind, listening is not a casual enterprise. Psychiatrists are supposed to be good listeners. Listening is an active craft that is honed by years of training and clinical experience. We also know that *being listened to* is highly therapeutic for patients. Implicitly, mental health professionals must learn *how* to listen and *what* to listen for. The level of concentration, discipline, and art involved in listening can be compared to the expertise required for a professional golfer to line up and execute a long putt on an undulating, unlevel green.

Ms. Anthony's sentence "I can't tell you how much I hate him" immediately caught my attention for several reasons. As I knew firsthand, Ms. Anthony was quite articulate in expressing negative affects. I asked myself, "Why can't she tell me? Is she hiding something?" As is often the case when patients use this expression or words such as "honestly," "really," "actually," or "to tell the truth," they are concealing painful thoughts and feelings from themselves and their clinicians. I was quite certain that, at that point in her therapy, she sufficiently trusted neither me nor herself to be able to deal with what was hidden. A panoply of hypotheses emerged in my mind, each of which would be discounted or corroborated by information that Ms. Anthony would share with me over future sessions—when she felt ready. I thus chose to wait for additional clues before I probed further.

An experienced surgeon does not "blindly" stick a patient with a needle. That is a form of torture. Rather, the surgeon wields a keen understanding of both anatomy and pathology to guide the needle into the pocket of pus. And the surgeon must also exert patience until such time that an abscess liquefies, or "ripens," so that it might be drained. Thus, a surgeon's informed and disciplined approach engenders relief and healing.

To operate on a knee or to recommend a diet before one knows the nature of the pathology or before a patient is ready to participate in the treatment is to be destined to fail. To do so is to be complicit in pointless acts of torture because neither having surgery nor dieting is very pleasant.

Pride and Poverty

> **Ms. Anita Anthony:** Both Kyle and I lived for school. It took us away from our abysmal home life and gave us a small modicum of pride.
>
> **Dr. Y.:** Pride?
>
> **Ms. Anthony:** I don't think you could ever understand what it's like to have *nothing*. The home that our father had bought us was the smallest one in a mostly white neighborhood. Our house became more and more rundown, while the neighborhood became rebuilt by replacing old homes like ours with much more expensive new ones. Our home stood out like a black eye, so to speak. No one ever took care of our lawn or landscaping. Eventually, it looked like we were living in the local dump. Of course, we were too embarrassed to invite any of our friends to our home.
>
> After Daddy's death, Kyle and I never had any idea of what we lived on. We were the poorest children in our school. Almost all of our African American classmates were actually quite rich. They were the children of doctors, lawyers, and professors, while for all practical purposes, we were orphans. We were ashamed of our clothes, which were never in style and usually falling apart. Kyle and I washed them ourselves. At school, we were on a special breakfast and lunch plan that provided us

most of our food for the day. I was always very hungry in the
mornings but tried not to eat too much. I had too much pride
to show my desperation and shame.

Given how big I am now, Dr. Y., you wouldn't believe how skinny
I was until my freshman year of high school.

Dr. Y.: What changed?

Ms. Anthony: I don't know. I just started to eat a whole lot more
in school. I also got an after-school job at the local library,
which gave me some pocket money to spend on snacks.

Dr. Y.: Where was Kyle at this time?

Ms. Anthony: Kyle went off to college when I began 10th grade.
After he left, I stopped making dinner at home, which I had
done for both of us. I ate out every night and began eating too
much junk food. That's really when and why I started gaining
a ton of weight.

During Ms. Anthony's discussion of her dietary habits and weight
gain, her use of language again caught my focus. First, when patients
use the expression "you wouldn't believe," they are alerting me to not
accept the premises that they are offering. Second, patients' use of
the word "just" is often a smoke screen. In this case, I was cautioned
by Ms. Anthony's language that her explanation of why she began to
gain significant weight during her sophomore year of high school
might be incomplete. When patients use the word "just" in such
phrases as "I just didn't want to go," "I just wanted to have a good
time," "I just didn't understand," or "I just didn't feel happy," they are
asking the psychiatrist to not probe further. They are trying to pre-
clude other possibilities. Under these circumstances, the therapist
must place a mental bookmark on the topic for further exploration
because there are likely critical unconscious conflicts and resistance
associated with the subject. Third, Ms. Anthony's usage of the word
"really" in her explanation as to why she started gaining weight again
signaled the possibility that she might not have been fully disclosive.
Nonetheless, I respected her reluctance and pursued another line of
investigation—while filing the topic away for another time.

Colonel Kyle Anthony

Dr. Y.: You mentioned that school was a source of pride for you.

Ms. Anita Anthony: And for my brother, Kyle. We both excelled
in our studies. I was good in math and the sciences, but he was
superior in every subject. He was also an excellent athlete but

chose to focus on his academic work. He graduated near the top of his class and was probably the best student in the school in math and science. I have always been in awe of Kyle.

Dr. Y.: Awe?

Ms. Anthony: "Awe" is an understatement. I have often thought that while my father was *killed* in action, my mother was *missing* in action. Kyle filled in the void for me after Daddy was gone.

The direction of Kyle's life and his career aspirations were well defined since the death of his father: he strove to be just like him. It was clear from his sister's account that Kyle wanted to achieve, through his own accomplishments, the unfulfilled potential of his father.

Kyle was told by the college counselor in his school that he would be competitive for admission to just about any school in the country. He chose to attend the United States Military Academy at West Point, where he continued to excel academically. Like his father, he was graduated with an engineering degree and with majors in both physics and chemistry. He was granted permission to delay his military commission and assignment for 4 years in order to earn a Ph.D. in chemistry and thereafter was deployed to both Iraq and Afghanistan, where he was engaged in active warfare.

Dr. Y.: Have you stayed in contact with Kyle?

Ms. Anita Anthony: More or less—but much "less" than "more." I missed him terribly after he left for West Point. At first, he would send me letters about once a month, but later, these came much less regularly. He was so busy in college and worked in laboratory jobs during the summers. He rarely came home, especially when he began graduate school and military duty. Although I now e-mail and text him quite a bit, I almost never see him these days.

Kyle married Margaret, the sister of one of his classmates, the year he graduated from college. I attended their wedding in the gorgeous chapel at West Point, but Mother couldn't get it together to come. I now have a niece and nephew, who are just wonderful. They live in a beautiful suburb near West Point. I worry every minute that something will happen to him before he gets back from Afghanistan.

Of Drama and Distrust

For approximately a year, Ms. Anthony saw me twice weekly for psychotherapy. She had returned to work, where she was functioning at her previous high level. Her mood remained stable, and her pain became so minimal that she rarely discussed it. She continued to live alone in her attractive apartment but with a limited social life, primarily involving occasional meetings with friends from work and attending professional meetings. She remained reluctant to discuss any aspects of her sexual feelings and related only that she had dated the occasional "unsuitable" suitor during nursing school.

> **Ms. Anita Anthony:** The reason I came to see you in the first place was for you to put me on a diet. I stepped on the scale this morning, and I weigh the same as I always have. You've been bugging me for over a year about practically everything else, Dr. Y., so how come you never ask me about my weight?
>
> **Dr. Y.:** We don't understand why you gained so much weight in the first place, and without that understanding, your going on a diet would be doomed to failure.
>
> **Ms. Anthony:** I told you I began to gain weight when I started eating a lot of junk food when I was 16. I eat it compulsively. I just can't seem to stop eating the stuff. That's the true and only cause.
>
> **Dr. Y.:** And that's the very mystery to which I was referring in our first meeting 2 years ago. If you know the "true and only cause," why can't you stop eating junk food?
>
> **Ms. Anita Anthony** (*expressing considerable irony and annoyance*): You're the famous doctor; you tell me!
>
> **Dr. Y.:** Let's start with what we know. We know that you began to gain weight when you were about 16. We know that this was a noteworthy time of transition for you: you began a new high school; Kyle left for college; you were left alone at home with your mother and Neil. One thing that we never discussed was whether or not you had reached sexual maturity by that time.
>
> **Ms. Anthony:** Are you asking about if I had reached puberty by age 16?
>
> **Dr. Y.:** OK, let's start with that.
>
> **Ms. Anthony:** I don't get the importance of this. For what it's worth, I do remember that I matured very late. I probably started developing at age 14 or 15. I was over 6 feet tall and thin as a broom handle. I was caught up with basketball at that time and probably looked more like a boy than a girl. It's been such a long time ago, I just don't recall.
>
> **Dr. Y.:** Do you have any photographs that were taken of you around that time?
>
> **Ms. Anthony:** After our father died, nobody took any pictures of Kyle or me. I guess it was too much trouble for our mother.

Dr. Y.: Since you played on your middle school and high school basketball teams, there must be some pictures of you in the yearbooks.

Ms. Anthony: Maybe, but I wouldn't know. We never had the money to buy yearbooks.

Dr. Y.: Would you object if I would try to find some of the yearbooks during the times when you went to middle school and high school? There might be some copies in the school libraries, or I might know someone who went to your school during the times that you were there.

Ms. Anthony: I don't see the big deal about getting pictures of me when I was little. But I don't object.

I distrust "dramatic moments" in psychotherapy. Rather, I believe that the wonderment and dramatic tension of discovery and impending change should suffuse *every* moment of *every* therapeutic session. No different from the art of a professional dance pair, the art of psychotherapy is to establish a trusting, relaxed, and comfortable interplay that, paradoxically, engenders immediate and ongoing tension.

Despite my skepticism regarding dramatic moments in psychotherapy, what happened after I had secured several yearbook pictures of Ms. Anthony during middle school must qualify as such. I began a session by showing Ms. Anthony a picture of her middle school basketball team. Placed in the center of the last of three rows of teammates, she looked like a towering pine tree amidst a patch of shrubs. She also looked much younger than her peers.

For a moment, as she stared at the photograph, she was mute and immobile. Then, like a muffled tremor in a deep ocean floor, she began to tremble. Thereafter, she began to wail and quake volcanically. A component of the drama was that neither she nor I had anticipated this eruption of emotion. Heretofore in her treatment—even in the emergency room after her suicide attempt—her feelings narrowly ranged from absolute composure to targeted irritation, and they always appeared to be firmly under her control. I had never before seen her shed a tear or lose herself in laughter. Ms. Anthony's vivid mental image of her emerging adolescence seemed to have slipped through a fissure in her defenses to set in motion a tsunami of feelings.

Other than handing her a box of tissues, I made no effort to console her. Ms. Anthony made several visible attempts to stop bawling, but wave after wave of emotions continued to crash through. Three times she managed to stop crying for a prolonged period, but, on trying to speak, she would succumb to tears. Finally, she spoke haltingly.

> **Ms. Anita Anthony:** I'm sorry for behaving like an idiot. I have no idea what came over me.
> **Dr. Y.:** Pent-up pressure of something that you have been trying to bury must have burst to the surface.
> **Ms. Anthony:** Jesus have mercy! Here you go again with the damned "surfaces."
> **Dr. Y.:** What *haven't* you been able to talk with me about, Ms. Anthony? I believe you know.

That question precipitated another bout of bawling. I stepped out of my office to ask my administrative assistant to cancel my next appointment. Eventually, Ms. Anthony was able to compose herself sufficiently to speak. Over the next hour she told me that she began to gain weight soon after becoming pregnant at age 16. She and Kyle had grown up sharing the only other bedroom in their small house. Shortly after Kyle departed for college, Neil started sneaking into her room late at night to molest her.

> **Ms. Anita Anthony:** I was young and totally inexperienced, but I knew exactly what he was doing. Neil is huge and very strong. And at nights he was always drunk and scary. Of course, I told my mother what he had done, and of course she didn't believe me. She never did anything to stop him. I don't think that she even tried to.
> I had no idea what to do. I was enormously ashamed and wanted to hide. I thought about calling Kyle, who had just started at West Point, but I knew that he would leave school in a heartbeat and come home to protect me. I was afraid he might kill Neil and ruin his own life. *My* life was already ruined. So I didn't do anything. Just like my moron mother, I didn't do a damn thing. I hate her, and I hate myself.

Ms. Anthony recalled that she was unaware that she was pregnant until about the fifth month following conception. She had thought that she was gaining weight from all the snacks that she had been eating.

> **Ms. Anita Anthony:** The only way I could get through it when Neil was raping me was by making my body go numb. I would lie still while he did his sick and disgusting things to me. But my mind wasn't still. I traveled to the space station that I was

reading about in school. That's where I hid at night in my head. During the days, I stayed away from home and tried never to think about that miserable pervert.

It was Neil who became suspicious that I was pregnant. I guess he figured out that I wasn't having my periods for several months. One Saturday he forced me to go with him to some scummy doctor. He examined me and gave me an abortion on the spot. I barely knew what was going on, but I knew. It was the second worst day of my life. Not only was I a slut, but I had killed a baby. You can't get any lower than that.

Something "snapped" inside me after the abortion. I wouldn't let myself be passive any more. I made up my mind that Neil would have to kill me before I would let him touch me again. When he came back into my room 2 nights later, I went ballistic. I screamed and fought against him like an insane person. Eventually, he stopped trying and left me alone. Once I got accepted to nursing school, I left that stinking dump, and I never came back. My mother still lives there with that pervert, which says it all.

The "Best" Defense...

Over the course of her ensuing treatment with me, Ms. Anthony and I discussed and analyzed the seemingly innumerable implications of what she had revealed. For all practical purposes, Anita had been on her own since Kyle departed for West Point. Although she had originally dreamed of going to Texas A&M as a premedical student, she accepted a generous scholarship to nursing school that supported all of her expenses, including housing and meals during the summers. The most attractive component of this scholarship was that she never again had to be around Neil or her mother. The psychological ramifications of the sexual abuse were even more profound. She became far more assertive and defensive. A tangible manifestation of this transformation was her weight gain.

> **Ms. Anita Anthony:** After being abused by Neil, I became horribly uncomfortable with my body. The boys in high school would stare at me. I believed that they could see right through me and could tell that I am a slut. I felt weak and vulnerable, and I hate that feeling. I felt like I was becoming my mother.

By gaining so much weight in high school, not only did Anita become less attractive to men, which "made me feel more comfortable," but she also felt formidable.

Ms. Anita Anthony: When I graduated from high school, I was over 6 feet tall and weighed 225 pounds. You can bet your boots that nobody was going to mess with me. And, as you know, Dr. Y., I'm not afraid to come on strong. In school and, later, at work, I also had my act together. I don't like being attacked for not doing my job.

Dr. Y.: There is no question that you are an impressive and imposing woman, Ms. Anthony. But your resolution has come at a considerable cost. You now weigh 275 pounds, which is making you physically vulnerable. In addition, both your weight and your aggressive personality push away many people who are not at all threatening to you.

Defenses are unconscious, only partially successful means to deal with conflicts. Two life experiences were key to Ms. Anthony's defensive structure. First, the sudden, shocking loss of her father and Kyle's leaving home left her terrified of further "abandonment" by loved ones and the associated vulnerabilities of painful feelings and loss of protection. Avoidance of intimacy by keeping people at a safe distance through her weight and aggressive manner "protected" her from the pain of future emotional loss and interpersonal exploitation. For Ms. Anthony (and probably everybody else), this protection from human connection comes at a high cost. We cannot escape being social animals. Ms. Anthony kept people at safe distances, but she was famished for closeness and connection. Hence the conflict: the fear and the wish. Second, her sexual violation by Neil was painfully confusing to her at the time of her emerging sexuality. She associated sexual feelings and behaviors with aggression, humiliation, and even infanticide. Responding with avoidance, she kept friends and suitors alike at bay with her weight and assertive personality and by numbing her feelings.

The bottom line: How could Ms. Anthony lose weight without resolving her conflicts involving abandonment, intimacy, and sexuality? The answer is that she could not. The solution was to work through these conflicts in psychotherapy.

Although a full explication of Ms. Anthony's psychotherapy is beyond the focus and scope of this book, a critical component of her treatment was to help her understand and reverse her confused and confusing feelings of responsibility for the death of her father and unborn baby and for the sexual violation by her stepfather. By blaming herself for these tragedies, Ms. Anthony gained magical control over future devastating events but at an enormous cost: guilt, anxiety, and avoidance of intimacy and sexual expression. Additionally, her misguided rage was internalized, which led to feelings of depression and self-loathing. She punished herself by both abusing and not caring for her body. How could she lose weight if she hated herself and her body that she felt was dirty and dangerous? The answer is that she could not. Ms. Anthony had to relearn how to love and care for herself.

The Case of Ms. Anita Anthony: D2 (Decision) Component

Ms. Anthony initially met with me for the expressed purpose of losing weight and approval for surgical treatment of obesity-related disabilities. Through psychotherapy, she gained an understanding of the role of her life experience and psychological reactions to this experience in her becoming obese. Ms. Anthony had gained clarity about how she had internalized her rage as well as the magical thinking associated with her self-punishing and avoidant behaviors. Just as important, she began to feel lonely and increasingly desired both psychological and sexual intimacy. She no longer felt protected by being obese; rather, it became a barrier to attracting suitors—in addition to engendering a myriad of associated health problems. In addition, there were biological factors related to her long-term dietary choices and habits. Among these biological factors was that she had become dependent on snack foods, fast foods, and processed foods that are high in fat, sugar, and salt. At the time she began her psychotherapy with me, Ms. Anthony weighed 275 pounds and was 6 feet 1 inch tall.

We both agreed that the time had finally arrived for us to consider a diet, which would mean her arriving at a *decision* (D2 component) and mustering and maintaining the *discipline* (D3 component) to lose weight and sustain weight loss on a long-term basis. These aspects of her care will be presented in Chapter 6, "Stuck in My Body, Part II (Decide and Discipline)."

References

American Psychiatric Association: Diagnostic and Statistical Manual of Mental Disorders, 5th Edition. Washington, DC, American Psychiatric Association, 2013

Ogden CL, Carroll MD, Kit BK, et al: Prevalence of obesity in the United States, 2009–2010 (NCH Data Brief No 82). Hyattsville, MD, National Center for Health Statistics, 2012. Available at: http://www.cdc.gov/nchs/data/databriefs/db82.pdf. Accessed February 1, 2014.

Roger VL, Go AS, Lloyd-Jones DM, et al: Executive summary: heart disease and stroke statistics—2012 update: a report from the American Heart Association. Circulation 125:188–197, 2012

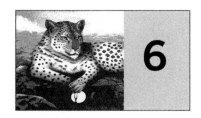

Stuck in My Body, Part II (Decide and Discipline): The Case of Ms. Anita Anthony

The Fatal Pauses 3-D Diet

With the sweat of your brow you will eat bread
Until you return to the ground;
For out of it you were taken
—*Genesis 3:19*

Don't dig your own grave with your knife and fork
—*After an old English proverb*

Did we devolve to need suspenders?
—*Stuart C. Yudofsky, "Pauses"*

"It's a war, and I always lose."

"It seems to me that you are treating one neurosis with another one."

Warning: Do not skip ahead to the rules of the 3-D Diet. Do not skip ahead to the sample meals of the 3-D Diet. Failure to savor and ingest the entire chapter slowly, thoughtfully, and completely places you at great risk of experiencing yet another "failed diet." It could turn out to be worth your effort this time.

Overview

People like Ms. Anita Anthony (presented in Chapter 5, "Stuck in My Body, Part I (Discover)") who are significantly overweight or obese are stuck in a state of *protracted pause*. Therefore, all of the principles and practices of *Fatal Pauses* that have been presented thus far in this book must be harnessed to help people who can benefit from dieting and sustained weight loss.

The Fatal Pauses 3-D Diet has three fundamental, interacting, and indelible components: *Discover, Decide, Discipline*. The D1 and D2 components of the 3-D Diet comprise the process of arriving at and then making the decision to lose weight. The D1 component is an approach and process to *discover* the conflicts and causes that underlie the disordered eating patterns. After you discover and understand why you have gained so much weight in the first place, you are finally in a position to *decide* (D2 component) whether you wish to choose to continue in your patterns of behavior that led to overeating and obesity or do the necessary work to change. What conventionally would be regarded as the diet component, D3, is, more comprehensively, the *discipline* that is required for you to establish and sustain the Fatal Pauses 3-D Diet, which is a highly informed and disciplined approach to calorie restriction, exercise, and a measured lifestyle.

The Case of Ms. Anita Anthony: D1 (Discover) Component

The D1 *(Discover)* component of the Fatal Pauses Method of Getting Unstuck has been presented in explicit detail in Chapter 4, "Stuck in My Job," and a case example of how this component can be applied to a person who is obese or overweight is portrayed in the case of Ms. Anita Anthony in Chapter 5.

The Case of Ms. Anita Anthony: D2 (Decide) Component

"Wanting" to Lose Weight Versus "Deciding" to Lose Weight

Why Do Most Diets Fail Most of the Time?

People embarking on a new diet will commonly say such things as "I know I am too fat, and I just hate the way I look." "I have tried to lose weight dozens of times since I was a teenager, but I never stick with the diet." "I think about not eating fattening foods all of the time—to the point of driving myself crazy. But I always give in to temptation; I just have no self-control." Clearly, the countless people who endure their lives as described above are enormously frustrated as they are stuck in pause.

An oft-repeated and published statistic is that 95% of diets fail. However, there are little hard data to confirm that statistic, which most likely derives from an article published more than 50 years ago by Dr. Albert Stunkard and Dr. Mavis McLaren-Hume. Reporting on a study of 100 patients treated for obesity at New York Hospital in the 1950s, they concluded the following: "Most obese persons will not stay in treatment, most will not lose weight, and of those who do lose weight, most will regain it" (Stunkard and McLaren-Hume 1959, p. 84). Although the success and failure rates of most diets are largely unknown and there are multiple factors—including criteria for subject selection and long-term follow-up care that would doubtlessly influence these outcome statistics—most experienced physicians today would agree with Stunkard and McLaren-Hume's disheartening conclusion.

I believe that it is not the diets per se that fail; rather, it is the dieters who ultimately fail to adhere to all current approaches to dieting. There are many reasons that this is the case. First and foremost, most people who initiate diets have not *truly* decided that they want to lose weight. They certainly *want* to lose weight, but they have not *decided* to lose weight. There is a huge difference between wanting something and making up your mind that you will attain it.

What Do Successful People Advise?

Lots of people want lots of things that they will never achieve: from being successful actors or athletes to writing a novel to losing weight. Few people succeed at any of these wishes, all of which require unremitting effort over time. They rarely understand or follow the advice that they receive from those who are successful:

> You really have to want it badly in order to do what it takes to be successful. Otherwise it won't happen.

There are three revealing elements in this concise advice about the fundamentals of success:

1. Accomplished individuals do not begin their advice by emphasizing the importance of such features as *creative genius, God-given talents,* or *physical gifts,* which may or may not pertain downstream.
2. What successful people do say is, "You have to make up your mind (i.e., *decide*) what you *really* want and then *do* everything it takes to get what you say you want." Please note the two parts of this component of the advice of the successful: *first decide, then do,* which parallel the last two vital components of the 3-D Diet.
3. The grammar of this succinct advice from successful people is also instructive. The first sentence is in the active voice—you must *decide,* and then you must *do.* The second sentence, "Otherwise, it won't happen," is in the passive voice, which warns against the true source of most failure: believing that some*thing*—such as a diet—or some*one*—such as an important advisor, coach, or "connection"— can be responsible for your getting what you say you want. *You* must decide and then *you* must do, and neither aspect is at all easy.

Clearing the Field to Build a Decision

What does it take to decide to do something that you believe that you want to do? To answer that question, let's review several of the fundamental elements in the case of Ms. Anita Anthony in light of the points summarized in Table 6–1. This review should help demonstrate what is required to remove the barriers to successful decision making. Please do not be put off by my directness (the fourth D).

TABLE 6–1. Why have I failed to get unstuck despite trying so hard?

Confusion: I am not clear or precise about *where* I am stuck

Ignorance: I do not understand *why* and *how* I became stuck

Superficiality: I have not discovered, gained insight about, or addressed my *underlying conflicts* that keep me stuck

Indecision: I have not *decided* that I want to get unstuck

Disorientation: I do not have a clear *direction* or *pathway* to get unstuck

---

Ms. Anthony's Confusion About Where She Was Stuck

Prior to her psychodynamically oriented psychotherapy, Ms. Anthony believed that her primary problems were that she ate too much of the wrong foods and that she possessed insufficient self-control. She was half right, but she also had several other related problems of which she was unaware. She was an angry person who kept most people at a distance. Consequently, she had few, if any, close relationships and spent most of her off-work time by herself in her apartment. She acknowledged being "a little bit lonely on occasions," and she had no sexual involvements: "I'm just not interested in sex. It's never been my thing." It was in her apartment, particularly at nights and on weekends, where she binged on salty snacks, candies and other sweets, pastries, hamburgers, fried chicken, milk shakes, French fries, etc. If, somehow, she were to manage to lose weight by sheer discipline alone, it would be unlikely that her problems with anger, loneliness, and repressed sexual drives would also be addressed or alleviated. Thus, she was confused about the fundamental source of her problems—it was not overeating per se; it was feelings and relationships.

Ms. Anthony's Ignorance About Why and How She Became Stuck

Ms. Anthony alleged that she could not lose weight because "I lack the necessary willpower to stick to a diet." Although she had "failed" in all of her many previous attempts to lose weight, her lack of willpower was more a *result* of her problem than a *cause or explanation* of the problem. Ms. Anthony's self-blame was an important clue for solving the mystery of why she could not lose weight even though she "knew" "my weight is killing me." After several months of psychotherapy it became clear to me that her self-blame constituted "neurotic" punishment for the unconscious sources of her obesity, and that clue led to her finally disclosing that she had been sexually abused by her stepfather. Prior to being abused, she had not exhibited problems with overeating or being overweight.

Ms. Anthony's Superficiality in Not Having Discovered, Gained Insight About, or Addressed Her Underlying Conflicts That Keep Her Stuck

Before she could commit to losing weight, it was necessary for Ms. Anthony to gain insight about and come to terms with her unconscious conflicts regarding her weight and the feelings associated with the sexual abuse that she had endured. As indicated by her angry, distancing behaviors toward me in our first meeting, her resistance to gaining insight into these unconscious conflicts was daunting. Unconsciously, she associated her enormous size with power and safety, and it also deterred the unsettling and confusing sexual attention that she had experienced at school and in the workplace. Psychoanalysts might also interpret that her aggressive feelings and her genital and appetite drives were displaced or redirected to "neurotic" oral fixations that included overeating and abusive language. At one point in her treatment, Ms. Anthony acknowledged, "Filling up with food probably helped to fill the void left after my father was killed and my brother went off to West Point."

Ms. Anthony's Indecision About Doing What It Takes to Get Unstuck

By its very nature, being stuck in a fatal pause requires inordinate efforts to reverse. A fundamental thesis of medicine and, therefore, of this book is that *diagnosis comes before treatment*. If a person does not understand how and why he or she has become stuck in the first place and does not understand and address the underlying conflicts that keep him or her stuck, it is highly unlikely that he or she will be able to muster the motivation or the discipline required to deal with the *symptoms* of being stuck. In the case of Ms. Anthony, obesity was a symptom of her problems, not her problem. Even if it were possible to make some progress in treating the symptoms of being stuck, sustaining symptomatic relief—i.e., staying on her diet over a protracted timeframe—would be even more unlikely without addressing the underlying conflicts. These principles could never be clearer than when applied to people who, like Ms. Anthony, are dangerously and painfully overweight or obese but whose diets ultimately fail.

Ms. Anthony's Disorientation in Discovering a Clear Direction or Pathway to Getting Unstuck

I had originally considered naming this diet *The Discovery Diet* by virtue of the central role of *discovering* the conflicts and other psychological influences that underlie the person's eating disorder in order that he or she will be able to *decide* to commit to a diet and mount and maintain the *disciplined* efforts required for sustained weight loss. Ultimately, however, I concluded that discovery, decision, and discipline are interrelated and are equally important for a person to lose weight and sustain the weight loss. After Ms. Anthony discovered that she craved companionship and intimacy, she could go about deciding what she wanted more: (what she mistakenly thought was) good food or good health.

Overcoming the Barriers Blocking Ms. Anthony's Decision to Lose Weight

Declaring a Truce in the War With Herself

The following discussion took place about a year after Ms. Anthony had begun psychotherapy:

> **Ms. Anita Anthony** (*ironically*): I think that I get it now, Dr. Y. My eating problems have to do with everything *except* what I put in my mouth. I still haven't lost a single pound since I have been in treatment with you. Am I finally ready to start on a diet, or should we wait until I die of a heart attack?
>
> **Dr. Y.:** What did you learn from your many previous attempts to diet?
>
> **Ms. Anthony:** The longest I stayed on a diet was for 2 months. I get the hungriest at nights and on weekends, when I usually do most of my eating. At those times, I fight with myself almost every moment not to give in to all the foods that I love. I never lose much weight, because eventually I always give up. I hate myself even more at these times because of my obvious lack of

willpower and self-control. My mother is such a weak person,
and I can't stand myself when I show weakness of any sort.

Dr. Y.: You describe your dieting as if you were at war with yourself.

Ms. Anthony: It *is* a war, and I always lose.

Exercising the Power of No

Ms. Anthony qualifies as a person who is stuck in pause, so she can
apply all of the principles of becoming unstuck that have been reviewed thus far in this book. Because D2 of the 3-D Diet involves
choosing *not* to do something Ms. Anthony likes to do, the five key
principles involved in exercising the Power of No to get unstuck (see
Table 3–6, p. 43) bear reviewing in light of her case.

Let's review these principles as they apply to Ms. Anthony.

1. You must *stop* something that you like in order to *gain* something
   that you like more.
2. You are saying "Yes!" to something that you fundamentally want
   by saying "No!" to something that you want less.

Ms. Anthony said repeatedly, "I really love food" (especially fried
foods and desserts). No surprise; most people do. In preparing her
to move forward to the severe restrictions of the *discipline* component of the 3-D Diet, I emphasized how her love of highly caloric
food seemed to "outweigh" the great danger to her health brought
about by her obesity. My responsibility was to help Ms. Anthony
raise her consciousness about the consequences of her dietary decisions without the "noise" and opacities brought about by her unconscious conflicts and other maladaptive psychological influences.
What this psychojargon boiled down to was my helping to make her
aware of the direct pathway from her current eating practices to her
physical ills and social frustrations. At length, Ms. Anthony realized
that she wanted to have a healthy, attractive body *more* than she
wanted the copious amounts of highly caloric foods that she had
consumed on a regular basis since high school. Because this approach places the emphasis on what she *wants more*, internal power
struggles resulting from so-called self-deprivation are reduced.

3. A *none or all* binary choice is required to achieve success. Moderation does not work in this case.

Similar to (but not entirely the same as) the *zero-tolerance approach* of specialized programs that treat people for alcohol and other substance use disorders, the 3-D Diet requires a *none or all* binary choice. However, this choice does not refer to food per se because one cannot stay alive without food. Rather, it refers to adhering strictly to the 3-D Diet. I emphasized to Ms. Anthony how she must exert the extraordinary discipline to stay on the diet *all* of the time, or she would certainly fail to lose weight. Only when Ms. Anthony was absolutely clear that she *wanted* to lose weight and maintain a healthful diet and lifestyle more than she wanted junk food could she *decide* to undertake and sustain the rigorous *discipline* required by the 3-D Diet. If staying trim were easy, the United States would not be faced with the current and worsening epidemic of obesity in children, adolescents, and adults. The 3-D Diet is everything but easy.

4. The Power of Go is *always* required to achieve the Power of No.

"Just saying no" to eating unhealthful, highly caloric foods would not be sufficient for Ms. Anthony to lose weight and sustain weight loss. To adhere to the 3-D Diet, she would have to change many critical aspects of her life, none of which would be easy and all of which would require the Power of Go. Primary among these changes would be for her to *actualize in her personal life the insights that she had gained in psychotherapy.* Important examples would include seizing the initiative to interact more frequently and closely with her brother and his immediate family, going out on a regular basis with her friends, making every effort to meet new people, being open to intimacy, and resisting being so interpersonally aggressive and confrontational. Additionally, she would have to rearrange and reorder her life so that she could exercise regularly and vigorously. The 3-D Diet is everything but easy.

5. A reprioritization of your time and restructuring of your schedule are usually required to become unstuck.

Since she completed nursing school, Ms. Anthony's daily schedule was quite rigid. On work days, she would arrive at the hospital at 5:00 A.M. for her shift that began at 6:00 A.M. and usually would not leave the hospital until 7:00 P.M., even though her duty hours were over at 3:00 P.M. Her self-loathing and deep-seated insecurities led her to work far longer than was expected or required. Of course, she simultaneously was furious for "being exploited and unappreciated." Her anger and sense of martyrdom fueled her feelings of deprivation, which, in turn, led her to feel "entitled" to treat herself to the foods she said she enjoyed. I ask my readers to recall that in my initial meeting with Ms. Anthony, she expressed her belief, shared by so many others, that all that transpires in psychiatry is "complaining and blaming others." When she transformed her *insights* from psychotherapy into such discrete *actions* as informing her nurse supervisor that she would no longer work additional hours without compensation, she no longer believed that myth about our field.

Ms. Anthony also had to make major changes to the types of food she ate and add exercise to her routine. Previously, on the way back to her apartment she would go to fast food outlets or to a supermarket where she would load up on foods to devour at home, alone in her apartment. Her pattern on weekends or days off was to spend most of her time alone in her apartment, punctuated only by trips to stores to purchase food and household items. Additionally, as with most people who *decide* to undertake the 3-D Diet, Ms. Anthony had to make extensive lifestyle changes that permitted *daily* vigorous, structured exercising for the first time since high school. The 3-D Diet is everything but easy.

Ms. Anthony's Central Conflicts

As has been presented in Chapter 5, many biological and psychodynamic factors were involved in Ms. Anthony's obesity. Ms. Anthony's protracted state of being stuck in pause was primarily a result of the central, unresolved conflict of her desire for intimacy and, concurrently, her fear of abandonment, an approach-avoidance conflict. Secondarily, she had become biologically dependent on foods with high caloric and salt content, which, as in the case of Dr. Holbrook's nicotine addiction (Chapter 3, "The Fatal Pauses 3-D Method of Getting Unstuck Through the Power of No and the Power of Go"), is an approach-approach conflict: the desire to eat foods high in fat, sugar, and salt while also wanting to be healthy and attractive to gain intimacy.

Key Features of Ms. Anita Anthony's Being Stuck in Pause

1. *How Ms. Anthony was stuck:* She was morbidly obese
2. *Goals for change:* Lose 115 pounds (from 275 pounds to 160 pounds)
3. *Central, unresolved conflicts:* Primary conflict (approach-avoidance): intimacy versus abandonment; secondary conflict (approach-approach): wants foods high in fat, sugar, and salt versus wants to be healthy and attractive
4. *Hallmarks of Ms. Anthony's being stuck:* Irritability, anger, depression, demoralization, isolation, self-deprecation, self-destructiveness, obesity, poor health
5. *Binary problem/solution:* Unhealthful diet and lifestyle/the 3-D Diet
6. *Critical decision points:* Adhere strictly to 3-D Diet (including daily exercise)
7. *Corollary factors required to achieve resolution:* Continued psychotherapy to learn how to express, emotionally and behaviorally, love for herself, how to care for her body, and how to develop openness to intimacy
8. *Resolution:* Continue to engage in psychotherapy; adhere strictly to the 3-D Diet; engage in a regular, vigorous exercise program

D3 (Discipline) Component (or, Know Thy Foe: An Evolutionary Perspective of What a Dieter Is "Up Against")

Sixty-Five Million Years Ago

The alarmingly high prevalence of American children and adults (approximately one-third of each population) being either significantly overweight or obese and the dire health-related consequences (from stroke and heart attack to breast and prostate cancer to Alzheimer's disease and depression) were summarized in Chapter 5. Over the entirety of the 65 million years of primate evolution, food and dietary patterns have driven the evolution of our bodies and digestive systems. For the vast, vast majority of this time, a great expenditure of energy was required to secure foodstuff from highly limited and seasonal nutritional sources. In temperate climates, primates would rely on natural cycles of fruits and seeds as well as the very few staples—such as nutritious roots—that were present throughout the year. Animal protein—insects, reptiles, fish, and the occasional mammals—was secured opportunistically and comprised a much smaller proportion of their diets. In arctic climates, animal protein from fish and sea mammals comprised the principal food sources. As in temperate zones, seasonal cycles of animals and the environment—such as salmon runs, whale migrations, and ice flows—dictated the availabilities of the respective food sources in arctic zones.

Table 6–2 summarizes food-related realities of our ancient ancestors prior to the discovery of cooking. These factors prominently influenced the evolutionary development of our digestive systems and our biologically based eating patterns.

TABLE 6–2. Food-related realities of ancient humans

Food *sources* and *quantities* were restricted to regional availability and seasonal cycles

Food *variety* was limited by and restricted to regional availability and seasonal cycles

Food *preparation* did not involve cooking

Food *stability* and *portability* were limited by the unavailability of preservatives and by competition with predators and rivals

Significant expenditures of effort and energy were required to secure, transport, and defend food sources

---

Because our bodies and digestive systems developed and evolved under these environmental circumstances—which are quite different from our current conditions—each of these factors must be considered in designing a dietary approach that will be safe, healthful, and effective in our present, postindustrial revolution circumstances and realities.

Two Hundred Fifty Thousand Years Ago to Today

Two monumental changes have occurred that have impacted radically the relationships among food, society, and our bodies. The first change, *cooking foodstuff*, was discovered by humans approximately

250,000 years ago—which comprises a mere instant in 65 million years of primate evolution. Cooking had far-reaching effects for both individuals and society. Cooking enabled the addition of such vegetables as grains, potatoes, and beans to our diets, and this permitted the greatly enhanced concentration of calories as well as improved preservation, transportation, and storage of provisions.

The accelerated growth of larger social systems eventually led to the second grand change: the *industrialization of food production, preparation, preservation, and distribution.* A by-product of this change was the rapid growth of large cities and nation-states, which is still occurring at an ever-accelerating rate. These massive social and industrial changes spurred a revolution in the variety, quantities, and availability of food over the past several hundred years, far too brief of a time period to have had even minimal, if any, positive influences on our somatic evolution. As a consequence, our evolutionarily derived biological appetitive drives and food-related behaviors remain constant in a world that is changing rapidly and is vastly different from the ancient environmental determinants of our bodies and bodily functions. One among many examples of the dietary implications of these recent changes is sugar.

Sugar is a generic term for sweet-tasting carbohydrates that are derived or *refined* from plant sources. Because sugars are present in minute quantities in plants, industrialized farming and processing that has occurred only over the past 300 years has been required to concentrate the sugars for commercial use. Sucrose is a disaccharide and comprises the primary type of granulated sugar that we use to sweeten food at our table or in our own personal cooking. The first major source of sucrose is sugarcane, which is a type of grass that is now grown on huge plantations throughout the world. The disaccharides in the stems of sugarcane are concentrated and crystallized through crushing the stems and boiling and distilling liquid residue into the form we purchase in grocery stores and sprinkle into our coffee and tea. The second major source of sucrose is from sugar beets, which is a root crop.

Monosaccharides are also a source of other forms of sugar that include glucose, fructose, and galactose. Many plant-based carbohydrates that we consume, especially potatoes, are converted into glucose by our bodies to be circulated as energy sources for our cells. Fructose is found in fruits, as well as in honey and in the stems and roots of some plants. Importantly, fructose can also be processed from grains—especially corn—to yield a highly concentrated syrup that is widely used to sweeten commercially prepared foods of all varieties.

Let us now look at the implications of each of the food-related realities in Table 6–2 in the contexts of overeating and the key elements of the 3-D Diet.

Food Sources and Quantities Were Restricted by Regional Availability and Seasonal Cycles

Evolutionary Influence

Because our appetitive drives evolved in eras of limited availability of foods, for most of our history it was adaptive for humans to consume everything physically possible that was currently available as rapidly as we could. For example, when the fruit on a particular species of tree ripened in season or when a large animal was killed, we would gorge until we could not hold any more. Of course, ancient humans would do their best, without methods of food preservation and processing, to hide and protect food from predators and from rivals within and outside their tribal systems. Fat stores would build up in their bodies during seasons or times of plenty in order to sustain them during the many times food would not be available. Episodic and prolonged periods of hunger and famine were a historical reality of the human condition.

Current Reality

Today, food is available in abundance nearly everywhere and at all times, whether in our homes, with jammed refrigerators and bulging pantries; en route to and from work or school with giant supermarkets, 24-hour "quickie marts," curbside vendors on sidewalks, or fast food outlets lining streets, highways, train stations, and airports; at work or school, with coffee and pastry shops, cafeterias, and vending machines dispensing candy, salty snacks, and sugar-sweetened soft drinks; at movie theaters, concerts, and sports events with snack bars and vendors selling ice cream, sodas, fast food, and alcoholic beverages; or even in the public areas of our museums and hospitals. And, as if this were not sufficient, we can use our cell phones to have nearly every type of food delivered to our homes, offices, and college dormitories and classrooms at any time.

Because we have evolved to be opportunistic eaters and because food is now available nearly everywhere, many of us eat relentlessly during most of our waking hours. Additionally, our hunter-gatherer instincts are channeled to shopping in food stores, choosing great restaurants, or calling for takeout. Most of us also believe that being hungry is an "unnatural state" that must be "cured" immediately by eating foods.

Disciplined response of the Fatal Pauses 3-D Diet: Predetermine times, places, and quantities of foods and beverages.

Food Variety Was Limited by and Restricted to Regional Availability and Seasonal Cycles

Evolutionary Influence

Before the advent of cooking and industrialized agriculture, the *variety* of food sources of our ancient ancestors was perennially limited by seasons and regions—but often the *quantity* was unlimited for brief periods of plenty. For example, the breeding runs of bountiful, egg-swollen salmon into the shallow freshwater streams of what is now known as northwestern Canada and Alaska provided an abundance of fresh protein for the ancient native hunter-gatherers of that region—far beyond any individual's capacity to ingest over the limited period of plenty. Without cooking, the intake and digestion of large quantities of animal protein was not possible. Similarly, the seasonal ripening of certain fruits in the tropics and more temperate zones could result in the same time-limited abundance. Complex biological functions evolved in humans to adapt to these cycles, such that intense hunger in the presence of food was, of necessity, limited in times of exceptional and singular availability of a particular food. Even gorging grizzly bears that are building up fat stores for winter hibernation become sated and take long breaks from devouring bonanzas of easy prey fish during the annual salmon runs.

Current Reality

Today, nearly every type of food is available in any quantity at any time of the year. For example, most people in New England and

Alaska can purchase fresh strawberries, watermelons, grapes, and pineapples, as well as fresh beef, chicken, fish, and pork, in the middle of the winter in nearly every supermarket. Processed foods of seemingly infinite varieties can also be accessed in abundance almost anywhere and at any time. Depending on the choices and decisions that individuals make, the nearly total availability of nearly infinite varieties of foods can be either helpful or harmful to one's weight or health. And the choices that far too many people make are fatal.

Today in America, most people lose interest in a particular food after eating it in what should be sufficient quantities to sustain normative weight and health. However, they override their disinterest, stimulating their dulled appetites by choosing foods from nearly infinite, omnipresent varieties.

Disciplined response of the Fatal Pauses 3-D Diet: Limit most foods to fresh and locally grown or regionally available varieties.

Food Preparation Did Not Involve Cooking

Evolutionary Influence

As has been reviewed previously, mankind's discovery of cooking about 65,000 years ago had several far-reaching ramifications. First, cooking increased the *varieties* and *quantities* of plants that people could safely ingest and digest. Primary among these vegetable sources were seeds, including grains (rice, corn, wheat, rye), and beans, as well roots and stems, including potatoes, sugar cane, and beets. Second, cooking exponentially increases the concentration of calories of plant-based food. Third, cooking makes animal protein far more digestible in much larger quantities while rendering food from plant and animal sources more savory and appealing to us. Fourth, cooking accelerated the development of progressively larger social systems that included farming and ranching that, in turn, gave rise to complex civilizations that developed industrialized agriculture and food processing and distribution. The net result was that these cooking-related "advances" vastly superseded the pace of our evolutionary somatic adaptations to these changes.

Current Reality

Imagine it is a crisp October Saturday morning and you are strolling on a commercial street in your town, going on an errand for your spouse at a large supermarket near your home or window-shopping at an upscale mall near your place of work. You have recently eaten breakfast, so you are not hungry. Now imagine that you walk by a bakery (or the bakery section of the supermarket) from which is wafting the fragrance of freshly baked breads, bagels, and pastries. You find yourself enticed to enter the bakery "just to have a look at what they have." You are tempted further by the almost irresistible sight of mounds of bagels of different compositions and flavors; of orderly trays of pastries adorned with glistening icings and sugared fruit preserves; and by a wide assortment of croissants, baguettes, muffins, scones, and the like. Fresh from the oven, a steaming batch of blueberry bagels is arranged under your nose in the glass case into which you are peering. You just can't resist purchasing a half-dozen of the bagels for your family to eat at breakfast the next morning. You also buy a container of freshly ground peanut butter "to go with" the bagels. En route home, the soft warmth of the bagels seeps through the paper bag to seduce you further, and by the time you arrive back at your home, you have eaten three of the bagels and half a cup of peanut butter.

Cooking was involved in nearly every aspect of this culinary seduction—from roasting the peanuts to baking the grains to boiling the fruits and fats that form the breads, cakes, butters, icings, and jams. Other than raiding a bee hive, there would be no way that our ancient ancestors could encounter this concentration and quantity of sugars and carbohydrates that were rendered immediately ingestible and digestible by cooking. Animal products, including dairy products, are rendered safer from harmful microorganisms by cooking, as well. And today, at nearly our every waking hour, we can hardly escape such culinary encounters.

Disciplined response of the Fatal Pauses 3-D Diet: Limit cooked grains and other plant-based carbohydrates.

Food Stability and Portability Were Limited by the Rapid Deterioration of Fresh Foods and by Competition With Predators and Rivals

Evolutionary Influence

As has been discussed, for most of mankind's 65 million–year history, plant- and animal-derived fresh foods that were collected, captured, or killed by our ancient ancestors had to be eaten immediately. Otherwise, the food would rapidly spoil, be stolen by human rivals, or be hijacked by countless other animal species ranging from maggots to carnivorous mammals. The plant-based foods were often fresh fruits that were highly perishable, as were the animal-based sources such as fish, small and large mammals, and dairy products.

Current Reality

As reviewed, the relatively recent advent of cooking enlarged our food sources to include grains, beans, potatoes, and other plant and animal products. Not only could their calorie values be concentrated by cooking, but in raw form, they could be stored safely for much longer periods of time. Recall from the Old Testament that Joseph predicted from the Egyptian pharaoh's dream that 7 years of famine would follow 7 years of plenty. Following the advice of Joseph, during the plentiful years the Egyptians stored grain in giant warehouses. This supply could be allocated judiciously over the 7 years of scarcity, although one cannot imagine fruits or animal products being stored safely over this long time period. Finally, by removing harmful microorganisms, cooking processes such as pasteurization enabled grain-based products such as beer and animal products such as milk and certain cheeses to remain safe and unspoiled for far longer periods of time.

Today, industrialized agriculture produces grains, beans, potatoes, sugarcane, and other sources of carbohydrates and sugars in vast quantities. Industries process these plant products into edible goods of nearly infinite variety, which then can be distributed nearly anywhere on the globe. Similarly, untold species and numbers of animals are raised on farms, ranches, ponds, and oceans or harvested in enormous abundance from our oceans, lakes, and streams. Preserving animal products with salts or refrigeration or by cooking processes such as pasteurization can maintain their digestible proteins for protracted periods of time, which enables their distribution—in fresh, frozen, or preserved forms—throughout the globe.

The benefits of food stability and portability resulting from cooking and industrial processing are offset by many serious liabilities, several of which most deserve our focus. First, as discussed, the increasing varieties, quantities, and appeal of and access to food combined with the augmented concentration of calories leads most individuals to consume too much food and thereby intake far more calories than we require for our daily physical activities. We preserve these calories in fat stores, which endanger our health.

Second, preserving foods with salt and industrial processing results in our ingesting too much salt and in the removal of many of the healthful elements of food. Industrialized mining as well as salt water evaporation technologies have made salt—once among the world's rarest and most highly sought-after commodities (the Latin word for *salt* is the etymological root of the English word *salary*)—inexpensively available in abundance to nearly every human being on our planet. As a consequence, modern man and woman's dietary intake of salt has soared, which has led to many human illnesses, the most prominent and dangerous among which are hypertension and related cardiovascular conditions, including stroke.

Third, heat-based processing of certain animal products, including dairy products, has resulted in our intake of far too much animal fat. This has resulted in a virtual epidemic of cardiovascular illnesses among men and women that include ischemic heart disease, hypertension, and stroke. Because animal fats are highly caloric, our currently unbridled ingestion of animal fat is also a primary source of obesity.

Fourth, our industrialized processing of sugar—particularly from sugarcane, sugar beets, and corn—has resulted in our deriving a disproportionate amount of our daily caloric consumption from sugar. The average American ingests nearly 160 pounds of *added* sugar per year, which works out to approximately 450 calories per day (Casey 2007). People who are overweight or obese often consume multiples of this amount. *Added* sugars mean that these processed sources in our diets are in addition to the sugars from fresh fruits and other natural sources.

Fifth, there are a myriad of dire consequences to our health from our overconsumption of sugars. Processed sugars consist of *empty calories*, which means that the energy content lacks the vital nutrients of fresh foods that include fiber, amino acids, vitamins, minerals, and the antioxidants that help resist inflammatory-based conditions including arthritis, certain types of cancer, and Alzheimer's disease. Additionally, too much refined sugar leads to insulin resistance, which is associated with type 2 diabetes, as well as impairing brain-based feedback mechanisms that control our hunger.

Disciplined response of the Fatal Pauses 3-D Diet: Limit the intake of processed sugars, animal fats, and salt.

Significant Expenditures of Effort and Energy Were Required to Secure, Transport, and Defend Food Sources

Evolutionary Influence

For most of humankind's evolutionary history, enormous physical effort and energy were expended in killing and gathering our food and, once acquired, in transporting that food and defending it and ourselves from mammalian and reptilian predators as well as human rivals. Hunger was an almost everyday reality of our ancient ancestors, and periodic starvation was commonplace. As reviewed in Chapter 2, "Getting Stuck," we were constantly in states of fight and flight, kill or be killed, eat or be eaten. Our periods of repose were rare and dangerous. The net result was that for almost the entirety of our evolutionary history, our bodies were in regular, intense states of physical activity; our daily expenditure of calories was enormous; and our daily intake of calories was minuscule, particularly as compared with today's average American.

Current Reality

Unlike Disney's Seven Dwarfs, most Americans do not march eagerly to and whistle while we work. Rather, we sit, fret, and eat while we work. We also sit, fret, and eat while we travel to and from work in crowded buses and subways, through rage-evoking traffic jams, and in congested airports and in stuffed and stifling airplanes. Additionally, we sit, eat, and often fret in our spare time, while we play, and while we watch other people play. Parked in chairs, we hunch and munch over computers most of our days and nights as we work and play on those captivating machines or while we spend untold hours each day watching TV or, on increasingly rarer occasions, while we read. Tragically, the identical scenario applies to a vast proportion of our young children and adolescents.

Disciplined response of the Fatal Pauses 3-D Diet: Exercise vigorously for a minimum of 1 hour *every* day.

The Fatal Pauses 3-D Diet

Guiding Principles

Table 6–3 summarizes the guiding principles of the Fatal Pauses 3-D Diet. Each of these principles was derived from the evolution-based dietary vulnerabilities outlined above. Each of these principles is associated with a set of rules that you must follow if you decide to follow through with the 3-D Diet. These rules are specifically designed to remove the "pause" from your weight loss experience. Your choices are either "no" or "go" but *never* "maybe..." and *never* "just this time...." The rules *never* include excuses and *never* include exceptions. You will find that by not having to renegotiate your decisions with yourself, you will remove the predominance of frustration and torture from your dieting and exercise experience. The keys to the Fatal Pauses 3-D Diet are *discipline, measurement, routine, honesty,* and *kindness*.

TABLE 6–3.   Guiding principles of the Fatal Pauses 3-D Diet

1. Predetermine times, places, and quantities of foods and beverages

2. Limit foods to fresh and locally grown or regionally available varieties

3. Limit cooked grains and other plant-based carbohydrates

4. Limit the intake of processed sugars, animal fats, and salt

5. Exercise vigorously for a minimum of 1 hour *every* day

6. Be truthful and honest with yourself

7. Be kind to yourself

I will now elaborate on each guiding principle as applied in the Fatal Pauses 3-D Diet.

1. Predetermine Times, Places, and Quantities of Foods and Beverages

Overview

As has been discussed, in contemporary America, all types of food are available in just about any quantity and at almost any time and in every location. And we take full advantage of this accessibility! In addition to eating our "regularly scheduled" breakfasts, lunches, and suppers, we eat between eating. We eat while standing, sitting, reclining in our beds, and while we are on the move. We eat while working, studying, and playing. Much of our so-called "between meals" eating is opportunistic: pizza and beer during halftimes of sports events, a giant bag of buttered popcorn and a 32-ounce Coke at a movie, cupcakes brought to work to celebrate Administrative Professionals' Day, a frozen treat and a bag of Doritos at the convenience mart while paying for our gasoline, birthday party leftovers and a half-quart of ice cream while watching "The Late Show" in bed, highballs and fried chicken wings while going out dancing with friends after classes and on the weekends. It seems like almost any event or so-called activity is also an occasion for eating. And the calories add up and up, as we become fatter and fatter.

Rules

1. Preplan all meals and snacks.
2. No eating while standing or walking.
3. No eating in your automobile or truck unless it is a preplanned meal.
4. No refilling the plate.
5. No "spontaneous" or unplanned eating.
6. No eating or drinking anything with calories between meals.[1]
7. No drinking alcoholic beverages during the weight loss phase of the 3-D Diet.
8. Limit drinking alcoholic beverages during the weight maintenance phase of the 3-D Diet to a single drink comprising *either* 3.5 ounces (one jigger) of hard liquor (gin, rum, vodka, or whiskey), 4 ounces of wine (small wine glass), *or* one light beer.

Discussion

> **Question:** Travel is an important part of my work. How can I preplan what I am going to eat when I am on the road?

---

[1]Preplanned snacks containing calories that are factored into the 3-D Diet's daily caloric intake are the exception.

Answer: You supposedly have made the decision to lose weight by adhering to the 3-D Diet. Your question indicates to me that you are not fully committed to your decision, and therefore, it is highly unlikely that you will stick to the diet. People who observe religious dietary laws travel all the time. It is far more challenging for many of them to find meals consistent with their dietary regulations than it is for you to follow the rules of the Fatal Pauses 3-D Diet. Yet they plan ahead and eat well. They are not frustrated or irritated with indecision because they have made firm decisions to keep their commitments to their diet. Unless you truly decide to lose weight, you will experience frustration, equivocation, and self-deprecation that far exceed the effort that it would take to plan ahead to stay on the diet while traveling.

Question: Why is alcohol prohibited from the weight loss phase of the Diet?

Answer: For many reasons. First, alcohol is a carbohydrate that is relatively high in calories. Specifically, alcohol contains 7 calories per gram, which is almost twice as much as most other types of carbohydrates and protein (approximately 4 calories per gram).

Second, with the possible exception of low amounts of red wine, alcohol has limited nutritional value. When you diet, your calories are best expended on foods that are not toxic to organs throughout the body—as is alcohol—and on foods that have vitamins, minerals, fiber, and protein, which benefit your body.

Third, alcohol stimulates your appetite and makes food taste better. You are prone to eat more when you drink.

Fourth, alcohol is a central nervous system depressant, which results in your being less active, and therefore, you burn off fewer calories. When you have alcohol with meals—particularly in social settings—you are much more likely to prolong your time at the table and, naturally, eat more food.

Fifth, alcohol acts in the brain to reduce inhibitions, which make it far more likely that you will break the diet when you drink alcoholic beverages. In an experiment that I observed as a medical student, a mouse was placed in an enclosure containing a saucer of water and a live cat in a cage that was placed about 5 meters away from the saucer. Predictably, because of its natural fear of the cat, the mouse stayed as far away from the cat as physically possible in the enclosure. It cannot be pleasant for a mouse to be eaten alive, and it appeared to understand that. Although the cat could not escape the cage to get at the mouse, the mouse nonetheless remained far from the feline. In the experiment, the mouse had been deprived of food, and slices of cheese were placed directly in front of the cat cage. Even though it was starving, the mouse did not risk approaching the cheese. Then alcohol was added to the saucer near the mouse. Not long after drinking the alcohol, the mouse ambled up and ate the cheese that was contiguous to the caged cat. If you drink alcohol, you will lose your resolve to stay on the diet and will give in to your "natural drive" to eat high-calorie and high-fat foods.

Question: May I eat noncaloric foods and drink noncaloric fluids in between meals?

Answer: Yes, if you like. Even low-calorie snacks are permitted when they are preplanned and the calories are calculated to be within the caloric limits of your diet. Certain high-fiber-containing vegetables such as celery and cauliflower have very few calories and are often acceptable to eat between (and during) meals. Just don't dip them into those fatty, high-calorie salad dressings.

Noncaloric beverages are also acceptable. There is great controversy about drinking beverages with so-called artificial or nonnutritive sweeteners such as saccharine (Sweet'N Low), aspartame (Equal, NutraSweet), sucralose (Splenda), or stevia (Truvia) when dieting. I believe that it actually is helpful to the rigorous diet process and have observed great success over the years with their use in the Fatal Pauses 3-D Diet. I have strictly adhered to this diet for more than 30 years and regularly drink iced tea that is sweetened by aspartame as well as the occasional diet cola. Despite a plethora of non-evidence-based contentions on the Internet, there is no firm evidence supporting the long-term harmfulness of these sweeteners—including neurological, carcinogenic, reproductive, or psychological conditions.

Question: What's wrong with eating while standing up or walking?

Answer: If you think about it, many of the occasions when you snack or eat impulsively in between meals are when you are standing. Examples include when you open the refrigerator and gobble down a leftover piece of pie; when you are tempted by chips, cookies, and candies in vending machines; when you buy a soft pretzel, hot dog, or falafel from a curbside vendor; when you go to the refreshment stand at a sports event or concert; when you grab a doughnut (or three) from a local bakery; and when you notice some goodies at your kitchen counter. We consume a tremendous number of empty calories when eating on our feet or "on the run." Many people who have adhered strictly to their diet for a week can undermine their great work in a minute or two of impulsive eating while on their feet. Also, for the same reasons, be very cautious about eating in your automobile or truck, unless this is a preplanned meal.

2. Limit Foods to Fresh and Locally Grown or Regionally Available Varieties

Overview

As has been discussed, 65 million years of diurnal and seasonal cycles shaped how our bodies and digestive patterns evolved. Our ancient ancestors ate mostly during the daytime when and where they could find food, and they consumed what was available at that particular time of year. Certainly, the absence of illumination, refrigeration, and preservatives made nighttime eating—the bane of many of our contemporaries who are overweight—far less convenient than it is today. We did not evolve to eat all types of food, all seasons of the year, at all times of the day and night—as is possible today. On the most practical levels, consistency of eating patterns and reduction of the varieties of food help to limit snacking and binging while facilitating our measurement of calories.

This principle has two primary advantages. First and foremost, a key principle of the Fatal Flaws 3-D Diet is to narrow choices and limit variability. We thereby liberate ourselves from the time wasted in arguing with ourselves about our approach-approach and approach-avoidance choices and decisions. By making these choices and decisions in advance, we no longer debate with ourselves about what we should or should not eat, about whether or not we should exercise that day, about what type of exercise we should do that day, or about how long or how intensively we should exercise. Thereby, we become free to use the time previously wasted in fruitless, frustrating deliberations for more creative, constructive, and productive pursuits.

I abjectly disagree with the oft-quoted adage of the Irish humorist Oscar Wilde that "consistency is the last refuge of the unimaginative." I also do not accept the "too clever for words" aphorism "Repetition is a sign of stupidity. Repetition is a sign of stupidity." Rather, I believe that consistency and repetition foster ingenuity and innovation—the productive uses of our imaginations and intelligence. For example, let us consider the taut rules that are fundamental to most competitive sports such as basketball, soccer, football, ice hockey, swimming, running, and even chess. These sports' strict limitations of space, time, and movements fertilize the estuaries of the inventiveness, creativity, and artistic expressions that define their athletes' gifts and training while at the same time captivating their fans.

A second advantage of limiting the choice and variety of foods is health related. Fresh, locally grown vegetable and animal products are more healthful and flavorful than frozen or processed foods. These days, "fresh" generally means that the food has not been frozen. For example, there are big differences in taste and protein chemistry between fish that are caught several days ago, put on ice, and shipped great distances to your grocer or restaurant and those that are locally caught and prepared and served that day. Likewise, chickens and cattle that are raised and grain fed in enormous, crowded, and confining industrialized farms; slaughtered and packaged in distant processing plants; and shipped on ice to your local food markets do not have the food value or taste of animals locally raised, grass fed, and slaughtered and consumed that day or the day after. Similarly, fruits and vegetables that are locally grown tend to have superior food value and taste than those that are grown, harvested, and packaged in large, remote, and superindustrialized agricultural enterprises. If you are going to limit your calories every day for the rest of your life, you deserve to gain health benefits from and enjoy each bite.

Rules

1. Prioritize fresh, locally grown, raised, and harvested vegetables, meats, and fish.
2. Limit variety in your food choices and preparations.

3. Eat the same number of meals every day (i.e., two or three meals).
4. Eat meals at around the same times every day.

Discussion

Question: I live in Kansas, not that close to any oceans or even great lakes. I love fresh fish like salmon and halibut that are caught in cold ocean waters. Is it OK for me to eat these fish regularly?

Answer: Yes, absolutely. Salmon and halibut are delicious, healthful (high in omega fatty acids), and relatively low in calories. Enjoy!

Question: Are you serious about my limiting the variety in my food choices? I don't see what's wrong with my enjoying all types of food, as long as they are not overly caloric and are good for me.

Answer: It is very difficult to regulate your caloric intake if you are constantly changing food choices and how you prepare your foods. Regularity of the types and amounts of food you ingest combined with weighing yourself daily will help you to establish eating patterns that enable measurement, regulation, and maintenance of weight loss. Fortunately, when you choose more locally grown fruits and vegetables, the changing seasonal availabilities of such produce usually can enhance variety without affecting calories significantly.

Question: I have difficulty finding and affording locally grown foods. Why should I go to so much effort to have to pay so much more?

Answer: I understand that fresh, locally grown meats and vegetables are simply not available in many neighborhoods and, when and where available, tend to be more expensive. This is unfortunate from so many perspectives, including compromising the diets and nascent dietary interests of children and adolescents. Nonetheless, I believe it is worth your while to spend the time and effort to locate affordable, high-quality fresh food sources and shop carefully for value. Farmers' markets are becoming more plentiful in many urban areas, and more and more supermarkets are prioritizing these products at competitive prices. Please keep in mind that the health care consequences of poor dietary choices can also be expensive, time-consuming, painful, and disabling.

Question: What's the point of my eating at the same times each day? It's a huge hassle, and I don't see why I have to if the calories add up to the same.

Answer: Although it might not appear so, neither I nor the Fatal Pauses 3-D Diet is mean-spirited or sadistic. Our remarkable digestive systems (which include our brain) develop memories for *what* we ingest and *when* we ingest it. If you drink coffee and eat breakfast at the same time every day, try skipping your coffee, orange juice, or breakfast a time or two. At your usual time for breakfast, you will crave the coffee, juice, and breakfast foods to which you—and your body—are accustomed. This craving has little to do with the time of day and everything to do with your body's memory for your eating patterns.

At the risk of losing any credibility I may have had with readers and dietary traditionalists, I confess that, with the exception of the occasional family celebration, I have not eaten breakfast in 40 years. And I almost never eat lunch before 1:30 P.M., yet I am *never* hungry before that time. My energy and mental alertness are unaffected by this practice. I do not recommend this mealtime pattern for anybody else, as I have adopted it to fit my work and exercise schedule. Rather, I am only making the point that if you vary your meal times and content, your brain and digestive system will "learn" that it is possible that they will be fed almost anything at almost any time. The result is that you are likely to find that you are hungry most of the time—even after you have just eaten. Try to adhere to the patterns suggested by the Fatal Pauses 3-D Diet, and you will find that it is much easier—and, *mirabile dictu*, much more compassionate—than your current mealtime and in-between-meals eating practices.

3. Limit Cooked Grains and Other Plant-Based Carbohydrates

Overview

As has been discussed, the advent of cooking 250,000 years ago made it possible for mankind to render grains far more edible and to concentrate their caloric contents. Cooking also made grain products much more savory with products such as breads, cakes, flakes, chips, syrups, and alcoholic beverages, as well as industrially processed plant-based sugars (which will be reviewed below in guiding principle 4).

Carbohydrates are our primary source of energy because they are converted into glucose, which our cells require for energy. It is not always understood or appreciated that carbohydrates contain fewer calories per gram (3.75/g) than fat (9.0/g), ethyl alcohol (7.0/g), and even protein (4.0/g). Ideally, we should derive slightly less than half of our calories from carbohydrates. Our bodies, which cannot store carbohydrates, rapidly convert into fat the carbohydrates that we consume but do not use right away. Complex carbohydrates, which are present in fresh fruits and vegetables, are released more gradually into our bodies than starchy carbohydrates such as potatoes or whole grains. Processed carbohydrates, including foods from white flours and sugars, are digested the most rapidly, which results in more extreme fluctuations in our blood glucose levels and increased cravings. People who are overweight or obese tend to consume higher amounts and proportions of carbohydrates—particularly simple and processed carbohydrates—in their daily diets.

Rules

1. No grain-based "sweets"—including cakes, cookies, muffins, pastries, pies, candies, and syrups.
2. Limit bread and bread-like products (e.g., bagels, pizza crusts, tortillas) to two measured servings per day.[2]
3. No grain- or potato-based chips such as potato chips, nachos, or tostadas.
4. No grain-based breakfast cereals such as cornflakes, shredded wheat, oat cereals, or bran cereals.

Discussion

Question: Are whole-grain breads or multigrain bagels permitted on the 3-D Diet?

---

[2]Two slices of bread maximum per day in weight loss phase; four slices per day maximum in weight maintenance phase of diet.

Answer: Although whole-grain and multigrain products have more fiber and vitamins than foods from processed grains, they are still highly caloric. You can secure the necessary vitamins and fiber from much more healthful fresh fruits and fresh vegetables. Regulating grain-based products tends to be especially difficult for people who are overweight or obese to manage—especially when we are dieting. Most people find it far easier to "do without" these foods during the weight loss phase of their diets and to regulate their intake during the weight maintenance phase. For once, the marketing of this category of foods is more revealing than misleading: "I bet you can't eat just one!"

Question: I thought breakfast cereals are good for me. Why are they prohibited by the 3-D Diet?

Answer: Breakfast cereals are more a tribute to the power of American food industry marketing than they are a good way to start your morning. I regard the vast majority of breakfast cereals as little more than morning time snack food. They are highly caloric with little, if any, food value. The addition of salt and sugar to many cereal products makes them irresistible to children and adults, and they are, thereby, harmful to our health. Adding vitamins and fiber to the cereal products are head fakes: these additives do nothing to change the high caloric contents of the products. Fresh fruit and vegetable products are far better sources of vitamins and fiber, and you won't feel as hungry after eating fresh fruits and vegetables as you will after eating cereals.

4. Limit the Intake of Processed Sugars, Animal Fats, and Salt

Overview

It is a Sunday morning and a family with four children, ages 11–16, maintains a weekly tradition of going to brunch at a local restaurant after early morning mass. Consistent with their tradition, the family orders the breakfast combination for which that chain of restaurants is renowned. In homage to binary symmetry, this breakfast, available at a highly competitive price, features two eggs, two pieces of toast, two sausage links, two pieces of bacon, and two pancakes. Thematically consistent, the parents and the children add insult to their future health injuries by adding two pads of butter to each slice of toast and to each pancake before they tsunami the pancakes with syrup and treat the eggs and toast to passing showers of table salt. We need to understand that this breakfast combination is the economy, stripped-down model, and, like the automobile business, restaurants count on "accessories" to enhance their profit margins. Obliging, both parents and three of the children order hash browns, which are essentially their morning dose of French fried potatoes. Ever accommodating, the restaurant concedes to the family's request to top off the hash browns with melted American cheese, and all marvel at the culinary creativity of the 11 year old, who creates a de facto grilled cheese sandwich with her allotment of buttered toast and melted cheese. In reply to their courteous waiter's thoughtful query, "And now what would you guys like to drink with your breakfast?" each of the children orders a large chocolate milk shake while the parents request large Cokes.

The scenario described above, which has been repeated by millions of Americans millions of times over many decades, would not have been remotely possible for all but the smallest fraction of mankind's evolutionary history. Beyond the wide range in the varieties and sources of food, the amounts and concentrations of fats, simple carbohydrates, sugars, and salts simply would not have been possible. As such, our bodies did not evolve to survive this edible assault, no matter how much we pray before or after the meals.

Each of the specific food items and their manner of preparation in the unhappy meal recounted above is not permitted in the weight loss phase of the Fatal Pauses 3-D Diet and are either prohibited or highly discouraged in the weight maintenance phase.

Rules

1. Limit animal proteins to fresh fish, fresh white meat poultry, and the leanest cuts of fresh beef and pork.
2. Limit dairy products to fat-free products.
3. No processed meat products—including hot dogs, sausages, bacon, sandwich meats, and salty beef and pork snacks.
4. No fried foods.
5. No fat-containing creams or sauces.
6. Limit salad dressings to small quantities of low-fat and low-salt preparations.

7. No candy, syrups, or sugared desserts.
8. No sugar-added, prepackaged, or prepared products or adding sugar to fresh foods.
9. No high-sodium prepackaged or prepared products.[3]
10. Limit adding salt to fresh foods.[3]

Discussion

Question: I love cheeses, and I thought they are good for me. Why are they restricted from the 3-D Diet?

Answer: As a rule, cheese is bad for your health. Most cheeses are high in fat, sodium, and calories, all of which are almost always a significant health problem for overweight or obese Americans. Even nonfat mozzarella cheese and most nonfat cottage cheeses contain too much sodium. It is best to limit dairy products to nonfat milk and nonfat, unsweetened, low-sodium yogurt. Nonfat Greek yogurt is a good choice. Oh, by the way, stay away from pizza—it is high in calories, sodium, fat, and processed grains.

Question: Why is the Fatal Pauses 3-D Diet so restrictive of fat? Don't we need to eat some fat to stay alive?

Answer: Yes, we do need fat to stay alive. Lipid is present and does important work in every cell and membrane of our body, but most of this can be manufactured by our livers. The majority of Americans consume and store far too much fat in our daily diets, and our fat intake likely leads to serious health problems ranging from obesity to cardiovascular diseases such as heart attacks, high blood pressure, and stroke, to some types of cancer, and to dementias such as Alzheimer's disease.

Human beings are highly drawn to prepared foods containing both sugars and fats, a combination that rarely occurs in nature. We love their tastes and textures. Examples in the American diet include ice cream, doughnuts, pastries, lattes, milk shakes, and many types of candy and sauce. In addition to their being highly caloric, combining fat and sugar interferes with the normal

---

[3]Maximum of 1,500 mg of sodium per day in the weight loss phase of the 3-D Diet or in people with elevated blood pressure and 2,000 mg sodium maximum in the weight maintenance phase of the 3-D Diet.

functioning of neurons in our brains that regulate our satiety, with the net result that we are unable to control our consumption of the particular sugar/fat concoctions in the foods that we are eating (Berner et al. 2008).

Question: Why is salt so restricted by the 3-D Diet?

Answer: Salt is restricted by the Fatal Pauses 3-D Diet primarily for two reasons. First, adding too much salt to our foods increases our blood pressure, which is directly associated with life-endangering heart and kidney diseases. High blood pressure also significantly increases the risk of stroke, which can lead to sudden death or to severe, chronic disabilities such as paralysis, speech and language dysfunctions, mood impairments, and dementias.

Second, adding salt to food affects its taste in ways that often lead to our overeating those foods. Hence, excessive salt makes losing weight more difficult.

Question: Why are frozen and canned foods limited by the 3-D Diet?

Answer: Aside from fresh meats and vegetables being more flavorful and more vitamin- and fiber-rich than frozen and canned preparations of the same food types, frozen and canned fish and meat products often contain more salt, and canned fruit and vegetable foods frequently have more sugar. There are exceptions: some frozen fish, vegetables, and poultry do not have added salt, and some canned fruits and fish (particularly sardines and salmon) do not have added sugar or salt. Prepared foods such as frozen fruit salads and soups often have significant amounts of sugar and/or salt added. Stick with fresh and local foods, and you won't have to worry so much about sticking to the 3-D Diet.

Question: I am a gourmet cook who loves to eat, which is what helped to get me in so much trouble with my weight in the first place. I have about 50 pounds that I need to lose. I am committed to adhere to the guidelines of the 3-D Diet and to staying on an 1800 calorie a day diet—the amount recommended as safe by my internist and dietitian—until I lose this weight. Will you give me some suggestions for some savory meals and snacks that are consistent with the 3-D Diet?

Answer: Congratulations on your decision to achieve your goal! I have asked my wife, Beth Yudofsky, M.D., and my oldest daughter, Elisa Yudofsky Nord, who both are quite creative cooks, to provide you with some "savory" and healthful suggestions that follow the guidelines of the weight loss component of the 3-D Diet. Enjoy!

Breakfasts

- Nonfat Greek yogurt parfait with fresh berries and sliced almonds
- Oatmeal with fresh or frozen blueberries (with no sugar added)
- Tex Mex egg whites, scrambled with salsa and black beans
- Fresh fruit salad (or half of a grapefruit) with slice of whole wheat toast with almond butter
- Berry and nonfat Greek yogurt smoothie
- Scrambled tofu with tomatoes and vegetables

Lunches

- Caesar salad with tuna or salmon (grilled or canned)
- Egg white and spinach frittata
- Turkey, tomato, and butter lettuce sandwich on multigrain bread
- Baby spinach, kale, and pear salad with almonds or walnuts
- Green goddess vegetable soup
- Pasta primavera
- Italian chopped salad with grilled chicken with low-calorie, low-fat dressing
- Greek salad with half of a whole wheat pita with low-calorie, low-fat dressing
- Sliced turkey breast or tuna with fresh vegetables on whole wheat wrap or pita

Dinners

- Grilled salmon or chicken breast with Dijon asparagus or vegetables of your choice
- Slow-cooked jambalaya with chicken or mahi mahi
- Grilled tilapia with baked potato, side salad, and vegetable
- Grilled fresh chicken with broccolini and balsamic glaze

- Seafood chowder with whole wheat pita toasts
- Grilled turkey burger on a lettuce "bun" with baked sweet potato fries
- Turkey meatballs with whole wheat pasta and light marinara sauce
- Homemade whole wheat pizza with tomatoes, basil, and fat-free mozzarella
- Pasta with lean meat sauce and salad
- Large salad topped with grilled or baked chicken or fish and low-calorie, low-fat dressing

Snacks

- Banana with peanut butter (in moderate amount)
- Roasted, unsalted almonds or pistachios
- Fat-free frozen yogurt
- Crudités: fresh cut vegetables
- Nonfat string cheese
- Grapefruit and oranges
- High-fiber granola bar
- Nonfat frozen Greek yogurt pops

5. Exercise Vigorously for a Minimum of 1 Hour Every Day

Overview

There are few clearer examples of the fundamental, essential message of *Fatal Pauses* than the principle of combining exercise with a healthful diet. As discussed throughout this book, worried, unproductive pauses were something that our ancient ancestors could not afford. Their time and efforts were expended in securing and safeguarding their food, their shelter, and themselves. Ancient men and women's survival fears were starvation and safety and very little, if anything, in between. Survival depended on *immediate* fight and flight decisions, both of which required vigorous movement and significant expenditures of energy. Our bodies evolved to function optimally within this environmental and experiential reality. Any departures from these patterns most often are a source of somatic and mental dysfunction.

On the other hand, most Americans do not expend significant amounts of physical energy in securing our food or in defending ourselves, our families, our food, and our shelters. Nonetheless, this reality does not deter us from consuming sufficient calories and storing in our bodies ample fat reserves to be in full *physical* fight and flight mode every minute of every day of our lives. Our "survival" has become mental, not physical. We sit and worry, primarily about our social, interpersonal, and employment status and security. And when we don't resolve our perceived and misperceived survival-related problems, we become anxious and eat even more. And then we become even more worried and anxious about how much we have eaten, about how much weight we have gained, about how bad we look, and about how our appearance endangers our social aspirations and survival. So we eat even more. We are stuck in pause until—like our ancient ancestors—we can no longer afford to sit still. Unless we decide to take action, our pauses will kill us.

Rules

1. Prioritize exercise in your life.
2. Exercise vigorously for a minimum of 1 hour every day.
3. Develop and follow a recurrent, weekly schedule for your exercise program.
4. Develop and follow a recurrent, consistent exercise routine.
5. Choose an exercise regimen that you enjoy, that is safe, and that is not harmful to your body.

Discussion

> **Question:** How can I survive in my busy, highly competitive job world if I take so much time off to exercise?
>
> **Answer:** You would serve yourself better if you would revise your "survival" question as follows: "What good does it do me to work so hard and sacrifice so much in my work if I am not going to be around to enjoy the supposed benefits of my labor?"
> Scientific evidence consistently supports the health benefits of regular exercise and the health dangers of a sedentary life. Economic studies consistently support the financial benefits of regular, vigorous exercise to employers, employees, and society. Not only will you be more efficient and productive at work

if you exercise regularly, you will also have far less time away from work because of illness. Further, the costs of health care for yourself, your employer, and society will be far less if you exercise regularly. So my evidence-based answer to your question is for you to realign your priorities so that they will better serve you and others.

Question: Why do I have to exercise every day? Doesn't working out 4 or 5 days a week have about the same health benefits?

Answer: Again, I believe that you will be better served by revising your question as follows: "Why have I had such a problem sticking with my previous attempts to exercise regularly?"

Some people truly enjoy exercising. They are quite fortunate. However, if you are like me and so many others, there are scores of other things that you would much prefer doing than exercising. Like so many of us, you have to push yourself to exercise consistently. Given this reality, exercising daily—without exception—will free you from having to "obsess" about whether or not this is the day that you should take off. Or about whether you can trade a day of not exercising for another day when you routinely don't exercise. Or about whether or not a particular unexpected work or family issue merits skipping a day of exercise.

The Power of Go requires that you exercise every day that your body is able to do so. No exceptions. By scheduling your exercise regimen far in advance and by abiding no exceptions, you will find, paradoxically, that exercising isn't so bad. And to your surprise, you might even get to the point that you don't mind regular, vigorous exercise. However, looking forward to exercising is something I have never achieved in almost 40 years of daily exercise, so that might be too much to ask or expect of yourself at this point.

Question: How do I find the exercise program that works best for me?

Answer: This question indicates to me that you have decided to use the Fatal Pauses 3-D Diet to change and to sustain your gains.

First, select an exercise regimen, or exercise regimens, that you believe that you might enjoy and that will sustain your enthusiasm over a long period of time. You will not lose more weight by suffering through workouts that are painful and difficult and that you do not enjoy doing. Rather, you are more likely to give up exercising altogether if you choose one that you don't really like doing. Please note that this does not mean that there aren't things that you would prefer doing to exercising. Similar to your job, it would be great if you enjoy every minute at work, but that is rarely, if ever, a realistic expectation. People don't get paid to go on vacations.

Second, choose an exercise or exercises that are consistent with your physical abilities and that are safe. I encourage you to pursue professional advice on your options and choices from your family physician, medical specialists, and qualified coaches and/or certified fitness consultants. It is always good to begin with experts who will teach you the techniques for doing the exercise regimen correctly and safely. These experts also can be excellent motivators.

Third, choose a regimen that is practical and a good fit for your work demands and lifestyle. This might entail purchasing some equipment, joining a fitness club, or becoming a member of a specialized exercise group or team.

Fourth, begin slowly and build up over time to your target goal of excising vigorously for at least 1 hour per day. Many people become discouraged if they try to take on too much too quickly. The key is to develop a program that will continue over a prolonged period of time. This is not a time to become too competitive with yourself or others.

Fifth, understand that you will probably modify and fine tune your choices and regimen over time. Your exercise interests, physical abilities, and opportunities are highly likely to change over many years.

6. Be Truthful and Honest With Yourself

Overview

You catch it in her disapproving glance as she stealthily peers at her reflection in the store's gleaming window. Or in the futile, furtive downward tug at the hem of her billowing polyester chemise over her voluminous hips. As if choreographed by some satanic deus ex machina, she simultaneously purses her lips around the straw that pierces the chilled, tarry thickness of her giant chocolate milk shake. But does *she* catch it? That she is fooling herself...almost.

As discussed in Chapter 3, a fundamental goal of *Fatal Pauses* is to help you understand yourself more fully—particularly with regard to how you have become stuck and why you remain stuck in pause. Additionally, it is critical for you to be crystal clear about how you will go about becoming unstuck and how to monitor validly your progress with becoming unstuck. Insight, self-awareness, openness, honesty, objectivity, and clarity are essential to your success. Measurement is the key to your achieving these six indispensible objectives.

Rules

1. Time and measure your exercise output.
2. *Prior* to consumption of food or fluid, compute the caloric content.
3. Plan and compute the daily caloric content of your food and beverage intake.
4. Weigh yourself daily.

Discussion

Question: Why is the Fatal Pauses 3-D Diet so big on measuring everything?

Answer: *Fatal Pauses* is all about being honest with and true to ourselves. The 3-D Diet requires that you measure the calories contained in what you eat and how much you eat; that you measure how long and how hard you exercise; and that you measure, every day, how much you weigh. All so that you live in a world of reality. So that you will live happily and healthfully for a long time.

It is *so* easy for us to deceive ourselves. "What's the difference if I drink this one milk shake? One milk shake won't kill me." But it won't be just one milk shake, and those milk shakes won't kill you right away.

It is *not* easy for us to be true to ourselves. It takes insight, understanding, and discipline. And be sure, if you are stuck in pause with regard to your weight, you will be resistant to all three: to the insight about how you became overweight in the first place, to understanding what it takes for you to become unstuck, and to the discipline required to do what it takes to lose and remain at a healthful weight.

Achieving a healthful weight can be accomplished only through continuous measurement. If change can't be measured, change won't happen. We certainly don't want to believe that we are accomplishing something important when we really are not. When you see people submerge in Roquefort dressing the salads that they have selected as their entrees, they are fooling themselves. When you see people ordering Diet Cokes with their enormous breakfast combinations, they are fooling themselves. When you see people doing glacially slow breast-strokes (usually in the fast swimmers' lane), they are fooling themselves. We all love food. If we don't measure how much food we eat and how many calories are contained in what we do eat, we will eat too much of the high-calorie foods that we all crave. And we underestimate how much we have eaten. In the same vein, if we aren't consistent in our exercise routines and we don't measure our effort, our effort levels will vary widely. And we won't realize when we're "bagging it."

Question: Is it really possible to measure how hard I am exercising? If so, how do I go about measuring my effort?

Answer: Yes, it is not only possible but, as stated above, essential for your success. For example, if you decide to do 1 hour each day of vigorous walking, begin by selecting a route and timing how long it takes you to complete it. Try to build up to the point that you can walk your chosen route for an hour at a challenging but not painful pace. By measuring how long it takes for you to cover your regular distance, you will readily be able to determine your effort level.

If you regularly take a bicycle spinning class, build up to and measure the speeds and levels of the resistance for pedaling that are challenging but not painful for you. At the end of hour-long workouts that are consistent for resistance levels, measure on the bicycle odometer how far you have gone. The distance traveled will be an accurate indication of your effort.

Here's how I have done in my own swim workouts nearly every day for the past 30 years: When I don't swim in a coached class (in which the coach establishes the distances and monitors the effort levels), I swim exactly the same routine each day. A minimum of five sets of 600 meters or six sets of 600 yards, depending on the setup of the pool in which I am swimming (i.e., meters or yards). I work as hard as I can and time each set. I measure the time it takes for me to complete the entire workout, which is always the total of the same sets and distances. My total time is, therefore, an accurate measurement of my level of effort for that day in the pool. This total time usually varies less than 15 seconds over an hour's workout and 3,000 meters traversed. If I were to take 5 minutes longer for the whole work-out, I would know that my effort level had waned significantly.

Question: Don't the repetitive exercise routines of the Fatal Flaws 3-D Diet just replace obsessive eating with obsessive exercising? It seems to me that you are treating one neurosis with another one.

Answer: Your question is fair. I understand why you and many others who read about my own exercise routine—similar to the exercise format that I advocate for you—will believe that I am either a masochistic exercise zealot or just plain sadistic to my patients and readers. Hopefully, I am neither. I took my time to build up to this level of physical activity, which is just about right for my particular strength and abilities. Many of my peers swim faster and farther, and others go slower and cover less distance. That doesn't matter. We are neither competing with each other nor competing with ourselves. We all do what is right for our individual abilities and goals. My goals are 1) good cardiovascular and pulmonary fitness; 2) optimal mobility, flexibility, and physical strength; and 3) good self-esteem and mental health. This exercise regimen is what it takes for me to achieve my goal. Within the parameters of the Fatal Flaws 3-D Diet, you, also, can find what works best for you to achieve your goals. And a routine that you might even enjoy.

But please understand that *Fatal Pauses* is all about being honest with and true to ourselves. Do you really understand the health consequences of a poor diet and insufficient exercising? As a hospital-based physician for most of my career, I witness these tragic, often fatal consequences every day. All the more tragic because, in 90% of the cases, these consequences can be prevented.

Two time-worn aphorisms apply to and may help guide your potential choices:

1. You can pay now or pay later, but
2. You cannot have your cake and eat it, too.

Question: Why do I have to weigh myself every day? Aren't there daily fluctuations in weight? During my previous attempts at dieting, I became painfully discouraged after a day of hard dieting when I weighed myself and found that I had not lost an ounce. Eventually, I just gave up. Shouldn't I take the long view and weigh myself once a month or something like that?

Answer: A fundamental recommendation of the Fatal Pauses 3-D Diet is that you check your weight every day. I strongly recommend that you use a good digital scale and that you do it first thing in the morning. You are correct that, even when you have been adhering to the 3-D Diet, your weight can fluctuate. These fluctuations can be the result of many factors, usually related to water retention. I also understand that it can be enormously discouraging to you when, after a meticulous day of adhering to the 3-D Diet, you find the next morning that your weight has actually increased. Trust me that these occasions will be infrequent and will pale in comparison to the days that you find that you have lost weight.

My reasons for strongly recommending daily weighings are threefold:

1. Weighing yourself daily is preventative. It helps you stick to the 3-D Diet. If you know that you are going to weigh yourself the very next morning, you will be far less tempted to break the diet. This is especially true if you, like so many others, are a nighttime nibbler or midnight muncher who is subject to being enticed by dinner leftovers or open packages of cookies, chocolates, ice cream, etc., and know that you will have to weigh yourself several hours later.
2. Weighing yourself daily provides you both positive and negative reinforcement. Behavioral models demonstrate consistently that reinforcements of behavior work best when accomplished as soon as possible after the behavior. If you stick to the 3-D Diet, you will almost always gain positive reinforcement the morning following your positive behavior. If you break the diet, you will receive negative reinforcement shortly thereafter. If you weigh yourself monthly, consider how demoralizing it would be for you to have strictly adhered to the diet over 3 weeks prior to weighing yourself but find that you actually gained weight over that month. You may have forgotten that you had "let yourself go" during a vacation (or holiday) in the first week after you had weighed yourself.
3. The Fatal Pauses 3-D Diet is all about self-honesty. Self-deception is elemental to so-called failed diets. If, every day, you know how much you weigh, you won't deceive yourself.

Question: What's the best way for me to plan my diet and compute the calories?

Answer: Thinking about the principles and following all the rules of the Fatal Pauses 3-D Diet form the core of diet planning. To summarize, preplanning what you eat every day and having a consistent, easy-to-follow meal plan form the basis of all good diets. For sample meals, see pp. 160–161.

An approach to determining how much weight you might want to lose and how to calculate the calories that you should ingest each day will also be provided later in this chapter in the section "Calculating the Calories Needed to Lose Weight."

7. Be Kind to Yourself

Overview

Many of us use food as a "reward" for having to do or experience things that we don't like having to do or experience. High-energy containing foods—such as those rich in sugars and fats—stimulate the release of dopamine in the central nervous system that, in turn, activates the pleasure centers of our brains. We like what we are eating and want more of the same. What we are actually doing is hijacking the brain's dopamine-mediated biological reinforcement systems that motivate us to eat ravenously for energy and survival. For example, we might "treat ourselves" to ice cream after sitting at a computer for 2 hours at work on our taxes or writing a paper. We might even use the reward of ice cream beforehand as an incentive to motivate ourselves to do these tasks in the first place. The problem is that our biological systems for energy use and storage are so efficient that we expend only a fraction of the calories in a bowl of ice cream that is required for sitting at a computer for 2 hours, and our bodies rapidly transform the unexpended calories into fat. Another problem is that we begin to use food to motivate us to do or experience almost anything that we might find unpleasant or, shall we say, *distasteful.*

Because any diet requires the restriction of calories and, therefore, the denial of immediate pleasure, it is understandable that we might experience the strict limitations and demands of the Fatal Pauses 3-D Diet as punitive. Rather, we must take the long view and keep reminding ourselves that we are doing the opposite of punishing ourselves, but the rewards we gain are not immediate. Every time we resist eating something that is tempting and every time we push ourselves to exercise a bit harder, we are actually being kind to ourselves. And we must repeatedly remind ourselves that we are being kind to ourselves by doing what we want for ourselves, not what some authority figure demands of us to do or not do.

Rules

1. Savor the foods that you do eat.
2. Savor the pleasure of having worked out.
3. Don't get angry with yourself if you break a rule of the 3-D Diet.

Discussion

Question: I really love food and gourmet cooking. What's the point of eating at all if so many of the foods that I love are not permitted by the diet?

Answer: I know that you realize that we all must eat to stay alive, but I also get the point that you are making. You do not believe that the Fatal Pauses 3-D Diet is, in any way, compatible with gourmet cooking and your enjoyment of food and eating. Au contraire; I expect you to derive even more pleasure from your meals once you recover from the withdrawal symptoms of your current diet and become adapted to the 3-D Diet.

I regard the prototypical American diet as a culinary cluster bomb of sugars, salt, fats, and alcohol. The result is that the sensory receptors for taste in our tongues and palates and, thereby, in the pleasure centers in our brain that these excite are drastically overstimulated. As occurs in neuronal receptors throughout our brains, when they are overstimulated they become what is termed *down regulated*. What this means in practical terms is that we must continuously ingest ever-greater quantities and varieties of foods and drinks with sugars, fats, and alcohol to feel sated and satisfied. After several months on the 3-D Diet you will be surprised to find that you will enjoy and savor more healthful foods that, previously, had tasted bland. Although I expect you to be highly skeptical about this, after a year or two on the diet, the fat-infested and sugar-suffused foods that you had previously relished will seem almost nauseating. As they should: nausea and disgust are natural, protective responses to dangerous foods.

Question: I always feel sore, tired, and sweaty after exercising. How do you expect me to exercise for an hour every day when I hate the feeling?

Answer: When I first began my clinical practice, I shared office space and a patient waiting area with about several dozen other academic psychiatrists. Many of these doctors saw their patients several times per week over protracted periods of time. Because most of us were on hourly schedules according to the clock, we began and completed our sessions at about the same times. I couldn't help but notice that several regular patients seemed more upset on leaving their sessions with their therapists than they had been before their appointment. Understandably, this can and probably should occur occasionally, but these patients seemed to have this response repeatedly, and, moreover, they did not seem to be improving over the ensuing months and years. On the basis of this experience, I hypothesized that something was amiss. Either the type of treatment was not suited to the patient's needs, the psychiatrist was incompetent, or the therapeutic fit between the practitioner and patient was far less than ideal. I never once believed that the patient could not be helped significantly by the appropriate treatment or clinician.

Similarly, if you feel worse after exercising than you did before you began, something is wrong. But it's not "exercising" per se. Perhaps the exercise that you are doing is not well matched with your physical capacity or athletic abilities; perhaps you are working too intensely; perhaps you are not doing the exercise correctly; or perhaps you just don't like that particular exercise. Try to find an activity that you truly enjoy or even ask a professional fitness trainer to make suggestions and help you get started. Although I do not expect you always to enjoy exercising, I have every confidence that when you finally find the appropriate workout, you will enjoy how you feel after exercising. Be kind to yourself.

Question: In the past, I became furious with myself when I broke my diet. Usually, I dropped the diet altogether not long afterward. How can I prevent this from happening again?

Answer: This is a wonderful question, and I assure you that you are not the only one who has had this experience. I also believe that you have answered your own question. Although it is understandable that you would become angry with yourself if you go off the diet, resume the diet immediately thereafter. Breaking the diet (which includes the exercise regimen) is not the end of the world; staying with the diet after a setback is what is important. Be careful not to use a few dietary indiscretions or skipped workouts as an excuse to give up. Also beware of using your anger with yourself as a cover up or smoke screen to hide your quitting something so important to you and your mental and physical health. If possible, you might consult a competent therapist to help you discover a conflict about which you are unaware. Anger at yourself is a symptom arising from conflict and being stuck. Recall that although Ms. Anthony was angry with herself for not being strong enough to stay with a diet and lose weight, she also felt less vulnerable and weak when she was much heavier. Her discovery that these conflicting feelings were connected to her being abused sexually when she was much younger ultimately enabled her to remain on a diet and lose weight.

Question: Doesn't all the focus that the Fatal Pauses 3-D Diet places on diet, exercise, and "being kind to yourself" constitute a recipe for a narcissistic lifestyle?

Answer: No, just the opposite. I believe that narcissism is excessive focus on oneself as a result of low self-esteem. Most overweight people who are stuck in pause are quite self-absorbed. They spend inordinate amounts of time thinking about themselves, usually in disparaging ways: How do I look in my bathing suit? Do you think that he would ever date someone so fat? I can't stand the way I look in that photograph, etc. They also are preoccupied with food and eating: How did I let myself eat that other dessert? I ate so much at lunch, I should try to skip dinner, etc.

More importantly, the harmful health consequences of obesity occupy a disproportionate amount of their attention. They consume significant amounts of time tending to their own health needs and physical disabilities, and they require substantial attention of others, ranging from their own family members to health care professionals.

On the other hand, people who follow the Fatal Pauses 3-D Diet establish patterns of eating and exercise that promote an efficient and healthful lifestyle that enables them to focus on and meet their responsibilities to others. These behaviors are far different from diets and exercise regimens with the purpose of enhancing a person's physical *appearance*. Examples include body builders and fashion models who seek to be whisper thin. Antipodal to narcissism, taking care of your miraculous body with a healthful diet and regular exercise and not abusing alcohol has a spiritual dimension, which will be amplified in Chapters 8 and 9, "Stuck in a Bottle."

Rules to Diet By

Table 6–4 includes the rules that are derived from the guiding principles that form the basis of the Fatal Pauses 3-D Diet. The rules have been arranged according to the Power of Go and the Power of No. If you follow these rules, not only will you be successful at losing weight and sustaining your weight loss but you will also be healthier, happier, and more productive. I know that this is promising a great deal, but I also know that what is being promised is true. Promises are easy; the hard work is up to you!

How Much Should I Lose?

Establishing Your Weight Loss Goal

> **Question:** How many psychiatrists does it take to change a light bulb?
>
> **Answer:** One. But the light bulb must want to change itself.

I realize that many health care professionals and others who are reading this chapter are quite familiar with this light bulb joke, but it bears an important message for weight loss goals that is worth reemphasizing at this point. The Fatal Pauses 3-D Diet is all about what *you* want and decide to accomplish for yourself. So, in the Fatal Pauses 3-D Diet, *you choose how thin you want to be and, thereby, the amount of weight you must lose to attain that goal.*

No person other than you can determine the weight at which you feel attractive and comfortable, and no other person can make the decision or do the work required for you to reach and remain at your preferred weight.

That being said, experts can help. Medical and behavioral health care professionals can be good guides and support to assist you in gaining insight and clarity about how much weight to lose and how to go about doing it. *One caveat is that many health care professionals and dietitians fail to address the psychosocial predeterminants of your weight gain—i.e., the "discover" component of the 3-D Diet.* You cannot

TABLE 6–4. Rules of the Fatal Pauses 3-D Diet

The Power of Go

1. Preplan all meals and snacks

2. Prioritize fresh, locally grown, raised, and harvested vegetables, meats, and fish

3. Eat the same number of meals and snacks every day (i.e., two or three meals)

4. Eat meals and snacks at around the same times every day

5. Prioritize exercise in your life

6. Exercise vigorously for a minimum of 1 hour every day

7. Develop and follow a recurrent, weekly schedule for your exercise program

8. Develop and follow a recurrent, consistent exercise routine

9. Choose an exercise regimen that you enjoy and that is safe and not harmful to your body

10. Savor the foods that you do eat

11. Savor the pleasure of having worked out

The Power of No

12. No eating while standing or walking

13. No eating in your automobile or truck unless it is a preplanned meal

14. No refilling the plate

15. No "spontaneous" or unplanned eating or snacking

16. No eating or drinking anything with calories between meals, except for preplanned snacks

17. No drinking alcoholic beverages in the weight loss phase of the 3-D Diet

18. Limit drinking alcoholic beverages in the weight maintenance phase of the 3-D Diet to a single drink comprising *either* 3.5 ounces (one jigger) of hard liquor (gin, rum, vodka, or whiskey), 4 ounces of wine (small wine glass), *or* one light beer

19. Limit variety in your food choices and preparations

20. No grain-based "sweets"—including cakes, cookies, muffins, pastries, pies, candies, and syrups

21. Limit bread and bread-like products (e.g., bagels, pizza crusts, tortillas) to two measured servings per day

---

TABLE 6–4. Rules of the Fatal Pauses 3-D Diet *(continued)*

The Power of No *(continued)*

22. No grain- or potato-based chips such as potato chips, nachos, tostadas

23. No grain-based breakfast cereals such as cornflakes, shredded wheat, oat cereals, or bran cereals

24. Limit animal proteins to fresh fish or fresh white meat poultry and to the leanest cuts of fresh beef and pork

25. Limit dairy products to fat-free products

26. No processed meat products—including hot dogs, sausages, bacon, sandwich meats, and salty beef and pork snacks

27. No fried foods

28. No fat-containing creams or sauces

29. Limit salad dressings to small quantities of low-fat and low-salt preparations

30. No candy, syrups, or sugared desserts

31. No sugar-added, prepackaged, or prepared products or adding sugar to fresh foods

32. No high-sodium prepackaged or prepared products

33. Limit adding salt to fresh foods

34. Don't get angry with yourself if you break a rule of the 3-D Diet

---

skip this step; otherwise, you will not be successful with sustained weight loss. Recall that Ms. Anthony had to discover the psychological determinants of her obesity before she could be in a position to want and decide to lose weight.

Calculating the Calories Needed to Lose Weight

There are several excellent Web sites that can help you calculate the number of calories that are required to sustain your current weight and to lose the precise number of pounds (that you determine) each week to reach your ultimate weight goal. The best of these sites take into consideration such factors as your gender, age, height, current weight, and level of exercise. Here's how Web-based weight loss calculators work:

1. Determine the number of calories required to sustain your current weight by entering into the calculator your gender, age, height, current weight, and current level of exercise or physical activity.
2. The Web-based calculator will then compute the number of calories per day required for you to maintain your current weight. Let's call this element your *maintenance calories.*
3. The Web-based calculator will also determine the number of calories that you must *eliminate* each day from your maintenance calories in order to lose 1 pound or 2 pounds per week.

Thus, if you wish to lose 25 pounds by losing 1 pound per week, it will take you approximately 25 weeks, or half a year, to achieve your goal. The Web-based calculator will compute the number of daily calories required for you to lose 1 pound per week. After you get to your goal, the Web-based calculator will help you compute the number of daily calories required to remain at your self-determined ideal weight. These will be your new maintenance calories.

Let us consider the example of a 35-year-old man who is 5 feet 8 inches tall and weighs 210 pounds. He is able to engage in moderately vigorous physical exercise. He wants to weigh 185 pounds, which means he will need to lose 25 pounds. The calorie calculator at www.calculator.net computes that this individual requires 2,886 calories per day to maintain his current weight and 2,386 calories per day to lose 1 pound per week. Thus, he will need to reduce his maintenance calories by 500 calories per day for about 6 months to achieve his goal of 185 pounds. At that point, he will need to take in 2,710 calories per day to sustain that weight.

Now let's see how this approach would apply to Ms. Anita Anthony.

Ms. Anita Anthony's Diet

When Ms. Anthony began the Fatal Pauses 3-D Diet, she was 34 years old, 6 feet 1 inch tall, weighed 275 pounds, and, because of her obesity-related physical disabilities, was able to engage only in light exercise. Her personal goal was to weigh 160 pounds, which meant that she had to lose a whopping 115 pounds.

The Web-based calorie calculator at www.calculator.net estimated that she required 2,853 calories per day to maintain her current weight and 2,353 daily calories to lose 1 pound per week. By eliminating 500 calories per day from the amount required to sustain her weight, it would take Ms. Anthony well over 2 years to reach her ideal weight. However, if she were to remove 1,000 calories per day, or take in 1,853 daily calories, she would lose 2 pounds per week and reach her goal in 1 year. She chose to do the latter.

> **Dr. Y.:** How did you decide to set your goal to weigh 160 pounds?
> **Ms. Anita Anthony:** That's what I weighed when I was 16 years old, before I began to gain so much weight. I felt good about my body and about myself at that weight.
> **Dr. Y.:** That was your weight before you were abused sexually.
> **Ms. Anthony:** For one moment, I'll stop being a surgery nurse and admit that there is a psychological significance to that weight.
> **Dr. Y.:** And I will stop being a psychiatrist for a minute and project that you will certainly be quite attractive at that weight.
> **Ms. Anthony:** You mean "hot," don't you, Dr. Y.?
> **Dr. Y.:** That is not an official term in either psychiatry or surgery, Anita.

Two-Year Follow-Up on Ms. Anita Anthony

Ms. Anthony exhibited determination (i.e., *decision*) and consistency (i.e., *discipline*) in following the Fatal Pauses 3-D Diet. She also continued to work with me in weekly psychotherapy (i.e., *discovery*). Initially, because of her many obesity-related physical problems, her exercise options were limited. She chose to begin her daily exercise regimen with water aerobics, a low-impact workout. An excellent athlete, she improved her proficiency and increased the intensity of her workouts progressively. She also began to make friends with other participants in her group. For the first time since high school, Ms. Anthony began to develop a circle of friends with whom she interacted on a regular basis. A few friends from her water aerobics group introduced her to indoor cycling spin classes and, thereafter, to outdoor road biking. She found that she "really enjoyed" and was very good at biking, and she soon joined a local cycling group. She went to advanced spin classes on work days and, on her days off, went on long biking excursions with her cycling group. She also continued to do water aerobics as well. The net result was that the increased intensity of her physical activity put her ahead of schedule on her weight loss goal. Remarkably, after a year on the 3-D Diet, she had lost 130 pounds and looked and felt like a different person. Subsequently, Ms. Anthony's weight remained stable at her revised, preferred weight of 145 pounds.

After not having danced in 20 years, Ms. Anthony also rediscovered how much she enjoys and how accomplished she is at dancing. She is now taking dancing classes and has been asked out on several dates. She feels uncomfortable dating men, primarily because she knows that this will likely lead to physical intimacy. In her psychotherapy, she is working diligently on addressing her conflicted feelings over her desire for intimacy and her fear of abandonment. More importantly, as her insight and self-confidence have grown, she has changed and is changing her behavior. No longer does she push men away with hostility or with an unappealing appearance. At this point she is beginning to permit a degree of physical intimacy with her suitors, but, understandably, she also is experiencing considerable discomfort, which she is addressing in her psychotherapy. Recently, she made the following observation about psychotherapy:

> **Ms. Anthony:** I have lost almost half of my body weight in a year. Don't you find it interesting, Dr. Y., that I find the psychotherapy part so much more challenging than the dieting part?
> **Dr. Y.:** There's a difference?

References

Berner LA, Avena NM, Hoebel BG: Binging, self-restriction, and increased body weight in rats with limited access to a sweet-fat diet. Obesity 16:1998–2002, 2008

Casey J: The hidden ingredient that can sabotage your diet: do you know how much sugar you're eating? WebMD, 2007. Available at: http://www.webmd.com/diet/features/the-hidden-ingredient-that-can-sabotage-your-diet. Accessed May 2, 2014.

Stunkard A, McLaren-Hume M: The results of treatment for obesity: a review of the literature and report of a series. AMA Arch Intern Med 103:79–85, 1959

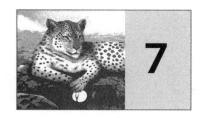

7

Stuck in My Marriage: The Cases of Helen and Blaise Hartman

When Traumatic Brain Injury Is Complicated by Narcissistic Personality Disorder

Behind every great fortune lies a great crime.
—*Honore de Balzac*, Le Pere Goriot

"I feel trapped."

The Cases of Mrs. Helen and Mr. Blaise Hartman: D1 (Discovery) Component, Part I—Assessment

Preliminary History and Presenting Illness

Congenitally congenial and characterologically gifted, Mrs. Hoffman, my administrative assistant, peered into my office and whispered plaintively, "Your new patient with traumatic brain injury decided to cancel his appointment this morning, but his wife came instead. I hope that you will agree to meet with her. She seems quite distressed."

If gold and diamonds are metaphors for sinew and muscle, Mrs. Helen Hartman could have been an Olympic weight lifter. Bejeweled and attired in opulence more appropriate for the coronation of royalty than for a visit to a commoner doctor, she nonetheless appeared anxious and vulnerable.

Mrs. Helen Hartman: I must apologize for my husband's not coming. He changed his mind at the last minute. I'm embarrassed to say that Blaise believes that psychiatrists are more troubled than their patients—but he would use a different word.

Dr. Y.: Would that word be "crazy?"

Mrs. Hartman: Yes, that's the word. But I could not disagree with him more.

Dr. Y.: Has he ever seen a psychiatrist?

Mrs. Hartman: No. But for many years before his skiing accident, I had asked him to go with me for couples counseling, but he always refused.

Mrs. Hartman proceeded to disclose that she had been married for 23 years to Blaise Hartman, whom she had met when they were both students at Dartmouth College. A native of Incline Village, Nevada, Blaise Hartman was not only captain of the Dartmouth ski team but also an excellent student majoring in business and president of the senior class. They married right after college and moved to New York City, where Mr. Hartman worked as a securities analyst for an investment banking firm while Mrs. Hartman attended medical school and graduate school in neuroscience.

Eighteen months prior to his scheduled meeting with me, Mr. Hartman was seriously injured while helicopter skiing in British Columbia. Not wearing a helmet, he suffered severe brain injury when he careened, at high velocity, into an ice-hardened snow bank. After 3 weeks he emerged from a coma with manifestations of prefrontal and left brain injury, including right hemiparesis, a severe expressive aphasia, and neuropsychiatric symptoms including impulsivity, impaired social judgment, affective lability, and depression. His intellect and cognition were spared for the most part. Over the next year and a half, he worked diligently with his team of rehabilitation professionals and made excellent progress. Nonetheless, his speech remained somewhat garbled and not fluent, his balance was impaired, and he ambulated slowly with a pronounced limp.

Mr. Hartman spent almost all of his time at home, where he would have temper tantrums elicited by seemingly minor frustrations in which he would scream expletives and throw and break objects. He reacted especially vehemently to Mrs. Hartman's efforts to assist him when he lost his balance and fell. On such occasions he would wrench away from his wife's grasp while screaming, "Stop putting me down! I'm not an invalid!"

> **Mrs. Helen Hartman:** For years I begged Blaise to wear a helmet when he was skiing—particularly because he always went down the most dangerous slopes. He kept telling me that he was not like other skiers, that he never had accidents and never even fell down. I blame myself for believing him and am angry with him that our lives have been destroyed unnecessarily. All of this heartache could have been prevented.
>
> **Dr. Y.:** How was your marriage before Blaise's accident?
>
> **Mrs. Hartman:** I confess that we had a troubled marriage before my husband's accident. With his brain injury, it has become much worse. Now I feel that I am walking on eggshells every minute, lest I set him off. He will explode in rage over almost anything, and it takes hours for him to calm down. I have grown to hate being in my own house, but I'm afraid to leave him by himself for more than a few hours. I feel trapped.

Preliminary Recommendations

I routinely schedule 2 hours for initial consultations for patients with traumatic brain injury. Cognitive slowing and difficulties with articulation can make history taking proceed more slowly. On the basis of the information above that Mrs. Hartman had provided in that initial session, I made the following preliminary recommendations:

1. Supportive psychotherapy for Mrs. Hartman's situational and family-related stresses
2. Insight-oriented psychotherapy to enable Mrs. Hartman and me to understand more about herself, her priorities, and the range of her options going forward
3. Neuropsychiatric education to help her understand the neurological and psychiatric bases for and implications of her husband's cognitive, behavioral, and emotional dysfunctions
4. The development of strategies—interpersonally and in the home environment—to reduce her husband's neuropsychiatric symptoms and symptomatologies
5. Encouragement for her to share with her husband what was relevant and constructive in our treatment sessions and to invite him to join her at any time to participate in our treatment

Mrs. Helen Hartman

"Angels are probably unaware of their luminosity," I thought on looking through the childhood photographs that Helen Hartman had brought, at my request, to her third session. Especially in pictures where she was among her school-age friends, one's focus was irresistibly drawn to her image—unposed, oblivious, surpassing beauty. Constitutionally shy, ineffably modest, selflessly generous, and gentle, Helen has always been a true believer. The Catholic faith is her lodestone. From kindergarten she was blissfully immersed in the religious spirit of the Catholic schools that she had attended, with her full being embracing and exemplifying the expressed value of Schenectady's Notre Dame Girls' High School: "Learning is a lifelong process, and Christian commitment never ceases."

Helen inherited her gifts for kindness and spirituality from both of her parents, but her dominant gene for science and math doubtlessly came from her father, an electrical engineer who worked his entire career at IBM. With Helen's younger brother, who grew up to be a priest, the small Byrne family lived modestly, enriched by their love of the Church, for one another, and for others in their community, particularly the disadvantaged. From all accounts, Helen's childhood was remarkable only for its "other era" simplicity, for its protectedness, and for its happiness. Christian youth groups and summer math and music camps were her passion, and she managed to graduate from high school without ever having kissed or missed having kissed a young man. So shy and modest was Helen that she asked the principal of her high school not to recognize her at her graduation as valedictorian of her high school class. "Only if you will let me announce your perfect scores on your SAT examinations," the priest twinkled. Who could resist loving Helen? Certainly not Blaise.

Mr. Blaise Hartman: Act 1

Blaise was born into the aristocracy of American alpine skiing: both of his parents were members of the U.S. national and Olympic ski teams. With his parents' marriage lasting little longer than a record downhill run, Blaise grew up bearing the rapid successions of his mother's one-night stands, insignificant others, fleeting spouses, and sour stepchildren. His father "wasn't around very much." His ski club buddies, his exceptional coordination and balance, and the potentials and perils of gravity formed the constancies of his childhood. So intensely competitive was young Blaise that he sped past without noticing or appreciating the sapphire beauty of Lake Tahoe and swaying dignity of the snow-bent pines that framed the slopes of Heavenly, Squaw Valley, Northstar, and Incline Village, where he raised himself. Often not knowing where he would sleep or if he would eat dinner from night to night, he learned to endear himself to wealthy families, who took him into their magnificent vacation homes in exchange for ski lessons and his engaging companionship. From the 10th grade, Blaise was among the nation's top-ranked high school downhill skiers, in addition to being a nationally ranked freestyle snowboarder. Not surprisingly, he was heavily recruited by many of the leading colleges with alpine ski teams, and he chose to attend Dartmouth College in Hanover, New Hampshire.

Helen and Blaise at Dartmouth

Helen's life at Dartmouth revolved around the Aquinas House Catholic Student Center, where she rarely missed an evening Mass and devotedly participated in many spiritually based campus activities. With seemingly effortless grace, she excelled in her twin majors of biology and chemistry. The only dissonance that marred her beatific college experience was her troubling indecision about her career direction—whether to become a basic scientist or a physician. The high-class dilemma was solved when one of her professors recommended that she become a physician/scientist, an M.D., Ph.D.

> **Helen Byrne:** Oh, I didn't realize that people could do both.
> **Professor Horace Hoff:** Most people can't, but *you* can.

Blaise's Dartmouth world was no less intense but far more diverse than was Helen's: ski team, campus politics, fraternity, alcohol, and coeds. Perennially among the best Division 1 collegiate skiers, he followed in the tracks of his parents with his selection to the national ski team. A business major, he chose academic courses at the graphic intersection of least work demanded with highest grades awarded. Not that skiing was Blaise's only skill: He was a great salesman, and his number one product was himself. He sold himself to important people, and the most compelling to Blaise was his fraternity brother,

Leighton Albright Jr. Leighton was the fourth generation of Albrights at Dartmouth, but more compelling to Blaise than Leighton's academic heritage was that he was rumored to be the scion of the wealthiest family of all current Dartmouth undergraduates. Over time, Blaise endeared himself to Leighton's father, the president and CEO of his family's privately held commodities trading company.

In the first semester of her sophomore year, Helen found her first boyfriend. Evan Walters was a junior and as shy and religious as Helen. Founded on shared religious values and interests, their relationship was closer to a friendship than an infatuation. Familiarity and companionship trumped attraction and romance. Evan majored in philosophy and comparative religion, and he took a position with Teach for America in New Orleans after his graduation. Over that summer, Evan and Helen gradually tapered their letter writing and phone calls. Helen was "unattached" when she returned to Dartmouth for her senior year. She was far more concerned about her applications to medical school than she was about having a boyfriend.

When he first saw Helen in November of his senior year, Blaise had come to Dartmouth's Baker-Berry Library to hang up posters for his campaign for student governing body president. Certain that he knew every beautiful female upperclasswoman on campus, Blaise assumed that Helen was a freshman. Because Blaise didn't spend as much time in bioscience laboratories or at the Aquinas House as he did at his fraternity house and in the local pubs, Helen's and his paths had never crossed. With the confidence based on skills honed and rewarded since his childhood, he strode up to the carrel where Helen was working to introduce himself.

Blaise Hartman: Where are you from?
Helen Byrne: Schenectady, New York.
Blaise: Are you a freshman?
Helen: No, a senior.
Blaise: Are you a transfer or an exchange student?
Helen: Neither. I am a senior at Dartmouth College; what about you?
Blaise: I'm also a senior. I'm running for student government president; do you have a few minutes so that I can solicit your support?
Helen: I apologize, but I don't. I have a genetics midterm tomorrow, and I am a bit behind schedule in my studies.

> **Blaise:** Then you should have some time after your midterm to be my guest this Saturday night at the homecoming weekend party at my fraternity house. It won't get started until about midnight, so you'll have plenty of time to do other things beforehand.
>
> **Helen:** No, I'm sorry, but I can't make that, either. Thank you for asking me, though.
>
> **Blaise:** Oh, I think I'm catching on. You're either married or have a steady boyfriend.
>
> **Helen:** I think it is best that I get back to my work now. Good luck with your election.

Although, by almost any standard, Blaise Hartman's track record with women was formidable, this was not the first time that he had been "blown off." In the past he reasoned that rejection "was just an inescapable cost of doing business. There always would be plenty of other opportunities to hit a homer with someone else just as hot." This time, however, striking out was different for him. As a consummate competitor, Blaise recognized an unusual strength and confidence in Helen's responses; it was a quality that he admired. And she was beautiful. He decided to go against one of his fraternity brother's rules: "Never take anything personal about getting laid or about not getting laid." Helen had affected him in a deeply personal way, and he did not have a clue as to why. It was a new feeling; it was uncomfortable, but he liked it. He was drawn to her.

Blaise Hartman: Psychodynamics of a Salesman

Blaise Hartman's considerable talents as a salesman can be traced to his childhood. The following are his skills and their psychodynamic sources.

Understanding the Product

Blaise's product was himself. With a disinterested father and a self-absorbed, overwhelmed mother, by necessity, he had been selling himself since childhood. He came to understand that his differentiating feature would be his skiing excellence. From observing his parents, however, he also understood that skiing would take him only "to the next level."

Fierce Competitiveness

Given that Blaise initially had to sell himself through his skiing excellence, he became fiercely competitive. There were three components to his competitiveness: 1) He was *proud*. Not only would he not tolerate defeat, he refused to accept that anyone could be better than he was—whether on his own team or an opposing team. He attacked every downhill run. Regardless of whether he was in practice or in a tournament, he skied flat out. 2) He was *fearless*. Unafraid of injury, he would always be on the edge of wiping out by going too fast for the construct of a particular course or for that day's snow and ice conditions. He took dangerous falls many times and was injured occasionally. But these setbacks never altered his all-out competitive approach. 3) He was *persistent*. Blaise usually knew what he wanted, and he would not give up until he got what he wanted. He did not take it personally, nor was he not put off by people saying no to him; rather, he perceived a "no" as a challenge. He reasoned—sometimes correctly and sometimes incorrectly—that if he were getting too many "easy yeses," he was playing it too safe; he was not being sufficiently aspirational. Too many easy wins could also mean that his competition was weak, which could dull his competitive edge. He had made up his mind that if he did not get what he wanted, it would not be for lack of trying. Giving up was not permissible to Blaise Hartman.

Analytical Nature

Because he perceived himself as having so little, there were many, many "things"—from objects, to opportunities, to positions, to people—that Blaise wanted. Before going after anything he wanted to get, or to which he aspired, he would think through carefully what would be required for success. For example, he wished to be the preeminent downhill skier of his generation, so he broke down championship skiing into the distinct elements that he believed were necessary for him to achieve this goal. He sought out the best coaches, worked out tirelessly to maintain his optimal physical condition, raced against the top-tier skiing competition, and researched and managed to procure and use the most advanced ski equipment. Most of all, he was relentless about detecting and overcoming any technical deficiencies that he might have. With the goal of self-improvement, he would watch and critically analyze tapes of his own runs, those of his competitors, and those of the all-time champion skiers. Like all great skiers, he was always looking for "an edge."

Attractive Persona

Blaise inherited not only athletic skills from his parents but also their attractiveness. Both of his parents were striking in appearance. Had they not been accomplished athletes, they could have been models. Tall and blond, Blaise's body was well proportioned and muscular from countless hours of conditioning. Consistent with his balance and nimbleness in skiing, he held himself and moved with a dancer's grace. He knew that people liked to be around him and to be seen by others in his company. Keenly aware that women were attracted to him, Blaise clearly understood the value and power of his physical attributes. He used his attractiveness as lure and payoff to get what he wanted—be it a sandwich, sex, or a recommendation for a scholarship to Dartmouth.

"Reading" People Well

Growing up without the benefit of his parents providing even the bare necessities for survival, Blaise realized early on that he would have to "depend on the kindness of strangers" to get "things" and to get by. This entailed the following: 1) identifying those who had sufficient resources or knowledge to fulfill his needs; 2) recognizing those who were likely to give him what he wanted, if he were to approach them in "the right way"; and 3) figuring out what these people wanted or needed from him in return and how best to give it to them. Blaise learned to size up people rapidly and accurately.

Blaise's Baggage

Blaise Hartman could sell himself to other people, but could Blaise sell himself to Blaise?

Self-Esteem

Positive self-esteem is multidetermined—including a person's temperament, life experience, and accomplishments. A major determinant of self-worth is how a person was prioritized and treated throughout childhood by his or her primary caregivers, most often

the parents. One only has to observe toddler-age children's independent play to gain a sense of the power and importance of their relationships to their caregivers. For example, as a two-and-a-half-year-
old child plays, periodically he or she will look over to the caregiver
for signals of her involvement and her approval. If, when the toddler
looks over, the mother smiles and communicates back to the child
how wonderful she believes her child's activity to be, the toddler will
immediately refocus on his or her play. If, however, the caregiver appears upset or disinterested, the toddler will desperately try to engage the caregiver to engender positive signals. The toddler will
become frustrated and will not return to independent play without
succeeding in doing so. In fortunate circumstances, an involved
caregiver communicates love and approval to a child hundreds of
times each day.

Those who do not receive such attention during critical phases
of their childhood often carry, indefinitely, unconscious beliefs and
pervasive feelings that they are less worthy, valuable, and valid than
their peers. They often feel more comfortable *pursuing* love and affection than *receiving* such. Because Blaise did not believe himself to
be worthy of love, he harbored only one fear of which he was
aware—a vague, ephemeral dread that always stalked him. The fear
of being "found out," of being exposed as a fraud.

Crossing the Edge

Despite his many gifts and accomplishments, Blaise could not escape
the effects of his deficient parenting. He tended to hide his family
heritage and inflate his accomplishments. For example, he was less
than honest about his academic record, his family's financial situation, and the important people who were among his friends.

In alpine skiing, small fractions of a second discriminate between
the winners and the losers, between the famous and the forgotten.
Accordingly, *all* world-class downhill racers look for the competitive
edge. Small advantages in technique, strength, and equipment determine success or failure. Blaise realized that the early acquisition
and application of information about technical breakthroughs—
both in equipment and technique—helped him gain advantage over
his rivals. Razor-thin lines often divided what was within or outside
the rules. For example, which ski waxes are permissible and which

ones are prohibited because they are unsafe or lead to unfair advantages? Which dietary supplements and drugs are allowed and which are disallowed because they are determined to be performance enhancers?

To Blaise, these rules—*all* rules—seemed arbitrary, and bending the rules became just another aspect of sport and life. *Breaking* a rule was never his concern, but *getting caught* breaking a rule was a form of defeat. Blaise never was caught breaking a rule, but, as in all competitions at the highest levels, whether sports or business, other competitors suspected him of doing so. They, too, knew the limits.

Exploitation of Others

Although artfully masqueraded, Blaise's sole "cause" was himself. His unswerving attention to himself was his response to receiving so little from his parents. He sought out relationships solely on the basis of their benefits to him. And when the benefits ran out, so did he.

Blaise had no idea as to why he was so attracted to Helen. Yes, she was beautiful, but Blaise had little trouble attracting other beautiful women. At first, he did not even know whether or not she came from a wealthy, well-placed family, which he had "forever" strategized to be an important consideration for any long-term relationship with a woman. What Blaise also did not know was that he had correctly "read" Helen, particularly her powerful, elegant, effortless self-presence. He sensed that she knew who exactly she who was, which was totally consistent with the type of person that she wanted to be. She was self-possessed in a way that was inexplicably attractive to him.

Subliminally, Blaise also sensed from how Helen responded to him in their first encounter that she did not rely on the opinions of others for her self-definition. (How different from him, whose self-definition was entirely reliant on how others valued him.) He would later discern that her power came from within and was based on internalized values of Christianity and her family. It was a form of power that he perceived intuitively in Helen, and he also instinctively knew it to be a power that he did not himself possess. He envied Helen for that power and wanted to "possess" that power. In a primitive, unconscious fashion he strived to capture and extract Helen's moral potency for himself by winning her. It was the primeval, primary-process blood lust of ancient warriors who would eat the hearts of lions in their efforts to become braver. But would he have to kill this gentle lion? Perhaps, in a spiritual sense.

All these longings were distant from Blaise's consciousness. What he *did* know was that he *wanted* Helen, and, as he had done since childhood, he would wield all of his skills as a consummate competitor and salesman to get what he wanted.

Blaise Hartman's Pursuit of Helen Byrne

Planning the Attack

Although fearless, Blaise Hartman was by no means reckless. Notwithstanding his expertise and confidence as a skier, he rarely descended a challenging slope without first carefully studying the course. He took great care of his product: himself. After having gently been rebuffed by Helen in his first foray, he sought to learn what he could about her before approaching her a second time.

Daniel Webster, who was graduated from Dartmouth in 1801, was famously quoted to have said about his alma mater, "It is, Sir, as I have said, a small College, and yet, there are those who love it." Little had changed over the succeeding two centuries. Dartmouth admitted only a relatively small number of undergraduates and had only begun to admit a modest number of women in the early 1970s when Helen attended. Given the small number of coeds at Dartmouth, Blaise was confident that he could find out a great deal about Helen from his fraternity brothers and his friends on the various athletic teams. He was wrong: no one seemed to have heard of her. Characteristically, he remained persistent in his search until he came across a senior premedical student from another fraternity who knew her:

> **Elliott Irving:** She is quiet, very studious, and very intelligent. I was her lab partner in organic chemistry, and she was always well prepared and unruffled. She was super polite and never talked about herself. All the other premeds thought that she did especially well in her sciences classes, but we were never certain *how* smart she was until we read in *The Dartmouth* that she was elected to Phi Beta Kappa as a junior. She might be the first woman in the history of the college to get in Phi Beta Kappa as a junior.

Blaise Hartman: So she's smart. I've got that. But what about her personal life? Do you know if she dates anyone seriously?

Elliott: If she does or ever did, she never talked about it. She doesn't give off vibes that she is someone who is that interested in being asked out, however. Someone told me that she is very religious and spends a lot of time at the Catholic Student Center. Maybe she is a lesbian.

Blaise: Trust me on this one, Elliott, she might be a religious freak, but she likes men. That is definitely a vibe that I picked up.

Blaise next approached a former girlfriend who had spent some time at the Catholic Student Center, and she confirmed how devout, modest, and studious Helen was. He also learned that she was currently unattached and very likely "inexperienced with guys," which Blaise interpreted to mean that she was a virgin.

Although both of Blaise's parents were nominal Protestants and although Blaise had never attended a church service in his life, he was aware that his maternal grandmother was Catholic. After carefully researching the history and customs of the Catholic religion, Blaise decided to wait 3 weeks until Advent Sunday to attend morning Mass at the Aquinas House. Predictably, Helen was also in attendance. After the services, Blaise approached Helen for the second time.

Blaise Hartman: Hello again, Helen. This is my first time at Mass since I came to Dartmouth. I am seeking to learn more about my spiritual roots. Do you come here often?

Helen Byrne: Yes, I do.

Blaise: I have been reading up on the Catholic religion. Although I experienced very little religious training at home, somehow I feel drawn to the Catholic faith. I would love to become more active at Aquinas House. But because I'm on the ski team, I won't have a whole lot of time to spare over the next 4 months. Could you recommend someone who would orient me to the activities here?

Turning Points

Every life has its critical moments when the most significant life-altering decisions are made, and this was one such moment for Blaise and Helen. Both Blaise and Helen departed significantly from their customary patterns of self-definition and decision making. As fate would have it, both decided *not* to play it safely.

Blaise

Always the accomplished salesman, Blaise's usual practice was first to "read the customer" and then to alter his sales pitch according to what he had picked up about that individual. Because Helen gave off so few clues about whether or not she had any interest whatsoever in what he was selling (i.e., himself), initially, he was uncertain how to frame his "pitch." In a creative leap that augured his future brilliance and success as a deal maker, Blaise spontaneously decided to do something diametrically different from "business as usual": he would tell the *truth* about his family, his past, and himself! Well, almost.

Helen

Helen and her life were not complicated: Church, family, and studies. Each came with its own clear rules and values, which she followed with the honesty, earnestness, and ability that obviated her need to take risks or to exaggerate. For example, even though she was applying to the most competitive programs at the top-ranked medical schools, she had no need to embellish or even highlight her achievements in her application essay. When one has the highest grade point average of any science major in her Ivy League college, has near-perfect scores on her Medical College Admission Test, and is universally adored by her faculty, one can afford to be understated. Helen's best defense against her shyness and modesty was that she had no reason whatsoever to call attention to herself.

But, as any gifted competitor understands, with great strengths come great vulnerabilities. For example, strength is a vitally important asset in college wrestling. When a skillful, accomplished wrestler competes against a stronger opponent, he will find a way to use his adversary's strength to his advantage. After all, wrestling is not a weight lifting contest. Blaise understood this principle, as well.

Helen's deep belief in Christian charity led to vulnerabilities: 1) She felt it to be her duty to reach out to help those who are materially and spiritually bereft. 2) Helen's intense devotion to her parents made it difficult for her to distinguish herself or to separate from them. 3) Her unalloyed work ethic in school left little spare time for her to date young men or to become worldly, psychosexually. Blaise would exploit each of these vulnerabilities.

When Blaise asked Helen to recommend someone to introduce him to Christian life at Aquinas House, she did not recommend the pious Monsignor William Nolan (Father Bill), who was its first director and was actively involved in Catholic student life there. Instead, she volunteered to do so herself. She instinctively knew that Blaise was very different from the members of her family and, somehow, he seemed more exciting than the few fine young Christian men whom she had dated previously. In the most stimulating and unsettling way, it was Blaise's novelty as an outsider that she found most attractive about him. In the contemporary parlance among young women, he was a "bad boy." So, for the first time in her life, Helen took a risk. However, Helen did not appreciate what every experienced investor knows: with significant risks come steep downside consequences.

> **Helen Byrne:** There will be a full-day retreat at Aquinas House next Sunday. Do you think that you can make it? You can have the opportunity to meet and ask questions of the religious staff and to meet some of the student regulars.
> **Blaise Hartman:** I wouldn't miss it for the world. I'll be here next Sunday in time for Mass. By the way, Helen, you look so beautiful in your purple dress. I learned in my reading about Catholicism that purple is a holy color for the Advent.

Blaise and Helen

Blaise immersed himself in Catholicism while simultaneously spending more and more time with Helen. She became not only his religious guide but his girlfriend. After dating each other for about 2 months, they had the following conversation:

> **Blaise Hartman:** Growing up, I had no sense of family. I could never depend on my parents to be there for me when I needed them. Because they seemed to neglect nearly everything, I did not appreciate how inattentive they were to my spiritual growth. Can you imagine, Helen, a little boy being alone in the world without even a connection to a faith?
> I always dreamed that someday I would get married and have a family of my own. That I would *belong* somewhere in this wide universe. I am passionate about having children and giving them the love and attention that I never received myself.
> **Helen Byrne:** If you would want me, I can be your "connection." I will *always* be there for you. I would *never* let you down.
> **Blaise:** If this is a proposal, Helen, I accept with all of my heart.

Blaise's fraternity brothers and teammates could not believe the transformation in him. He no longer chased women or got drunk every weekend. He became a regular at church. Although they missed his exciting companionship, they believed that Helen was the best thing that ever happened to their friend. One recurrent refrain was "If you have to give up the good life, Blaise, Helen is the only chick we know who is worthy of doing it for."

Helen and Blaise planned to visit her parents on Easter to announce their engagement.

The Love of a Father

Blaise did not ask Patrick Byrne for his daughter's hand in marriage. On Easter morning he and Helen simply announced to her parents that they were engaged and planned to be married at the end of the coming summer. Almost as surprising for Mr. and Mrs. Byrne as the engagement announcement was that Blaise had declined sleeping on the convertible sofa bed in the den. Instead he slept in Helen's bedroom, which had only one bed.

> **Mrs. Louise Byrne:** You should be ashamed of yourself for looking so glum, Patrick. We've never seen Helen happier. It's just not right for you to drag around looking like someone died.
>
> **Mr. Patrick Byrne:** Don't you think this is all a bit too fast? What's the big hurry?
>
> **Mrs. Byrne:** I think the timing is perfect. Helen will be going to medical school in New York City next year. I'd be worried to death if she were in that big city all by herself. Blaise will be there when she comes home late at night to take care of her and protect her.
>
> **Mr. Byrne:** And just how do we *know* that? And how on Earth would he know *how* to do that?
>
> **Mrs. Byrne:** He's a man, Patrick, and a great athlete to boot. I don't follow what you're getting at.
>
> **Mr. Byrne:** You heard what Helen told us about his family life. What kind of role models were his father or his mother? Call me old-fashioned, but I believe that every son needs both a mother and a father.
>
> **Mrs. Byrne:** Oh, I understand now. Of course it's so hard for you to see Helen grow up. To build her own life apart from us. I know how close the two of you are. You have always been her role model, and now a new man has come into her life. It's only natural, Patrick, but if you're worried about something, why don't you just talk to her?

Mr. Byrne: You know that I'm much better with numbers than I am with words, but I will try.

The evening before Blaise and Helen were to go back to Dartmouth, Mr. Byrne asked Helen if he could speak to her privately.

Mr. Patrick Byrne: Sweetheart, I'd like to ask you to put off marrying Blaise for at least 1 year.
Helen Byrne (*bursting into tears*): I thought you would be happy for me, Daddy. I love Blaise with all of my heart.
Mr. Byrne: You are so inexperienced with young men, Helen. He's practically the first person you have ever dated. How do you know that he is right for you?
Helen: I know my own heart, Daddy. Please don't do this to me. It will destroy me if you and Mom don't love Blaise as much as I do. I know he's much smarter than I am, he's a better person than I am, and he's learning to love Jesus just as much as we do. What possibly could you not like about him?
Mr. Byrne: What are you saying? On what basis can you say that he is more intelligent than you are? Are you a better athlete that he is? I know my daughter. No one is a better person than you are. I can't put my finger on it, sweetheart. But I just don't trust him.
Helen (*now hysterical*): You're ruining everything for me, Daddy. I don't want to talk about it anymore. This is supposed to be one of the happiest days of my life, and you've made it the very worst day. What's wrong with you? Why can't you just be happy for me and just leave us alone?

A sick, panicky feeling overtook Patrick Byrne after this conversation with his beloved daughter. He sensed that Helen was in danger and knew that he was powerless to help her. He was unable to put into coherent thoughts or words what was troubling him about Blaise. He could not understand how a person could love and respect God if he didn't love or respect his own parents.

In the companion text to this book, *Fatal Flaws* (Yudofsky 2005), I included a rating scale whereby people could assess whether or not they are in an important relationship with someone who might have a personality disorder. If Helen had completed this scale at the time of the Easter visit to her family, Blaise would *not* have been rated as "likely" to have a personality disorder. In Table 7–1, the bold number indicates Blaise Hartman's score on the Fatal Flaw Scale during the courtship phase of his relationship with Helen. (Questions for which she did not have personal knowledge were left unscored.) He would have rated only "1" on the 10-point scale. The one question in the Fatal Flaw Scale for which a negative answer would have placed him in the "possible personality disorder" category was "Do *other* people whom I love and trust the most believe this person is good for me?" (question 10). Helen's father and several of her friends did not believe so. They did not trust Blaise. They were uneasy about his family background, about the rapidity of his behavioral transformation, about the fit of his values and personality with Helen's, and about how soon they were getting married after first meeting each other. The bottom line is that there was insufficient time for Helen or her family to secure reliable information. Table 7–2 indicates how Helen filled out this scale when in treatment with me several decades later.

A scientist, Helen's father believed in gathering and analyzing data with deliberate caution before arriving at conclusions and making decisions. Intuitively, he felt that when people are moving too rapidly toward an answer, they are likely not collecting sufficient data to arrive at a valid conclusion. In my clinical practice of psychiatry I have witnessed the unbearable anguish of parents who are powerless to rescue their children from destroying their lives through their relationships with people with severe, persistent, untreated personality disorders. As a parent myself, my heart goes out to you, one and all.

Married Life

Transitions

Blaise

Selected since his freshman year of college by the U.S. Ski Association (USSA) as a member of the U.S. national ski team, Blaise received notification in his senior year that he was chosen to be on the Olympic ski team. His selection to participate in the Winter Olympics was not a surprise to anyone who followed the sport closely, but his response was shocking. He declined. For nearly everyone who competes at Blaise's level, skiing in the Olympics is the dream that

TABLE 7–1. Fatal Flaw Scale for Blaise Hartman, completed by Helen Hartman, courtship phase

The following scale is in the form of a questionnaire that will help you determine whether or not a person with whom you have an important relationship has a fatal flaw of personality and/or character.

Please check the best answer, "yes" or "no," to the following questions regarding the person with whom you have an important relationship. If you are not sure, mark that answer "No."

1. Do I trust this person?	**(Yes)**	(No)
2. Has this person "come through" on important commitments?	**(Yes)**	(No)
3. Do I feel better about myself as a consequence of this relationship?	**(Yes)**	(No)
4. Does this person consider my needs equally to his or hers?	**(Yes)**	(No)
5. Is this person sensitive to and supportive of me?	**(Yes)**	(No)
6. Will this person communicate with me honestly on significant issues affecting our relationship?	**(Yes)**	(No)
7. Is this person honest with other people and trustworthy in his or her other relationships?	(Yes)	(No)
8. Do I and, if applicable, my children always feel physically safe with this person?	(Yes)	(No)
9. Does this person respect rules and obey laws?	**(Yes)**	(No)
10. Do *other* people whom I love and trust the most believe this person is good for me?	(Yes)	**(No)**
Helen's total score for Blaise Hartman before marriage:	(7 Yes)	**(1 No)**

Directions: Total the number of "No" answers that you checked.

Scoring

0 "No"—*Highly unlikely* that this person has flaws of personality and character.	
1–3 "No"—*Possible* that this person has flaws of personality and character.	
4–5 "No"—*Probable* that this person has flaws of personality and character.	

TABLE 7–1.	Fatal Flaw Scale for Blaise Hartman, completed by Helen Hartman, courtship phase *(continued)*
5–10 "No"—*Highly likely* that this person has flaws of personality and character.	

Source. Yudofsky SC: Narcissistic personality disorder, in *Fatal Flaws: Navigating Destructive Relationships With People With Disorders of Personality and Character.* Washington, D.C., American Psychiatric Publishing, 2005, pp. 11–15. © 2005 American Psychiatric Publishing. Used with permission.

has motivated them since childhood. Being on the Olympic team is a pinnacle—with winning a medal being the only peak that is more lofty. Few competitors are asked to be members of an Olympic team, and almost no one who *is* asked turns down the opportunity. Speculation ran rampant in the ski world and among Blaise's friends about the reason for his decision to demur. Was he injured? Was he suffering from some sort of medical condition, like cancer? Did he violate a USSA rule by taking performance-enhancing drugs or by using illegal equipment in the trials? Did he have a psychiatric problem? Revealingly, no one who knew him well conjectured that he was fearful of the competition or of failure—which was not even remotely the case. Nor did anyone guess his real reason.

For Blaise, skiing at his level of international excellence was neither an avocation nor a vocation. Competitive skiing at the international level demands too much work to be fun, and, as Blaise learned full well from the example of his parents, it led almost nowhere as a profession. His goal was not to train the children of the big shots who lived in the enormous houses in Lake Tahoe; he aspired to *be* one of those big shots and to *own* one of those houses. Blaise had long accepted that, for him, skiing was no more than a means to an end.

Blaise chose to go to Dartmouth not because of its outstanding ski team but rather because it was a sturdy platform from which to launch his business ambitions. Through Mr. Albright, the wealthy father of a fraternity brother, he had secured a prime job in New York City as a commodities trader, and he had no further need to waste time on a frivolous sport. For Blaise, skiing had petered out before what others might have regarded as the "finish line" of a long, steep slope.

The salesman in Blaise would not permit a dramatic moment to pass unexploited. When he received a letter from a reporter from a

TABLE 7–2. Fatal Flaw Scale for Blaise Hartman, completed by Helen Hartman, several decades later

The following scale is in the form of a questionnaire that will help you determine whether or not a person with whom you have an important relationship has a fatal flaw of personality and/or character.

Please check the best answer, "yes" or "no," to the following questions regarding the person with whom you have an important relationship. If you are not sure, mark that answer "No."

1. Do I trust this person?	(Yes)	**(No)**
2. Has this person "come through" on important commitments?	(Yes)	**(No)**
3. Do I feel better about myself as a consequence of this relationship?	(Yes)	**(No)**
4. Does this person consider my needs equally to his or hers?	(Yes)	**(No)**
5. Is this person sensitive to and supportive of me?	(Yes)	**(No)**
6. Will this person communicate with me honestly on significant issues affecting our relationship?	(Yes)	**(No)**
7. Is this person honest with other people and trustworthy in his or her other relationships?	(Yes)	**(No)**
8. Do I and, if applicable, my children always feel physically safe with this person?	**(Yes)**	(No)
9. Does this person respect rules and obey laws?	(Yes)	**(No)**
10. Do *other* people whom I love and trust the most believe this person is good for me?	(Yes)	**(No)**
Helen's total score for Blaise Hartman after marriage:	(1 Yes)	**(9 No)**

Directions: Total the number of "No" answers that you checked.

Scoring

0 "No"—*Highly unlikely* that this person has flaws of personality and character.	
1–3 "No"—*Possible* that this person has flaws of personality and character.	
4–5 "No"—*Probable* that this person has flaws of personality and character.	

TABLE 7–2. Fatal Flaw Scale for Blaise Hartman, completed by
Helen Hartman, several decades later *(continued)*

5–10 "No"—*Highly likely* that this person has flaws of
   personality and character.

Source. Yudofsky SC: Narcissistic personality disorder, in *Fatal Flaws: Navigating Destructive Relationships With People With Disorders of Personality and Character.* Washington, D.C., American Psychiatric Publishing, 2005, pp. 11–15. © 2005 American Psychiatric Publishing. Used with permission.

national sports magazine asking him to explain why he decided not to compete in the Olympics, he issued the following press release:

> I wish to express my gratitude to the U.S. Ski Association and to the United States Olympic Committee for affording me the great honor of being chosen as a member of the Olympic ski team. I also wish to thank my many outstanding coaches and teammates, especially those on the national ski team and at Dartmouth, for your hard work, support, and friendship that resulted in my having this unparalleled opportunity in the first place.
>
> Respectfully, I am declining the offer for two reasons. First, prior to my being invited to join the Olympic team, I accepted a job offer to work next year in New York City for Mr. Leighton Albright Sr. at Enterprise Capital Investments. This is also a once-in-a-lifetime opportunity, and I am compelled to honor the commitment that I have made to Mr. Albright. Second, I am engaged to be married in several months to a lovely young woman with whom I will graduate Dartmouth this spring. Helen will begin medical school this fall at Columbia College of Physicians and Surgeons in New York, and I will spend any free time that I might have away from Enterprise Capital Investments to support her in her new life adventure.
>
> Competitive skiing is a jealous taskmaster that requires full-time involvement. After a wonderful lifetime of fidelity to this incredible sport, I am moving on to new commitments.
>
> This winter I will join all of you as an enthusiastic fan at the edge of the slope to cheer on our U.S. Olympic ski team to victory.

The sports magazine published Blaise's press release in its entirety, and a delighted Mr. Albright republished the release in his company's weekly newsletter. Blaise also saw to it that a copy of the release was sent to Helen's parents, who, on reading the release, had the following conversation:

Mrs. Louise Byrne: Now doesn't this make you feel much better about Blaise, dear? Look at how much he is giving up in order to take care of our daughter.

Mr. Patrick Byrne: These are pretty words; but actions speak louder than words. Let's wait and see what he *does*, not what he *promises*.

Helen

Helen was accepted by every medical school to which she applied. During the previous two summers, she had worked in the molecular genetics laboratory of a neuroscientist at Harvard Medical School. Originally, the Harvard M.D./Ph.D. program was her first choice. Although Columbia College of Physicians and Surgeons had outstanding programs in her primary areas of interest, Helen chose to attend Columbia because Blaise's new job was also located in New York City. However, she issued no self-serving press release about her decision. Helen understood and accepted that sound relationships involved give and take, and she was led by Blaise to believe that he was *giving* a great deal. He had agreed to convert to Catholicism, had stopped his weekend binge drinking, and had told her that the main reason that he passed up the Olympics was to build a life and a family with her. He had even met her "halfway" about sex. In junior high school, Helen took a chastity vow that she would not have sexual intercourse prior to getting married. Blaise tried in vain to convince Helen that because they intended to get married in the future, she could have sex with him without breaking her vow. He also made it clear to her that it was quite a sacrifice for him "to give up having sex for such a long time." Nonetheless, Helen would not consider violating a solemn oath. One of the reasons that Helen had agreed to marry Blaise so soon after having first met him was so that he would not be "unduly deprived" (as he put it) for too long. Although Helen was completely unaware of such, Blaise's early signs as a master negotiator and deal maker were evident and operant throughout their courtship.

Two Young Lives in New York City

Helen

For Helen, medical school and New York City were "business as usual." Organized, disciplined, motivated, maturely involved, and profoundly interested, Helen thrived, seemingly effortlessly, in the combined medical and graduate school program at Columbia. Her routine was to arrive at the medical school at about 6:00 A.M. and to leave by 6:00 P.M. in order to get home in time to make dinner for Blaise. Commuting by subway on the A-train and then taking a bus to their apartment took about an hour each way because they chose an apartment in southern Manhattan, near the Wall Street firm where Blaise worked and the athletic club where he worked out. Mr. Byrne, however, did not fail to notice that his daughter had to travel in the dark to and from Washington Heights through what he considered to be dangerous areas of the city "in order to accommodate Blaise."

Blaise

Although commodities trading was new to Blaise, the same qualities that led to his success in alpine skiing turned out to be well suited to his new position at Enterprise Capital Investments: hard work; intense focus; careful analysis; ability to spot trends and patterns and to make instant decisions; and a delicate balance of fearlessness and careful, rapid risk assessment. As in skiing, trading and investing have winners and losers, and finding an edge to apply to the throats of competitors is fundamental to victory. The commodities company for which Blaise worked specialized in metals and minerals trading, with a smaller subdivision that traded in agricultural products. Soon recognizing that he was relatively deficient in the sophisticated quantitative skills that formed an important tool of this trade, Blaise arranged to work under the tutelage of Neil Kahn, Ph.D., a 38-year-old minerals trader who was a whiz in mathematics and statistics. The pair had complementary assets, with Blaise exhibiting special talents for information acquisition, strategic thinking, and developing and exploiting professional relationships, while Dr. Kahn was exceptionally proficient at data analysis. Information must be accurate, but the big money is made by securing key information before other investors do. Right up Blaise's alley.

Their Marriage

First Four Years

It certainly is not unusual for newlywed spouses who are beginning their careers to have limited time together. Both Blaise's vocation and Helen's profession are notorious for their time demands. It is the rule, not the exception, that young commodities traders work 7 days a week for long hours each day. Additionally, when traders deal in international markets, as is the case with rare metals, their working hours occur at irregular times of the day or night. Blaise frequently traveled internationally and remained at work until late at night or all night much of the time that he was in New York. The net result was that, for the first several years of their marriage, Blaise was almost never home during the times that Helen was there.

Not that Blaise's quality of life was that lacking. He regularly entertained clients at New York's most exclusive restaurants. When he traveled, he flew first class and stayed in five-star hotels. He developed an interest in and facility for golf "because that's where lots of business contacts are made and deals get done." Dutifully, he played golf nearly every weekend on some of the finest courses in Westchester County, southern Connecticut, and northern New Jersey. He also developed another new hobby: collecting and enjoying fine wines.

Although it upset Helen that she rarely was able to be with her husband, she was understanding and never complained. She believed in him and therefore believed him when he told her how much he disliked entertaining, traveling for business, and being away from her. Helen worried incessantly about how hard Blaise worked and the job pressure to which he was subjected. From preparing elaborate meals to doing his laundry to managing all the household chores and expenses, she did everything possible to support and encourage him. Little was reciprocated, however. Blaise never asked Helen about her courses in medical school or her research in graduate school, nor did he demonstrate interest in getting to know her classmates or faculty mentors. Consequently, her closest friends at Columbia never met Blaise, nor was Helen invited to join her spouse when he entertained for business.

> **Blaise Hartman:** Sweetheart, there is no need for you to join us for dinner. All we do is talk about business—numbers, markets, and finance. You couldn't follow a thing that we were saying.

As her father had pointedly mentioned to her several years earlier, Helen was at least as proficient with numbers and statistics as Blaise was with skis, but she did not object to being left out of Blaise's business entertaining.

The only cards or gifts that Helen received on her birthdays and their anniversaries were from her parents and brother. But Helen always understood and never complained: Blaise was a busy man.

Year Five

While yearning to spend more time with her husband, Helen took full advantage of her time alone to devote to her study of basic science and medicine. She was identified early on as a rising star by the Columbia faculty, particularly as a gifted and creative hypothesis-driven scientist. During years three and four in her combined M.D./ Ph.D. program, Helen pursued her research in the molecular genetics of neurodevelopmental disorders of children. She loved children and was passionate about conducting relevant research that led to easing the suffering and increasing the potentials of disabled children. She also decided to take a residency in pediatrics after graduating from medical school.

Many years later during a psychotherapy session, Helen described this period in her life as follows:

> **Helen Hartman:** I became pregnant with our older daughter during my fourth year at Columbia and gave birth to her right before I was to begin my clinical rotations. Although I was approved to take 3 months off from school, I never went back. I had very mixed feelings about returning. On one hand, I loved school and remained passionate about science and becoming a physician. Since Blaise was away so much, my medical career had become much of my identity. On the other hand, I wanted to be with our new baby almost every moment. I had been commuting to and from medical school every day on crowded subways and was wasting 2 hours each day that I could have otherwise been with our daughter. You spent years at Columbia, Dr. Y., and must have taken the A-train many times. You know that the train is far too crowded and noisy to study on. I was torn, but Blaise made the ultimate decision. He told me, "Since I am so busy, our daughter needs one of us with her at all times. I don't want her to be abandoned by her parents like I was. You're it. Besides, medical school makes no sense for us: You will waste tons of time to make piddling amounts of money. Let me take care of that part, and you take care of the baby."

Blaise Makes His Move

Moving Out: An Immodest Proposal

Blaise and Neil became widely known as innovators in investing and trading in the rare metals that are essential to certain components in cellular phones and other mobile devices that were just beginning to gain wide usage at that time. Soon their division became a strong profit center of Enterprise Capital Investments. By almost any standard, the pair was highly compensated for their accomplishments, but not by Blaise's standard. In fact, he resented being paid such a small fraction of what he believed that he was bringing in by himself. Hardly mindful of the fact that the Albright family had been in the financial business for nearly 100 years, that their company had built up significant capital and had earned a spotless reputation for integrity and reliability—qualities that are the lifeblood of their industry—Blaise considered himself as central to their current and future success.

He had been at Enterprise Capital Investments for 6 years when he scheduled an appointment to meet with Mr. Albright.

> **Blaise Hartman:** I have a proposal to make to you, sir.
>
> **Mr. Leighton Albright:** Go for it.
>
> **Blaise:** Our industry is changing, and we are missing out on the big money. As you know, 6 of the top 10 commodities firms trade in global oil and other energy products. There is also huge money to be made in hedge funds. We don't do either, but we could easily.
>
> **Mr. Albright:** So how do you propose that we address that?
>
> **Blaise:** Let's establish new divisions of both. I'll head them up; do a lot of the trading myself; and recruit and train a group of young, bright, competitive-as-hell other traders. I'll need about $250 million of Enterprise capital to start off with—before we are in a strong enough position to go to outside investors to raise money for the hedge fund.
>
> **Mr. Albright:** A quarter of a billion dollars is nearly half of our cash reserves. That's a huge gamble for something that we haven't done before. And what's your piece, Blaise?
>
> **Blaise:** I'd want total control of both divisions and 75% of all the profits that we bring in.
>
> **Mr. Albright:** There is no denying that you have done a great job for us, Blaise. As you know, however, your proposal is a total

departure from how we do business and how we pay our traders. You've been at this for only about 6 years and still have a lot to learn. Both you and the company are making good money doing what we are doing now, and we have no need to take on such a huge risk. Perhaps we should start off more modestly. Perhaps you can gradually fit in some energy trading along with your rare metals work. Just to get a sense of how it might go.

Blaise (*shocked and noticeably enraged*): It won't work unless we do it as I proposed. One needs lots of capital to be players in the energy markets. It's either all or none.

Mr. Albright: In that case, the answer is "no."

Blaise: Then in that case, I resign. I'll clear out of here today!

Moving On

Once more, Blaise brandished the skills that he had learned during his impoverished childhood to further his business ambitions. Taking quite naturally to the concept of the expense account, he managed to live quite lavishly in one of the world's most expensive cities while rarely spending his own money. From restaurant bills to his health club membership, from golfing tee fees to the rent for his apartment ("home office"), Blaise denoted almost every dollar that he spent as a so-called business expense covered by Enterprise Capital Investments (doubtlessly, a practice that did not go unnoticed by Mr. Albright). Consequently, he spent very little of his mid to high six-figure income and had accumulated several million dollars over the first 6 years of his employment. This, however, is "chump change" in the high-stakes world of energy trading.

Relatively deficient in resources, Blaise was never wanting in resourcefulness. Perennially industrious on his own behalf, Blaise had combined his personal attractiveness with his position and access at Enterprise Capital Investments to establish a strong network of friends and colleagues among international commodities traders. One consistent piece of advice he received was that if he wanted to be in the "big leagues" of energy trading and energy-related hedge fund deals, he would have to move to Houston.

> **Blaise Hartman:** I have been thinking about our children, Helen. I don't think that Manhattan is the best environment for them to grow up in.

Helen Hartman: What makes you say that?

Blaise: The values are so superficial here. Everything boils down to how much money you have. Also, it's a dangerous place for children. It's not safe for little girls to play by themselves outdoors with so many perverts and drug dealers everywhere. I would like them to grow up in a place like we did, a place with safe, green neighborhoods where they can run and play outside without their lives being endangered.

Helen: Where do you think would be better? The suburbs of Boston or New Haven?

Blaise: I was thinking Houston.

Helen (*in shock and disbelief*): Houston, *Texas?* We'd be so far away from my parents and from our church. Also, I had hoped someday, when the girls are on their own, that I could go back to my research and medical studies at Columbia, Harvard, or Yale.

Blaise would never go into an important negotiation unprepared. He had anticipated Helen's concerns.

Blaise Hartman: That's the beautiful part, Helen; Houston is the perfect place for children *and* medicine. We could live in a beautiful, safe neighborhood called Bending Brook, and the girls could attend a wonderful Catholic girls' school, St. Mary's Academy. I looked into it carefully, and it's very much like the Notre Dame Girls' School where you attended—small, with outstanding academics.

And when you are ready to go back to school, Houston would also be perfect. It's the up-and-comer in medicine. Baylor College of Medicine is supposed to be developing one of the strongest genetics and neuroscience programs anywhere, and Texas Children's Hospital is absolutely first rate. And guess what they're strong in? Developmental disorders of children! Of course, I will have to leave my job at Enterprise and find something related to commodities trading to do down there. But we've saved up some money, so we'll be OK. Most importantly, our kids will be safe and grow up with good values.

Moving In

Blaise left a highly paid, secure position in New York to move with Helen and their two daughters, ages 4 and 1, to Houston, where he had neither a job nor firm prospects for one. A paradoxical asset that Blaise had gleaned from the harvest of deprivations of his childhood was his familiarity and comfort with uncertainty—including how he would use his own ingenuity on a day-to-day basis to come up with the necessities of life. On their plane ride to Houston, Blaise recalled his first flight from San Francisco to Boston en route to Hanover, New Hampshire, where he was to begin his freshman year at Dartmouth. Other than his ski equipment, his one suitcase contained the entirety of his possessions. He had spent all of his money on the airfare. But mostly, he recalled that he was going to a place where he had never been before and that he had no place to go back to. His father had moved to Switzerland to live and work in a resort as a ski instructor. Additionally, Blaise was told in no uncertain terms that he was unwelcome in the household of his mother and her third husband. By comparison, his sojourn to Houston was a veritable cakewalk to a fertile garden of opportunity where he was absolutely confident that he would sink deep and sturdy roots into oil- and gas-enriched ground.

True to his word to Helen, Blaise purchased a spectacular home on Forrest Drive in Bending Brook, one of the best addresses in one of the most exclusive neighborhoods of Houston. Given that neither he nor Helen knew a thing about interior decorating, he commissioned an interior design firm to furnish the home as well as the spacious suite of offices that he had leased in downtown Houston. He then persuaded Neil Kahn to join him, offering a high salary, a generous package of incentives, and potential bonuses from his newly founded company, Alpine Capital Enterprises (ACES). On his first day at work, Dr. Kahn looked up at Blaise, who was seated at a huge, empty desk in his spacious, oak paneled office amidst a suite of 15 other furnished, vacant offices and asked,

Dr. Neil Kahn: And now what, Blaise?

Blaise Hartman: And now we begin. Remember this moment, Neil; I'm going to make you very rich.

Moving Up

Anchored for the first time in his life by a sense of place and independence, Blaise began making the rounds to every oil titan, energy trader, and venture capitalist in Houston who would agree to meet with him. Essentially, he made the same proposal to them as he had to Mr. Albright, but this time, most listened attentively and several were interested. The salesman had found his customers, and the products cost millions of dollars. Blaise thought confidently to himself, "I now know that I made the right move getting away from the self-righteous, risk-aversive Northeast and going to Houston, where it's still the Wild West. I can work with these gunslingers, and we'll carry the future of energy trading with us."

Within 6 months he had raised sufficient capital to begin trading in energy futures and related investments as well as to establish an energy-based hedge fund, for which he had also landed several significant investors. Blaise was now ready to recruit traders and analysts, to set up his infrastructure, and to shape his company's culture. Once more he planned to apply the lessons he had learned about winning from competitive downhill skiing to Alpine Capital Enterprises:

Lesson 1: He would hire only the best, which, in commodities trading and investment analysis, meant the most intelligent, prepared, competitive, and cutthroat people.

Lesson 2: There are winners and losers; for every dollar that ACES makes, someone else loses a dollar. For every dollar that some other firm makes, ACES loses that dollar. ACES would be a place that was hospitable only to winners.

Lesson 3: The traders at ACES should compete with one another to bring in the best deals. The winners would make the most money, which could be astronomical. The losers would be fired—usually unceremoniously, on the spot, after bad trades.

Lesson 4: Every day is a new race. What you did yesterday—no matter how profitable—doesn't matter today. The money that you bring in today is the only thing that counts.

Lesson 5: *Every* investment decision would be made by Blaise. Others might load the gun, but only Blaise was permitted to pull the trigger.

Blaise cultivated a stressful working atmosphere, which he believed kept his team sharp and on their toes. Reasoning that each trader should be racing flat out for gold, and lots of it, every day (and night), he wanted the office to radiate with the tension and anxiety of the final run for an Olympic gold medal. Hardly the absent or passive CEO, Blaise spent his days in front of a colossal bank of computers in search of information, trends, and market opportunities. His instinct for edges paid off, and his trades and purchases vastly surpassed those of any other member of his team. On those nights when Blaise wasn't at his desk in the pursuit of international trading, he hosted dinner meetings with institutional investors in his hedge funds or spent the evening in negotiations with partners in joint ventures.

Blaise's intensity, competitiveness, and cutthroat business practices were controversial. On one hand, he was respected, liked, and trusted among those for whom he made large sums of money in brief periods of time. On the other hand, he was feared, despised, and distrusted by his competitors and by many of his own employees, who felt abused, exploited, and/or cast aside. In addition, because he was delivering returns that considerably exceeded his industry's averages, rumors abounded that Blaise was violating accepted business standards and probably violating federal laws regulating financial transactions. Although there were fact-finding investigations by federal regulators of several of his most profitable transactions, no violations were uncovered or lawsuits filed. Blaise's business practices were an extension of his values and narcissistic personality disorder, as will be amplified later in this chapter. Table 7–3, which is taken from the companion book *Fatal Flaws* (Yudofsky 2005), highlights 20 common characteristics of narcissistic managers.

Life in Houston

Helen's Adjustment

Although Helen did not know a single person in Houston and was uncomfortable in her palatial new home in Bending Brook, she adjusted to her new life far more easily and rapidly than she had anticipated. To her surprise, she found the people in her fashionable neighborhood warm and inviting to her and her children. The mothers of young children in the neighborhood found commonality in Helen's values as a parent and were drawn to her understated warmth and modesty. Helen enrolled her oldest daughter in the prekindergarten program of St. Mary's Academy and was immediately connected into the school's familiar, comfortable, comforting, and confining spiritual network. Although she missed the intellectual stimulation and gratifications of medical school and although Blaise was rarely at home, Helen felt less lonely and disconnected in Houston than she had in New York.

TABLE 7–3. Twenty common characteristics of narcissistic managers

---

1. They value the loyalty of their subordinates more than their competence or productivity

2. They overestimate their own knowledge about nearly every area of the business or organization

3. They do not appreciate the important contributions of others

4. They take personal credit for the accomplishments of others

5. They are competitive with and threatened by peers and competent managers

6. They micromanage competent subordinates in areas in which they themselves have little expertise

7. They insist on making all decisions—even minor ones—themselves, often with insufficient information about and understanding of the relevant issues

8. They overstate their own and the organization's successes—to the point of bragging

9. They never admit to making mistakes

10. They blame others for their own mistakes and failures

11. They distrust, intimidate, or fire subordinates who make independent decisions or raise concerns about their questionable decisions or business practices

12. They surround themselves with "insiders" who constantly praise and never disagree with them

13. They do not mentor their subordinates or advance their careers

14. They pursue highly visible (i.e., flashy) short-term successes at the expense of supporting solid, long-range strategic plans

15. They misappropriate the organization's resources for their personal benefit and self-aggrandizement

16. They devalue and underestimate the achievements of competitors in similar businesses or enterprises

17. They miss out on important opportunities by not recognizing their own lack of knowledge in some areas

18. They display great deference and respect for their superiors to their faces yet criticize, devalue, and undermine them behind their backs

TABLE 7-3.	Twenty common characteristics of narcissistic managers *(continued)*

19. They respond to constructive criticism of their work with anger, defensiveness, and thoughts or acts of retribution

20. They prioritize their own ambitions for advancement over the needs of the organization

Source. Yudofsky SC: Narcissistic personality disorder, in *Fatal Flaws: Navigating Destructive Relationships With People With Disorders of Personality and Character.* Washington, D.C., American Psychiatric Publishing, 2005, p. 106. © American Psychiatric Publishing, 2005. Used with permission.

Blaise's Adjustment

Blaise had dreamed since childhood of owning and living in one of the mansions that clung to the steep mountainsides of Incline Village, Nevada. He had also understood early on that the singular key to the stately doors that guarded those manors was as cold and deep as the mountain snow that surrounded them in January: cash. In his first 5 years in overheated Houston, he amassed an ever-increasing fortune that rivaled those of many with houses on the mountains stretching above Lake Tahoe or in his live oak–shrouded Bending Brook neighborhood. No longer a pretender or aspirant, Blaise was well on his way to wealth and power, but he still did not feel that he had arrived.

Beyond wealth, he longed for what he believed to be the two measures of having "arrived" in Houston: acceptance and access. Memberships in the Houston chapter of the Young Presidents' Organization (YPO) and in the Bending Brook Country Club would provide both. YPO is an international organization of business leaders under 50 years old, and there are stringent requirements for eligibility. Among these requirements are that members must lead a company with at least 50 full-time employees and with a net worth of at least $10 million. If the company is a financial institution, the average annual assets managed must be at least $160 million. One additional requirement is that the total compensation of all employees, excluding the compensation of the candidate, must be greater than $1 million per year.

By year five, Alpine Capital Enterprises exceeded YPO's minimum membership requirements manyfold. For example, 11 of

Blaise's traders earned more than $3 million that year. The Houston chapter of YPO is particularly strong, and its membership, which is by invitation and application only, provides invaluable access to business and avocational opportunities. Blaise's home in Bending Brook was literally around the corner from the main building of the Bending Brook Country Club. The windows of many of the grand rooms in his home framed the meticulously tended, verdant fairways of its golf course, which he could play only by invitation of a member. This was a daily reminder to Blaise that, despite his growing fortune, he still was not on the inside. Not yet where he had to be.

The family of Charles Coverdale was among the original members of the Bending Brook Country Club. Mr. Coverdale was also one of the first major investors in Alpine Capital Enterprises' energy hedge fund, from which he had earned enormous returns. Blaise and Mr. Coverdale developed a personal relationship, and Mr. Coverdale had taken Blaise under his wing to introduce him to some of Houston's and Texas' most able investors. Mr. Coverdale had been a member of the YPO until he turned 50 years old, whereupon he transitioned to the World Presidents' Organization. Blaise was not shy about asking favors from those whom he had enriched.

> **Blaise Hartman:** I was checking out the requirements for the Young Presidents' Organization, and I believe that I now qualify. Can you advise me, Charles, how I should go about applying? I also would like to look into becoming a member of Bending Brook Country Club. Many of the friends of my daughters go there to swim and for tennis and golf lessons. It's like the neighborhood playground for them, but we don't belong.
>
> **Mr. Charles Coverdale:** As you may know, I was a member of YPO until I got too old. And a long, long time ago I also was one of those little kids splashing around in your neighborhood pool. You should be a slam dunk to get into YPO, but Bending Brook Country Club may take some doing. Most of the members of Bending Brook have known each other since *they* were kids. You are relatively new to town, so we have to work on getting them to know you. I'll do everything in my power to help. And having lived here all my life, Blaise, I know a person or two in this town, and some of them owe me big favors.

To Mr. Coverdale's surprise and to Blaise's fury, the membership committee of YPO did not approve Blaise's application. Mr. Coverdale speculated that he was passed over because too few of the members of YPO knew Blaise or Helen personally.

> **Mr. Charles Coverdale:** YPO is less important to you and your family than becoming members of Bending Brook Country Club. I think that some people at Bending Brook may know about you through your business accomplishments, but they will also want to know about your spouse. My wife and I will help Helen get better known in town.

Mr. and Mrs. Coverdale decided to do a makeover on Helen so that she would fit in better with the women members of Bending Brook Country Club. They believed that her hairstyle, makeup, wardrobe, and accessories were too pedestrian and had to be made over. They also thought that Helen spent too much time "with the wrong people," which meant her friends from church, which, along with her children's school, was located in a section of Houston quite distant from the Bending Brook area. Mrs. Coverdale especially believed that Helen's jewelry could "use an upgrade." At Mrs. Coverdale's direction, Blaise purchased an 8 carat diamond engagement ring with a matching diamond necklace, bracelet, brooch, and earrings. Given that he rarely acknowledged special occasions or gave Helen gifts, the "girl's best friends" were certain to be unexpected arrivals.

> **Blaise Hartman:** I have a surprise for you, Helen.
>
> **Helen Hartman** (*opening her gifts*): Oh my heavens, Blaise. What on Earth are these for? What has gotten into you?
>
> **Blaise:** You have never had an engagement ring. I always wanted to get one for you, but we never could afford it. Now we can, and I want you to have this one. And Helen, I want you to wear it every day.
>
> **Helen:** Oh Blaise, I have always been happy wearing my grandmother's wedding band. It has great sentimental value to me, and it's really all that I would ever want. What matters most to me would be if you could find the time to spend more time with our girls and with me.
>
> **Blaise:** You've just cut yourself a deal, Helen. You're a tough bargainer. You wear the jewelry—the ring and earrings every day—and I'll carve out more time to spend with the family. In fact, let's start by going to the Houston Grand Opera Ball this weekend with the Coverdales. It's about time we started supporting

the arts. Mrs. Coverdale knows all about that stuff, so she will take you to Neiman's and get you all fixed up for the fun.

The jewelry was just the beginning of Helen's "upgrade." Mrs. Coverdale was insistent that the children be transferred from St. Mary's Academy, where they were very happy, to a private, nonsectarian school near Bending Brook: "It is absolutely essential that your children become schoolmates and friends with the kids whose parents belong to Bending Brook Country Club. That's the best way for 'the right people' at the club to get to know you." Accordingly, Blaise tried to convince Helen that it would be in the best interest of their daughters, who, like their mother, were gifted in mathematics and science, to attend a private school in Bending Brook that was especially strong in these academic areas.

> **Helen Hartman:** Our daughters have wonderful teachers and friends at St. Mary's, so why do they need to change, Blaise? I am more interested in our girls being happy and having a good Christian education than I am in their learning math and science.

Always prepared, Blaise presented to Helen a dossier of comparative data that included standardized test results, National Merit scores, faculty educational backgrounds, and college selections of graduates.

> **Blaise Hartman:** Helen, you are being purely emotional and not rational. If this did not involve our children's futures, I would let it go. But I will have to insist for once. I have already made arrangements for their transcripts and tests scores to be collated by St. Mary's, and I have enlisted an educational consultant to assist us with their application process.

As usual, Blaise prevailed. However, Helen held the line with respect to Blaise's assertions that Helen change churches to a larger one in Bending Brook that Mrs. Coverdale advised would advance their social status in Houston.

Blaise's Fury

Blaise does not compete to lose. He spent 3 years of preparation before asking Mr. Coverdale to put up the Hartman family before the

Membership Committee of Bending Brook Country Club. From being the omnipresent sponsor and host of a wide array of charitable events to learning to shoot deer, pheasants, and wild pigs to purchasing a ranch at which to entertain his Bending Brook neighbors and their children, Blaise invested inordinate amounts of his time and treasure in advancing his candidacy. Without question, he knew far more about the history, members, and admissions guidelines of the country club than many of its long-time members. Always confident in his charm and salesmanship, Blaise thought that the face-to-face meeting with the Membership Committee went well. He had not appreciated, however, that his reputation for ruthlessness, arrogance, and possible dishonesty was well known to the members of that committee and had influenced their decision. He would have been stunned had he known that the strongest factor weighing in his family's favor was Helen, who was beloved by her neighbors, many of whom were members of the club.

> **Charles Coverdale:** I got bad news, Blaise: the Membership Committee did not approve your application. When I asked them what the problem was, they said that they didn't believe that you would fit in well. I don't have a clue what in hell that means. You got more money and class than that whole damn committee put together. Sorry, buddy.
>
> **Blaise Hartman:** You did your best, Charles. And I thought that I did too, but apparently I am mistaken. Anyway, thanks for all your help.

While managing to maintain his composure with Mr. Coverdale, Blaise was enraged. His blowtorch fury flared in three directions: toward the club; toward the business community of Houston, which he was certain had undermined him; and toward Helen.

> **Helen Hartman:** I know how much this meant to you, Blaise. But these things work out for the best. We have to respect that the committee knows what's best for all concerned.
>
> **Blaise Hartman:** Are you too dumb to get it, Helen? This town has just told me, you, and our children what they think of us. They think we're shit! And you did more than your part to convince them that they're absolutely right. I know that you could care less about being a member of that club, but did you ever think for one minute about supporting me and your children? If I cared, you should care. End of story. But all that you

care about is your church. Where do I come into the equation? I promise you this: our relationship will never be the same.

Blaise did not keep this promise to Helen, entirely: their relationship was more of the same.

Blaise's Revenge

Shift

Releasing a tectonic plate of seismic force that had been building up pressure for each of Blaise's 43 years, the rejection by Bending Brook Country Club set in motion a destructive fury from which there was neither resolution nor return. Deep in his being, Blaise had always believed that life's race had been fixed against him from the starting gate, and, although frustrated and furious, he felt strangely liberated. Never having trusted the rule makers, at long last he was free to run the course his way. At the end of the day, he was the only member of any team, club, or family on whom he could rely. Everyone else was either against him, holding him up, or holding onto the stuff—and the access to the stuff—that he wanted for himself. And when he got what he wanted, he would take delight in rubbing all their faces in his winnings.

Bending Brook Country Club

Blaise never again cast his eyes on the forbidden fairways of the Bending Brook Country Club, nor would he enter the club's premises. Immediately on learning of the decision of the Membership Committee, he ordered that paper sheeting be fitted over the windows of his house that faced the club, and shortly thereafter, he sold the estate. He purchased and moved into an even more extravagant home on a nearby road that rivaled Forrest Drive in its exclusivity.

Business

Determined to beat the Houston business establishment at its own game, Blaise pulled out all the stops in building Alpine Capital Enterprises. First, he bought out every Texas-based investor who had stock in his company: "I don't care if I have to overpay them; no more free rides on my back for these ingrates," he fumed. Next, he established political, personal, and business relationships with selected leaders of foreign nations with mammoth oil and gas reserves and other energy-related interests, opened several offices abroad and in the Caribbean region, and transformed ACES into a multinational corporation.

Honore de Balzac's oft-quoted aphorism "Behind every great fortune lies a great crime" is actually misquoted from the French. The true lines and their English translation are as follows:

> *Le secret des grandes fortunes sans cause apparente est un crime oublié, parce qu' il a été proprement fait.*
>
> The secret of great fortunes without obvious source is a crime that is forgotten because it was done properly.

Crouched in the shaded difference between the Balzac quotation and its translation is a fragile "safe zone" between riches and ruin where Blaise began to operate his company and guide his personal business dealings. Slalom skiing was never Blaise's best event because his love of speed and victory too often led to infractions from cutting the boundary poles too closely. Nevertheless, he was irresistibly drawn to shortcuts, risks, and stratospheric payoffs. Through bribery of international political leaders, through shady stock transfers, through cleverly disguised violations of U.S. trade agreements and trade embargoes, Blaise amassed enormous capital, which he then invested legally for his own account. One among many examples was based on his early recognition of the game-changing potential of combining the fracking process with horizontal drilling to open up gigantic, previously inaccessible reservoirs of North American oil and gas. He surreptitiously "borrowed" large sums of money that others had invested in his energy-based hedge funds to purchase for himself, at bargain rates, immense stakes (i.e., leases) in energy and mineral rights in the Eagle Ford, Marcellus, and other shale oil and gas plays in Texas, Louisiana, Ohio, West Virginia, Pennsylvania, North Dakota, Colorado, Alaska, and Canada. Others who tried such schemes were discovered and prosecuted, usually because market fluctuations in the prices of oil and natural gas resulted in their running out of money before they could repay the vast sums that they had secretly "borrowed" from investors in other deals. But this did not happen to Blaise.

The key words in Balzac's actual quotation are *properly* and *forgotten*. Blaise built for himself a "great fortune" by executing his shady dealings so adeptly that they remained undiscovered and eventually forgotten. By age 50, he had moved entirely back into legal investments and business practices. Once again clean, the urine of the champion skier could now be aimed safely and squarely at those whom he believed had betrayed, excluded, and humiliated him. And Helen was on that list.

Helen

Blindsided by Blaise's blaming and punishing her for their not getting accepted to Bending Brook Country Club, Helen searched her soul for what she had "done wrong." She struggled to make changes in herself to salve her husband's wounds and repair their marital relationship. She confided to a close, well-intended friend that Blaise no longer was interested in her sexually. Her friend advised Helen to hire a personal trainer "to get her body back in shape" and to pay more attention to her grooming and attire. Her friend opined, "How we look is so much more important to some men than who we are." Dutifully, Helen obliged, but Blaise continued to ignore and belittle her.

> **Helen Hartman:** I worry that we spend so little time together, Blaise. I thought that, with our girls growing up and needing less of my time and with your business doing so well, we could have more time to be together.
>
> **Blaise Hartman:** And what would you suggest that we do together with all that freed-up time? Go to church? Or would you like to join me this Thursday at Smuggler's Notch to ski the triple-black-diamond Black Hole run? The truth is, Helen, that we have nothing in common and that you bore me to death.
>
> **Helen:** We're married, Blaise, and we are meant to be together. Maybe it would help if we talked to a couples counselor.
>
> **Blaise:** You mean a priest or some crazy shrink? Not in my lifetime.

Over the next several years Blaise was rarely at home. Devoting most of his time to business and recreation, he rarely demonstrated interest in or involvement with his wife and daughters. He traveled internationally to watch sporting events and to go on skiing, hunting, and fishing expeditions with business associates and friends. He even missed his older daughter's graduation from high school in order to attend a World Cup soccer match. When he was home, he was pitilessly critical of Helen's appearance, intelligence, and shy temperament.

The Cases of Mrs. Helen Hartman and Mr. Blaise Hartman: D1 (Discovery) Component, Part II—Treatment

Pseudoindividuation

Engaging in her biweekly psychotherapy with the same openness, dedication, and intellectual curiosity that, three decades before, she had applied to her studies, Helen posed the following question in her third week of treatment:

> **Mrs. Helen Hartman:** Dr. Y., why do you think that Blaise married me in the first place? I never could figure that out.
>
> **Dr. Y.:** That's a better question for your husband to answer, Mrs. Hartman. To paraphrase John Lennon, I hope, someday, that he'll agree to join us in treatment so that we might ask him that very question. My supposition, however, is that he will not readily be able to answer your question without some help. But I have a related question for you.
>
> **Mrs. Hartman:** Yes?
>
> **Dr. Y.:** Why did you marry Blaise?
>
> **Mrs. Hartman:** Oh my heavens! Can you believe it, Dr. Y.? I have never asked myself that question. I'm not sure right off. Please help me start.
>
> **Dr. Y.:** Do you remember your feelings when you *first* met Blaise at the library at Dartmouth?
>
> **Mrs. Hartman:** That was so, so many years ago. I know that I found him interesting, but, again, I am not certain as to why.
>
> **Dr. Y.:** Were you attracted to Blaise?
>
> **Mrs. Hartman:** He was a most attractive young man, and I'm sure I noticed that. It would have been impossible not to. But I was so shy and inexperienced with men that if I were sexually attracted to him, I might not have admitted it to myself.
>
> **Dr. Y.:** And his personality?
>
> **Mrs. Hartman:** He was assertive and very self-confident. That hasn't changed. Do you think I was attracted to those qualities, Dr. Y.?

Most things that are significant to us come with "trade-offs." Even the most selfless, supportive, nurturing parents and families breed special challenges. Under these beatific circumstances, children may have difficulties separating and individuating from their parents, particularly with being able to determine whether important life choices and decisions are truly their own or their parents'. Power struggles and adolescent rebellions may occur that are terrifying and painfully confusing to the caring parents. Sometimes, our children learn from and are strengthened by the experiences associated with their rebellions, but, all too often, our children make self-destructive interpersonal choices with tragic long-term consequences.

Frequently, young adults who are trying to individuate from their caring parents do, indeed, select friends and spouses whose values and capacities for reciprocal, lasting, mature relationships are diametrically opposite of those of their parents. What remains the same, however, is that their self-agency remains overly influenced by others—but this time people who are self-serving. I term this dysfunctional, often dangerous, state *pseudoindividuation.*

Knowledgeable and skillful mental health professionals can be of invaluable help to children and families in traversing these troubled waters or, less desirably, in repairing the wreckage that occurs when our children do not cross, unscathed, the battering torrents of their rebellions. Most often the mental health professionals arrive at the same conclusions and make identical recommendations as the caring parents. However, adolescents and young adults will accept from their therapists the identical advice that, time and again, was bitterly rejected when offered by their parents. When treating young adult patients and their families in these circumstances, I watch as the parents glance at one another in frustrated disbelief when their children regard and grasp onto my recommendations as if they were etched into stone tablets that had come down from Mt. Sinai. At the appropriate time in the future, I explain to the loving parents that, paradoxically, it is precisely because they (the parents) are so important and authoritative to their children that their progeny *cannot* and *will not* accept and follow their advice. Their children incorrectly perceive that to do so would be for them to lose their sense of individuation and agency.

Few seniors at Dartmouth were more devoted to and influenced by their families than was Helen. As angelic as she might have been at that time, Helen also was not immune to the more liberal influences of college, to her concerns over finding a suitable young man to marry and with whom to have children, to her sexual attraction to Blaise, and to her family-based psychodynamics. Recognizing and taking full advantage of her inexperience, ingenuousness, goodness, and conflicts, Blaise sold himself to Helen as a lost soul who was searching for intimacy and personal meaning. She was attracted to the "bad boy" for whom she could serve as a bridge to a life of commitment, intimacy, and spirituality. And because Blaise was not the young man whom her parents would have chosen for their daughter, he was all the more attractive to her. What Helen could not possibly have understood at the time was that Blaise was not predisposed to growth and change and that she merely had transferred her agency from her parents to him.

> **Mrs. Helen Hartman:** Next to my children, the most important thing in my life has been to make Blaise happy, but I am never able to do so. In fact, he always lets me know how much I am disappointing him. Over the course of my marriage, I have lost most of my self-confidence.
>
> **Dr. Y.:** And much of yourself.
>
> **Mrs. Hartman:** What do you mean by that?

In treatment, Helen became aware that she had traded away much of her professional ambition and self-definition—her career in science and medicine as well as her close relationship with her parents—for the illusory salvation of the soul of and intimacy with a man who was disinterested in both. She came to realize that such a bargain should not have been necessary in the first place. With great pain and at long last, Helen accepted the futility of her endless efforts to change herself to please Blaise: no matter how much she changed, it would never be sufficient.

> **Mrs. Helen Hartman:** So where do I go from here?
>
> **Dr. Y.:** Back to yourself, Helen. You can't aim higher than that.

Back to Herself

Helen devoted the next year of her psychotherapy to gaining further insight into the psychodynamics that led her to be attracted and committed to Blaise as well as to a realistic appraisal of her future options and opportunities. Blaise persisted in his refusal to join Helen in treatment and continued to be irritable and verbally abusive to her at home. On one occasion in therapy, she confided,

> **Mrs. Helen Hartman:** About 3 years before Blaise's accident and long before I began meeting with you, Dr. Y., my daughter Mary surprised me by asking how I could stand remaining married to her father. I was taken aback by her question. Mary finally told me, "All of my high school friends know that Dad is always cheating on you. They hear it from *their* parents. Don't you get it, Mom? He only cares about himself. He doesn't really care about you or about us."
>
> I then confronted Blaise with what Mary told me. He then told me that he was no longer attracted to me and added, "Don't ask me about other women, Helen. I learned in business never to ask a question when you don't want to know the answer."
>
> **Dr. Y.:** And then how did you respond?
>
> **Mrs. Hartman:** I have never again discussed Blaise's infidelities with him. I spoke to my priest, however. Ruling out divorce or separation, he said, "Two wrongs don't make a right." He made it clear that my moral duty is to remain true to my marital vows—no matter how my husband behaves. The motto of my high school was "Christian commitment never ceases." So I'm stuck.
>
> **Dr. Y.:** Not entirely.
>
> **Mrs. Hartman:** How so?
>
> **Dr. Y.:** You can go back to yourself, Helen. We can't aim higher than that.
>
> **Mrs. Hartman:** You said that once before, Dr. Y., but now I want you to be more specific. Are you saying that I should reapply to medical school?
>
> **Dr. Y.:** *You* are the world's authority on *you*, Helen. No one else is able to define you. Not your parents, not Blaise, not your children, and certainly not I. You have to decide what you want.
>
> **Mrs. Hartman:** How strange, Dr. Y., I just now remembered that it was my parents—not I—who first decided that I should become a doctor. They were practical people. They thought that I could always earn a good living as a practicing physician. However, in college and in graduate school I discovered my *real* passion is for research and the basic science of medicine. Do you think I should reapply to graduate school *and* medical school?
>
> **Dr. Y.:** Since I'm a physician, Helen, you probably assumed that I would prefer you to pursue an M.D. degree. But it's not about what I think....

Central Unresolved Conflict of Mrs. Helen Hartman

Helen was stuck in pause not only in her unhappy, disparaging marriage but also with regard to her actualization of her potential as a mature, independent professional. She learned that she had transferred her strong dependence on her parents' values and expectations of her to Blaise without going through a stage of individualization and self-agency. Until her treatment, she had failed to ask herself, "What do I want for myself?" and "How do I expect that I should be treated by my husband?" Her unresolved conflict related to dependence versus individuation. At its extremes, Helen's conflict is approach-approach: wanting to depend too much on the values and expectations of her parents or husband conflicted with her wanting to individuate from them and determine her own path and self-definition.

Key Features of Mrs. Helen Hartman's Being Stuck in Pause

1. *How Helen was stuck:* In a disparaging, destructive marriage
2. *Goals for change:* Become her own person
3. *Central, unresolved conflict* (approach-approach): dependence versus individuation
4. *Hallmarks of Helen's being stuck:* Demoralization, confusion, low self-esteem, amotivation, anxiety
5. *Binary problem/solution:* Abused, exploited wife/independent professional
6. *Critical decision points:* Reapply to graduate school in neuroscience; make decisions and act independently of the will of her husband
7. *Corollary factors required to achieve resolution:* Continued psychotherapy to gain insights into the psychodynamic reasons that she relinquished personal agency and permitted and tolerated marital abuse
8. *Resolve the problem:* Individuate from husband, pursue her career

The Power of No and the Power of Go

In Helen's case, the application of the Power of No and the Power of Go is more subtle than for most individuals who are stuck in pause—but no less important. As in all cases wherein this binary technique is implemented, both cognitive and behavioral aspects are involved. A component of Helen's psychotherapy was to learn how to recognize when she made decisions that were based on what other people wanted or expected of her while simultaneously working to identify what she would choose to do independent of the desires, expectations, and needs of others. For example, Blaise expected his wife to dress in a certain fashion that he believed reflected positively on him and his position—referred to in psychoanalytic terms as Helen's comprising a *narcissistic extension* of himself. For the entirety of her marriage, Helen chose clothing on the basis of whether or not she felt that her husband would approve. When looking at herself in the mirror while trying on a new dress in a department store, she would ask herself, "How would Blaise think I look in this dress?" If the answer were affirmative, she would purchase the dress without probing whether she herself liked it.

In treatment Helen was encouraged to pause before making any decision and ask herself whether the decision was being made to please others or to please herself. Given her altruistic nature and focus on pleasing others, the line between establishing personal agency and what she might view as "selfishness" was, at first, difficult for her to draw. In treatment, she learned to ask herself such questions as "Don't I have the right and responsibility to choose for myself clothes that I like and in which I feel I look the best?" After she determined what she wanted, the Power of No would be deployed to resist doing what others wished and the Power of Go would be utilized to move forward with effecting what she wanted for herself. This process proved more challenging than Helen had anticipated, but, always intellectually "open" and a hard worker, she improved substantially over time.

Another example of applying the Power of Go related even more fundamentally to her identity and how she would live her life going forward. After his injury, Blaise demanded that his wife spend most of her time at home caring for his physical needs. Given her profound sense of marital duty and responsibility, it was difficult for Helen to assay how she, herself, would like to devote her time, efforts, and intellect. Through treatment she realized that she wished to return to her graduate school studies but felt conflicted about "abandoning" her husband. She utilized the Power of Go to take the necessary steps to hire home health care workers to care for Blaise, despite his strong objections. She also utilized the Power of Go to take the steps required to reapply to graduate school and, once accepted, to make the many decisions involved in the intensive pursuit of a demanding career.

Neurodevelopment

Helen rigorously prepared for the examinations that are required for admission to graduate school in the biological sciences. Simultaneously, she studiously reviewed the revolutionary scientific advances in the neurosciences and molecular genetics over the two decades since she had left medical school—especially as these fields of basic science impacted pediatric neurodevelopmental disorders. To no one's surprise but her own, she was enthusiastically accepted into the graduate program in neurosciences at Baylor College of Medicine, where she excelled.

> **Mrs. Helen Hartman:** I had forgotten how much I love learning and love science. I also love being around people who are like me and who like me. I haven't been this happy since I was a junior in college.

Over Blaise's objections, Helen hired home care specialists to be with her husband on a full-time basis, and she leased a small office near the medical center where she studied when not in classes. She developed close friendships with her fellow students as well as with the Baylor College of Medicine Graduate School and Medical School faculties. Her energy, happiness, enthusiasm for life, and self-esteem increased progressively. After her daughters left home for college, she went home mostly to sleep.

Helen was beginning her second year back in graduate school when she scheduled an urgent meeting with me.

> **Mrs. Helen Hartman:** I am so sorry to impose on your time, Dr. Y., but I am quite concerned about Blaise. Over the last month or so, he has become much less irritable but much more withdrawn and negative. He talks about feeling hopeless and being worthless. As you know, this is so unlike him. He hasn't mentioned suicide, but I worry that he might do something to himself. Would you see him?

Dr. Y.: Of course I will, Helen. But will Blaise agree to see me?

Mrs. Hartman: I asked him that, and he said he would as long as he could see you by himself. You and I both know he will feel humiliated having to ask for help.

Dr. Y.: Are you OK with my evaluating Blaise without your joining us? At least to start.

Mrs. Hartman: As you know so well, Dr. Y., my problem isn't with trusting people too little but with trusting them too much. I have been working on that, but in this case, I'll make an exception.

Dr. Y.: If that's a compliment, thank you. I'll notify Mrs. Hoffman to schedule Blaise in as soon as we hear from him. You are correct to be concerned about his safety.

Before I see Blaise, I would like you to fill out a scale regarding Blaise's potential for having a personality disorder. The Fatal Flaw Scale is rated from the perspective of someone who is in an important relationship with that individual.

Helen's rating of her husband after 23 years of marriage is represented by the bold number in Table 7–2 (p. 199). On the basis of Helen's rating of Blaise on the Fatal Flaw Scale, 9 out of a possible 10, it is *highly likely* that he has flaws of personality and character. It is important to emphasize that had Helen filled out this scale prior to their marriage (see Table 7–1), Blaise would have scored only 1 out of 10 (p. 197). Blaise did not reveal these flaws at the time. People with narcissistic personality disorder characteristically hide unfavorable aspects of their personality during the courtship phase of relationships, but these flaws inevitably emerge over time. Table 7–4, from the companion book, *Fatal Flaws*, summarizes the three phases of marriage to a person with narcissistic personality disorder. Helen's experience is an example of the fact that when one rushes into making commitments for long-lasting relationships, one is all too often running away from painful truths.

Psychiatric Care of Mr. Blaise Hartman

Hitting Bottom

Mrs. Hoffman scheduled Blaise to meet with me one evening after his call to my office. As is my practice for initial evaluations of patients with neuropsychiatric disorders, 2 hours were allotted for this appointment.

TABLE 7–4.   Three phases of marriage to a person with narcissistic
personality disorder

Courtship phase

Is attentive to and considerate of prospective partner

Idealizes prospective partner

Exaggerates, embellishes, and lies about personal accomplishments to
appear unique and attractive

"Sells" himself or herself to family and close friends of prospective
partner

Marital Phase

Becomes progressively critical and devaluing of spouse and his or her
immediate family

Is competitive with spouse for the attention and admiration of others,
including the children

Tries to control the spouse though psychological and emotional
manipulation, such as by communicating anger and contempt when the
spouse acts independently or even expresses opinions that are different
from his or her own

Tries to control the spouse by making all important family-related
decisions, especially those related to finances

Becomes emotionally detached from spouse

Refuses to assume a fair and reasonable share of marital responsibilities

Either neglects his or her children or seeks to gain the attention and
admiration of others through the children

Engages in secretive, dishonest, and unsavory relationships outside the
marriage

Becomes emotionally and/or physically abusive to spouse

Dissolution Phase

Becomes enraged and abusive when spouse challenges his or her
exaggerations, embellishments, and dishonesties

Blames spouse for all of the problems in the relationship and the
marriage

Through lies and distortions, seeks to turn family members and mutual
acquaintances against spouse

Transfers dependencies from spouse to other parties outside the
marriage and family

TABLE 7–4.	Three phases of marriage to a person with narcissistic personality disorder *(continued)*

Dissolution Phase *(continued)*

Feels entitled to an undue proportion of the marital assets

Deploys distortion, coercion, and deceit to secure the material assets of the marriage

Wields children as a weapon to harm spouse and to leverage from the spouse an undue share of marital assets

Once divorce is finalized, is hostile with spouse and reduces involvements with children

Source. Yudofsky SC: Narcissistic personality disorder, in *Fatal Flaws: Navigating Destructive Relationships With People With Disorders of Personality and Character.* Washington, D.C., American Psychiatric Publishing, 2005, p. 130. © 2005 American Psychiatric Publishing. Used with permission.

Having learned from Helen of Blaise's cruelty to and abuse of her and exploitation of so many others, I had anticipated and was concerned that my feelings and attitudes toward him might be antipathetic. However, on watching the broken body of this once-agile athlete stagger before me into my office and sensing the broken spirit of this once-consummate competitor, I felt sadness and empathy.

Mr. Blaise Hartman: I can't get any lower than this.
Dr. Y.: How so?
Mr. Hartman: Needing the help of a headshrinker means I have hit bottom.
Dr. Y.: Sometimes the bottom has value. I've been to Incline Village, Nevada. The most awesome homes are around the lake, at the *bottom* of the mountain.

In and for an instant, Blaise Hartman's disheartened, disinterested, steel-blue eyes flashed a surprised competitor's stare directly into my eyes.

Mr. Blaise Hartman: Growing up in Incline Village, I got to spend a lot of time in the homes near the tops of the slopes. They were beautiful, but they didn't compare to the homes on the lake. I never once was invited into the guarded estates on the beaches of Lake Tahoe. I knew that the only way I could get past those gates and fences was to buy my own mansion. It's funny, Doc, now that I have the money to buy the best of those places, I have no interest in going there.

Dr. Y.: At this very moment, people are driving around the neighborhood in Bending Brook where you live and looking through the fences at the mansions. And do you know what they're thinking, Mr. Hartman? They're thinking, "The people inside those amazing places have so much money that they don't need to worry about a thing. If I could afford one of those, I'd have no worries. I'd be on easy street."
We know better, don't we?

Psychiatric Technique

Psychiatrists learn a great deal in our residencies, and we must unlearn a great deal of what we have learned to provide effective psychotherapy. As first- and second-year residents, most of us work in the busy emergency departments of large municipal hospitals. Given the large numbers of patients with emergencies who must be evaluated urgently and given the severity of their disorders, psychiatric residents must gain a great deal of information in a brief period of time in order to make safe and informed treatment recommendations and decisions. To do so, residents often rely on structured questioning formats or symptom checklists. Questions tend to be "dysfunction oriented" and quantitative, for example, "How long have you been hearing voices?" or "How many pills did you take when you attempted suicide?" Efficiency can come at the expense of our listening to our patients and may (or may not) interfere with our establishing trusting and respectful short- and long-term therapeutic relationships. By necessity in emergency settings, we focus initially on what's wrong with our patients rather than what's right. If we generalize and expand these practices to outpatient psychotherapy, our interactions with our patients can become routinized, impersonalized, and unoriginal. The poetry in what we should be doing will be lost. We are in danger of becoming caricatures spouting clichés: "And how did that make you feel?"

In treatment, all beginnings are important. Blaise had been in my office for less than a minute when he admitted that he felt demeaned by needing the help of a psychiatrist and declared that he had "hit bottom." Although I regarded Blaise's precise description of what he meant and was feeling by "hitting bottom" as critical and essential information, I also respected the timing wherein I would solicit these data from him. To offer him the standard response—"Please tell me what you mean by 'bottom'"—so early in our encounter would be to ask for information that, inherently, he would perceive to demean him further. Such initial responses would not address (in a creative, unexpected, and constructive fashion) the therapeutic relationship/alliance issue that he also raised in the first minutes of his initial session: "Needing the help of a headshrinker means that I have hit bottom." My primary goal in our first hour together was to establish a trusting, therapeutic alliance with Blaise. To do so, it was my responsibility to communicate that I cared about him as a unique and empowered human being *before* our endeavoring to address any problems, needs, and deficiencies that he might have. A secondary goal was to deliver the message that psychiatric treatment might be different, more interesting, more uplifting, and more useful than he had anticipated.

Given the clear possibility that Blaise might be suicidal and/or might require immediate psychiatric intervention, I utilized the second hour of the session and subsequent meetings to secure the information required to establish a diagnosis and treatment plan with Blaise (see the next section). A positive, respectful foundation set in the first hour would enhance our therapeutic alliance and relationship and increase the probability that he might trust me more and comply with my recommendations and our emerging treatment plan.

Diagnosis and Treatment Plan of Mr. Hartman

Blaise met the following DSM-IV-TR diagnoses (American Psychiatric Association 2000):

Axis I: l) mood disorder due to traumatic brain injury with a major depressive-like episode (293.83) and 2) personality change due to traumatic brain injury, aggressive type (301.1)

Axis II: narcissistic personality disorder (301.81)

These diagnoses would be termed the following in DSM-5 (American Psychiatric Association 2013): depressive disorder due to traumatic brain injury with major depressive-like episode (F06.32); personality change due to traumatic brain injury, aggressive type (310.1 [F07.0]); and narcissistic personality disorder (301.81 [F60.81]).

Early Treatment Response

Within 2 months, Blaise's major depression with suicidal ideation responded to antidepressant treatment, and his irritability and episodic dyscontrol were mitigated by a combination of a lipid-soluble β-blocker and an anticonvulsant. Nonetheless, he remained demoralized and disinterested in reengaging in work, recreation, family relationships, or friendships.

> **Mr. Blaise Hartman:** All of my life I have wanted stuff. I accomplished my main goal in life, which was to make a lot of money. I can buy anything I want right now. The things that I want now, I know I can't get—like a normal, functioning body. My problem is that I don't want anything anymore. It's kind of like I don't *exist* anymore.
>
> **Dr. Y.:** I see it differently, Mr. Hartman. Up until this very moment, you have existed entirely "inside yourself." It's now time for you to move beyond yourself. And I believe that you are ready to do so.

Key Features of Mr. Blaise Hartman's Being Stuck in Pause

1. *How Blaise was stuck:* No purpose in life
2. *Goals for change:* Find meaning in life
3. *Central, unresolved conflicts:* Control versus trust (approach-approach), intimacy versus abandonment (approach-avoidance)
4. *Hallmarks of Blaise's being stuck:* Demoralization, confusion, low self-esteem, amotivation, dysthymia, anxiety
5. *Binary problem/solution:* Aspirituality, alienation/altruism, involvement
6. *Critical decision points:* Giving of himself to Helen, his daughters, and others
7. *Corollary factors required to achieve resolution:* Continued psychotherapy to gain insights into the psychodynamic reasons that he is self-centered and disconnected from others
8. *Resolution:* Involvements in family, church, charity, and the lives of others

Discussion of Treatment Plan

People with personality disorders often have histories of childhood deprivations and mistreatment or are subject to biologically derived *mis*perceptions that they have been deprived and mistreated. In response to their senses of emptiness and unfulfillment, they become overly self-involved and self-absorbed. In other words, they are *stuck in themselves*.

People with personality disorders (and their families) are even more prone to become overwhelmed and "stuck" when afflicted with the sudden onset and prolonged consequences of neuropsychiatric disorders. The case of Blaise Hartman illuminates the five principles about the care of patients (and their families) in which traumatic brain injury (TBI) is complicated by a personality disorder. These principles are summarized in Table 7–5.

TABLE 7–5. Principles of treating patients with both personality disorders and traumatic brain injury

1. Comorbidity of personality disorders and traumatic brain injury (TBI) is common

2. TBI often intensifies the symptoms associated with personality disorders and the associated reluctance to accept help and support from family members and mental health professionals

3. TBI and many other neuropsychiatric disorders almost invariably place enormous stress on family members and caregivers of the identified patient

4. The psychiatrist must be eclectic and flexible in the treatments provided

5. Psychiatric treatment of patients with both TBI and a personality disorder is both essential and effective

---

1. Comorbidity of personality disorders and TBI is common. For a multiplicity of reasons, this comorbidity is common. First, both conditions are highly prevalent. According to the Centers for Disease Control and Prevention, each year approximately 1.7 million people sustain traumatic brain injury, which results in 52,000 deaths, 275,000 hospitalizations, and 1,365,000 hospital visits (Centers for Disease Control and Prevention 2003; Orman et al. 2011). For many of the survivors of TBI, there are chronic sequelae. The median prevalence of published studies of *all* personality disorders ranges from 11.55% to 12.26%, although narcissistic personality disorder comprises only about 0.61% of the population (Torgersen 2005). Second, personality disorders can increase the risk for sustaining TBI, with impulsivity, recklessness, irritability, and aggressiveness leading to physical altercations for people with antisocial personality disorder. The combination of Blaise's problems with intimacy and his low self-esteem led to his not achieving mature, relationship-based life satisfactions. He endeavored to compensate by calling attention to himself through participating in spectacular and dangerous sports feats including helicopter skiing, hang gliding, and bungee jumping. The disabilities engendered from TBI further diminished his self-esteem and aggravated his impulsivity, which could easily have led to further risk of injury.

2. TBI often intensifies the symptoms associated with personality disorders and the associated reluctance to seek help. Relatedly, as it does with mood and anxiety disorders, TBI often intensifies the symptoms associated with personality disorders and the associated reluctance to accept help and support from family members and mental health professionals. I am frequently asked by students and by family members of people with neuropsychiatric disorders whether or not the condition will improve personality disorder symptoms. My first response is to try to describe the unfathomable complexity of the human brain, as honed by tens of thousands of years of evolution, and then offer a metaphor: "If a new flat-screen, high-definition TV were to be dropped from the roof of a 20-story building onto the cement sidewalk below, would you expect its reception to be improved?"

3. TBI places enormous stress on family members and caregivers. The suddenness and multifarious deleterious consequences of TBI and many other neuropsychiatric disorders almost invariably place enormous stress on family members and caregivers of the identified patient (Silver et al. 2011, 2012). When TBI occurs in the context of personality disorder, the familial and caregiver relationships with the patient are exceedingly complex. Interventions must be understood and effected in the context of the nature of the pre-TBI and post-TBI relationships, which will be significantly influenced by the identified patient's personality disorder. For example, it is especially challenging to become a caregiver for a spouse who has a long history of being selfish, demeaning, hurtful, and rejecting. The good news is that our training as mental health professionals renders us well equipped to comprehend these complexities and intervene effectively for all parties involved.

4. The psychiatrist must be flexible in providing treatment. Given the complexities involved in the neuropsychiatric manifestations of brain injury complicated by personality disorder, the psychiatrist must be eclectic and flexible in treatments provided. In the case of Blaise, I provided psychopharmacology; individual, supportive, and insight-oriented psychotherapy for both him and his wife; neuropsychiatric counseling/education (related to brain-based aspects and implications of TBI) for him and his family; couples counseling; and family counseling.

5. Psychiatric treatment of patients with both TBI and a personality disorder is both essential and effective. As described, prior to his psychiatric care, Blaise was severely impaired by the concomitants of TBI and narcissistic personality disorder, which also adversely affected his wife and children. The identified patient and family unit were failing. Without psychiatric treatment Blaise was likely to become even more despondent, withdrawn, and alienated from his family and friends. My responsibility to engage Blaise in psychiatric treatment was no less vital than that of a surgeon to encourage a person with an inflamed and necrotic appendix to undergo an immediate operation. The symptoms and signs of Blaise's mood disorder and organic dyscontrol responded within 2 months to psychopharmacological treatment. Couples counseling with Mr. and Mrs. Hartman helped them reduce power struggles, identify and agree on strategies to reduce his risk-taking behavior, and avoid the unwieldy consequences of maternal transference by curtailing Helen's propensity to monitor and intervene in Blaise's risk-taking behaviors, ambulatory and balance disabilities, etc. These interventions helped improve their relationship to a point that it became vastly superior than it was before Blaise's TBI.

The Psychotherapies of Blaise and Helen Hartman

Individual, insight-oriented psychotherapy aided Blaise in gaining understanding of the implications of his childhood experiences with his parents and their effect on his low self-esteem, need for constant admiration, desire to be in "total control" of important relationships, unrealistic goals for a complete recovery from the TBI, and interpersonal problems with Helen and his children.

> **Mr. Blaise Hartman:** From as far back as I can remember, my father felt that I was a nuisance. He hated the fact that I needed things, like money for clothes and school lunches or someone to drive me to a ski meet. By the time I was 12, I could tell that

he just didn't want to be around me. I probably haven't seen him more than 10 times in the last 30 years.

My mother was different. She always wanted me to take care of *her*, even when I was a very young kid. The worst was when she drank too much, which was most of the time. She'd come home sobbing and drunk after some guy had mistreated her, wake me up, and start telling me all the lurid details. I didn't want to know, but that never stopped her. She reeked of the smell of booze and would get into bed with me. It always made me feel very uncomfortable. She didn't have much modesty, either.

After being all over me for weeks and weeks, she would meet somebody new and disappear from my life. She just wouldn't come back one night to wherever we were living. No calls, no explanations. Then, I wouldn't hear from her at all for months and months—until she got thrown out the next time.

Dr. Y.: Early in her treatment, Helen asked me why I thought you married her. I told her that only you could answer that question, Mr. Hartman. Do you know why?

Mr. Hartman: I asked myself that question many times over the years. It remains a mystery. We don't seem to have anything in common.

Dr. Y.: Well, that's the first clue to solving the mystery. Did Helen have something that you want and sensed that you didn't have?

Mr. Hartman: I always went after women for money and sex. I could have married plenty of women with a lot more money than Helen, and a few who were even prettier—although Helen was very good looking. I'm stumped, Dr. Y. Tell me what you think.

Dr. Y.: Do you know the Eagles song "Desperado"? Every word is about you.

Mr. Hartman: I have heard the song, but don't remember it. I certainly don't know if or how it applies to me and Helen.

Dr. Y.: Go back and listen to it. You always thought that you wanted the queen of diamonds, but you chose the queen of hearts. So what you have been doing is trying to change her into a queen of diamonds.

Helen has divine purpose. She cares deeply about things beyond herself. I believe that's what attracted you to her in the first place. But you have a pattern of chasing what you don't have.

Mr. Hartman: True enough. What am I supposed do with this so-called insight?

Dr. Y.: Change what hasn't been working for you. You have spent a lifetime caring for and about yourself. You have spent your lifetime wanting material things and going after power and position. Things you never had as a child. But what happens when you *get* those things—all those things that you have always thought that you wanted? Then what?

Mr. Hartman (*with irritation*): Be a businessman, for once! Get to the bottom line. I repeat myself: What am I supposed to do from here?

Dr. Y.: You learned how to *get*, but you never learned how to *give*.

Blaise gained further insight into how his emotional responses to his critical, detached father and episodically enveloping mother were directly related to his low self-esteem, constrained capacity for intimacy, poor quality of relationships, and impaired psychological adjustment to his physical limitations. All of these symptoms improved significantly over time.

To Helen's surprise, not only did her husband agree to include their children in family treatment but he also became motivated to engage in more intensive, psychodynamically oriented psychotherapy. This would mean that he would have several psychotherapeutic sessions per week—as compared to the current one session per week. Given that I was continuing to treat Helen in supportive psychotherapy and was conducting the couples and family treatment, I strongly encouraged Blaise to accept my referral to an outstanding psychotherapist for more intensive, individual psychotherapy.

Mr. Blaise Hartman: Even though you're a shrink, and you're weird, and can't even ski, I have come to *kind* of like you, Dr. Y. And even though you had plenty of ammunition, you never turned Helen against me. So I *kind* of trust you. I think I should stay with you. It wouldn't be good for me to see another psychiatrist.

Dr. Y.: And why is that?

Mr. Hartman: Didn't you hear me say that I kind of trust you? As you know, everyone in my life whom I have trusted—except Helen—has abandoned me. No matter how you dress this deal up, Dr. Y., if you make me see someone else, I will experience it as just another betrayal of my trust. Just another rejection. Just another abandonment.

Dr. Y.: You are a master negotiator and deal maker, Mr. Hartman. I'll continue to work with you until you fire me.

In treatment, Blaise came to realize that he did not accept his inherent value and worth, so he tried to gain and control the acceptance of others by accumulating wealth and power. On the occasions that he was defeated in competitions or felt excluded by others, he would become enraged and vindictive as his deep-seated feelings of worthlessness were confirmed. His previous response was to work harder to get ever more power, wealth, and control while simultaneously becoming increasingly ruthless and dismissive of the rules and the rights of others.

> **Dr. Y.:** We have talked about how you viewed the awesome homes around Lake Tahoe. We have also discussed how you thought the wealthy people who lived in those homes lived perfect lives. But do you care to speculate about how the people in those homes must have regarded you?
>
> **Mr. Blaise Hartman:** I have no clue what you are trying to get at, Dr. Y. Why don't you just make your point without having to drag it out of me? Do you realize that I pay you by the minute?
>
> **Dr. Y.:** The people in those mansions were just people. That means that many of them weren't tall, handsome, agile athletes like you were. I would guess that many of the people in those homes had infirmities or children with disabilities who weren't even able to ski safely down the mountain slopes. I surmise that to them, you were some blonde god—a veritable king of the mountain—and they would think, "If only I could look, move, and ski like him, I'd be happy. I wouldn't have a care in the world."
>
> **Mr. Hartman:** I get your point, Dr. Y. After my brain injury, I look at people with intact bodies and envy them. I wish I could be like them again.
>
> **Dr. Y.:** That's only part of my point, Mr. Hartman. A silver lining of your dark cloud of TBI is that you can begin to understand what *others* feel like when they are weak and anguished. When they can't compete with the strong. I believe that Helen's extraordinary selflessness and capacity to empathize are qualities that attracted you to her in the first place. You wanted to have *that* power, to be more like her.

The Power of No and the Power of Go

Far from coincidentally, Blaise's application of the Power of No and the Power of Go was the mirror image of that of Helen. Whereas Helen focused on being sensitive and responsive to her own needs and priorities as opposed to what people expected from her, Blaise's work was to become aware of and attentive to the needs and priorities of *others*. *Mentalization* is the capacity to keep *the minds of other people in your mind.* As a salesman, Blaise had learned to gauge in others how they were responding to him and what he wanted *from* them, but he never thought of people as multidimensional entities with their own needs and rights. Rather, people were vending machines, and his job was to figure out the right currency to put in them to get back what *he* wanted from them. Beyond that, human beings had no existence or value to him.

A component of Blaise's treatment was to work at trying to become aware of the value, needs, and purpose of *everyone* whom he encountered in his life—from his home care nurses whom he had treated as slaves to the president of a Middle Eastern country whom he was trying to impress for a business purpose. Concurrently, his job also was to become aware of 1) what he wanted or expected from these individuals and 2) whether or not what he wanted from them was appropriate, fair, and respectful to them and their needs and rights. The Power of No was to be exercised when he was tempted to influence them or gain advantage in ways that were not honest, fair, or respectful. Not surprisingly, Blaise's resistance to this alien concept was monumental.

> **Mr. Blaise Hartman:** With all due respect, Dr. Y., you have never run a business or competed in sports at the highest levels. You have been a cog in someone else's gear for your entire career. What you are telling me to do is antithetical to success, which is all about getting the advantage. You are asking me to become a communist, or worse, an academic.
>
> **Dr. Y.:** What I am asking you to consider, Mr. Hartman, is learning how to treat people *with all due respect.* Not tell them that you are doing that and then do the opposite—as you just did with me.

The application of the Power of Go with Blaise was to exert kindness and aid to others without it being a ploy to get something or having an expectation of their reciprocity. This was met with even more resistance. Couples counseling provided an excellent opportunity and fodder for Blaise to exercise this principle.

> **Mr. Blaise Hartman:** Dr. Y., I'd like to bring up an issue that's really bothering me. Ever since Helen went back to graduate school, she hardly pays any attention to me or her household responsibilities.

Dr. Y.: Please give a specific example.

Mr. Hartman: I'm upset with Helen for not calling that home care agency to have them replace that horrible nurse, Rebecca. I asked her to do that several times, but she is ignoring me. That nurse is lazy and incompetent.

Mrs. Helen Hartman: Blaise, you are just angry with Rebecca for not giving you pain medications. They were discontinued by Dr. Naifeh, and she's not allowed to give you any more.

Mr. Hartman: You and I both know that there are a lot more capsules left in the bottle. I paid for them, so they belong to me. I need the meds, and I want her out of our house.

Dr. Y.: Why do you think she is withholding the medication from you?

Mr. Hartman: You're supposed to be the mind reader, not me. I would guess that she's either sadistic or wants them for herself. Whatever the case, I asked Helen to call the agency to replace her, and she hasn't done it. I will do it myself in the morning.

Dr. Y.: It's illegal for her to administer a medication that a physician has discontinued. Not only would she lose her job, but her nurse's license would also be jeopardized. Try to put yourself in her place, Mr. Hartman. She doesn't want to upset you, but she also does not want to lose her livelihood by breaking a law.

Consider exercising the Power of No by *not* calling the agency and by *not* being rude to her and the Power of Go by doing something kind—like asking her about her family or thanking her when she has done something helpful.

Mrs. Hartman: Just try it, Blaise. You will feel so much better about yourself when you are kind and generous to the people who depend on you.

Current Status of Mr. and Mrs. Hartman

Through his treatment, Blaise gradually learned to elevate his self-esteem by caring about and caring for others. This included his taking an interest in Helen's work and the personal lives of their children. He joined the boards of charitable organizations—not just to donate money but to give freely of his time and expertise in their management and the investment of their endowments. As he became more interested in Helen's work, he became aware of the painful, challenging lives of children with neurodevelopmental disorders and the heartbreaks and sacrifices of their loving families. Given his own medical condition, he sensed their minute-by-minute, hour-by-hour, day-by-day struggles. With Helen, he formed a not-for-profit medical foundation that supported research, treatment, and political advocacy on their behalf. It was the first truly joint venture in their marriage. Blaise devoted as much time to advancing the foundation and its cause as he did to his own businesses, and to his surprise, these activities were as rewarding to him as adding to his fortune.

Continued individual psychotherapy with Helen helped her to understand further the vulnerabilities that led her to engage and remain in an exploitative, demeaning marital relationship and how to change herself in ways that enabled independent growth and actualization of her scientific potential and professional goals. Given the increasing demands of graduate school and her improved self-esteem and mental status, Helen reduced the frequency of psychotherapy to once or twice per month, depending on her schedule. She also began to spend a great deal more time with her husband. They now regularly attend church together and work on their charitable foundation. When Helen and the children are free, the family goes on elaborate, extended vacations. Both Helen and Blaise agree, "We are closer and love each other more today than we had ever thought was possible." At this time Dr. Helen Hartman reports feeling "happy and successful as a wife, mother, and in my work [as an assistant professor of neuroscience]." Interestingly, she tells me that she almost never wears jewelry these days.

References

American Psychiatric Association: Diagnostic and Statistical Manual of Mental Disorders, 4th Edition, Text Revision. Washington, DC, American Psychiatric Association, 2000

American Psychiatric Association: Diagnostic and Statistical Manual of Mental Disorders, 5th Edition. Washington, DC, American Psychiatric Association, 2013

Centers for Disease Control and Prevention: Report to Congress on Mild Traumatic Brain Injury in the United States: Steps to Prevent a Serious Public Health Problem. Atlanta, GA, Centers for Disease Control and Prevention, September 2003. Available at: http:/www.cdc.gov/ncipc/pub-res/mtbi/report.htm. Accessed December 3, 2011.

Orman JAL, Kraus JF, Zaloshnja, et al: Epidemiology, in Textbook of Traumatic Brain Injury, 2nd Edition. Edited by Silver JM, McAllister TW, Yudofsky SC. Washington, DC, American Psychiatric Publishing, 2011, pp 3–21

Silver JM, Yudofsky SC, Anderson KE: Aggressive disorders, in Textbook of Traumatic Brain Injury, 2nd Edition. Edited by Silver JM, McAllister TW, Yudofsky SC. Washington, DC, American Psychiatric Publishing, 2011, pp 225–238

Silver JM, Hales RE, Yudofsky SC: Traumatic brain injury, in Clinical Manual of Neuropsychiatry. Edited by Yudofsky SC, Hales RE. Washington, DC, American Psychiatric Publishing, 2012, pp 119–180

Torgersen S: Epidemiology, in The American Psychiatric Publishing Textbook of Personality Disorders. Edited by Oldham JM, Skodol AE, Bender DS. Washington DC, American Psychiatric Publishing, 2005, pp 129–134

Yudofsky SC: Fatal Flaws: Navigating Destructive Relationships With People With Disorders of Personality and Character. Washington, DC, American Psychiatric Publishing, 2005, pp 87–137

8

Stuck in a Bottle, Part I (Discover): The Case of Mrs. Lynda Jensen

When Alcohol Use Disorder Is Complicated by Generalized Anxiety Disorder

Drinking is a way of ending the day.
—*Ernest Hemingway*

It was like something you have dreaded and feared
and dodged for years until it seemed like all your
life, then despite everything that happened to you
and all it was just pain, all it did was hurt....
—*William Faulkner*, Intruder in the Dust

What is the late November doing
With the disturbance of the spring?
—*T. S. Eliot, "East Coker," in* Four Quartets

"Please pray for me."

Author's note: This chapter was cowritten by Mrs. Lynda Jensen and me. The process has been for each of us to write, independently, our impressions of the origins and repercussions of her alcoholism and of our treatment for this condition. Also included are my responses to and interpretations of what she submitted. Mrs. Jensen's first meeting with me was October 3, 2011, and her treatment is ongoing. I did not endeavor to influence nor did I alter what she so graciously has prepared and contributed to this chapter. Other than my changing identifying information, the chapter includes an exact replication of her employer's e-mails to me regarding the referral of Mrs. Jensen and my response to him.

The Case of Mrs. Lynda Jensen, D1 (Discovery): Part 1—Assessment/Diagnosis[1]

Referral

September 28, 2011 (e-mail from Mr. Clifford Bentsen)

Dear Stuart,

I trust this finds you well. Our company's Senior Vice President for New Product Development is having recurring issues with alcoholism. I value her highly as a person and the work in which she's engaged is particularly important to our organization.

She was in a rehab program in Minneapolis for one month about two years ago. Returning with a fresh start, she attended AA until, I believe, six months ago. She's now slipped back into problem drinking, which is impacting her life and work adversely. She no longer attends AA meetings.

Lynda, 60, received her Ph.D. from one of America's most prestigious science/engineering schools with highest honors and has been a lifetime high achiever. She had four children by her first marriage, and married again a number of years ago. Her husband is a retired attorney.

Stuart, if you could give her some assistance, either personally or with someone you recommend, I'd be most grateful. She's prepared to come to Houston from San Francisco, as needed.

Thank you for considering this.

Best wishes to you and Beth.

Clifford

September 29, 2011 (Reply from Dr. Y.)

Dear Clifford:

I hope that you are well and looking forward to the fall season.

Thank you for this important message and for the opportunity to help out professionally with Mrs. Jensen. Manifestly, she is altogether a remarkable person and professional, and it will be my pleasure to help out in every way that I am able.

I believe that the best way to begin is to have Mrs. Jensen call my office and speak with my Administrative Assistant, Mrs. Patricia

---

[1]Although Lynda Jensen received a Ph.D. in engineering and computer sciences, she prefers to be called "Mrs. Jensen" in her professional and personal lives and "Lynda" in psychotherapy.

Hoffman, who will set up an appointment as soon as possible. I will also call her before the appointment time to make certain she is safe and protected and to be as reassuring as is indicated.

My warmest regards,

Stuart

Presenting Illness: Trying to Stop (Lynda Jensen's Perspective)

"Now or never," "no matter what," "the time is now," "do or die." These phrases became my mantras upon entering a 90-day recovery program for alcoholism in October 2011. (My other mantra, "who gives a shit," also played prominently, which I'll explain later.)

This was not my first attempt to quit drinking; far from it. During the 4 preceding years I had participated in 30-day inpatient and evening outpatient programs. Before that I had bounced between abstaining for brief periods followed by attempts to moderate my drinking, efforts that became increasingly futile as my alcoholism intensified.

The net result of these efforts was that I was able to quit, sometimes for relatively long periods of time, but I was not able to keep it up, to persist in the effort. I just couldn't seem to stay on the high ground and repeatedly broke faith with my commitment to sobriety. I kept giving in to alcohol's siren call, which left me confounded, appalled, and at times terrified.

In late 2007 when I entered my first inpatient program, I finally came out of the closet and admitted to myself and my family, boss, and close friends that I had a drinking problem and I needed help. This was traumatic, but it was also a relief. I was revealing myself in a way that ran counter to my overachieving self-image. An image carefully built and protected over many years that included achievements in the academic, engineering, and business worlds: elected Phi Beta Kappa junior year, the only woman in my class to graduate with highest honors (I also had my first child the second year of graduate school), national reputation in my chosen engineering field, elected to the executive committee of a global consulting firm, and so on. When I set out to do something, I had generally succeeded through hard work, persistence, and determination. But, for some reason, I was not able to consistently marshal these attributes in my struggle with alcohol, which was both baffling and demoralizing.

It turned out that admitting I was a problem drinker, or alcoholic, was only a piece of the puzzle. It has taken me much longer to understand and accept there were other areas of my life I needed to examine and rewire. When I entered my first rehab program in

2007, I truly believed that alcohol was my only real problem and that if I could just quit drinking everything would be fine. I had a great family behind me, a good job and understanding boss, and all the other amenities such as a nice home and car. I just had this pesky problem with alcohol, which, once dealt with, would allow me to pick up and resume life where I had left off. Or so I thought.

It turned out that this myth "that everything else with me was OK" had to be shattered, along with the myth that I could learn to drink moderately.

Flash forward to the summer of 2011, when a number of forces for change began to coalesce. Over a relatively brief time in the months leading up to October, as I was stumbling my way through periods of abstinence and intermittent bouts of drinking, my children, husband, and boss all became aware of my situation despite my best efforts to keep it private and telling myself I would soon get things under control again.

My boss sat me down and clearly and directly addressed the situation. "What are you going to do about this?" he firmly asked. I didn't have an easy response, other than something along the lines that Alcoholics Anonymous (AA), which had been a long-term fallback position of mine, wasn't working for me, and that I really did not want to go back to rehab. He made it clear to me that he wanted to help and that he needed me as an employee. He was on my side, clearly, but I had to grab hold of the situation and work toward real and lasting change. He inquired whether I might benefit from psychotherapy. Although I had been seeing a therapist for more than a year, I had to admit to myself that it wasn't really working and that I hadn't been fully honest with her. I kept secret my recurring bouts of drinking partly because I didn't want to be a failure in her eyes.

What I didn't fully realize at the time of the conversation with my boss was that I was embarking on a process in which I'd be called on to become increasingly honest with myself as well as others. This was the first leg in a new road to freedom. My boss referred me to Dr. Y. and what ended up being a totally new therapy experience and relationship.

Presenting Illness: Trying to Stop (Dr. Y.'s Perspective)

Lynda brings to her treatment a baffling, unsolved murder mystery: Why am I killing myself with alcohol? I do not believe that her mantra, "do or die," is in any way overly dramatic or untrue. If she cannot win her battle with alcohol, she will lose all that she holds dear—her relationships with her husband, children, and grandchildren; her job and professional status; her health; her relationship with herself (sometimes called *self-esteem*); and perhaps even her life.

The fundamental question that Lynda poses—"Why can't I stop drinking despite how hard I have tried and how successful and disciplined I am in all other areas of my life?"—offers both a clue to her murder mystery and a "secret treasure map" to guide treatment. Perhaps her success comes at too high of a cost, and perhaps she is conflicted about both her success and the discipline it takes to achieve it. From the darkness of her mystery and confusion, Lynda has pointed her flashlight at two issues that we must address together: 1) Although we understand what alcohol does *to her*, we do not yet know what alcohol does *for her*. 2) From her successes in her academic career and engineering profession, we know that she has exceptional powers of discipline. Thus, it is unlikely that D3 *(Discipline)* is the key component of the Fatal Pauses 3-D Method of Getting Unstuck from alcohol dependence.

It was clear to me that the psychotherapy on which we were about to embark must provide *discovery* of the hidden, complex sources of Lynda's alcohol dependence that would complement the work of AA and her residential rehabilitation programs that previously had been insufficient in sustaining her sobriety. My first job would be to engage Lynda in working with me on this quest.

First Meeting (Lynda Jensen's Perspective)

I was extremely nervous at my first appointment with Dr. Y. I had never had an extended session with a "psychiatrist," and a prominent one at that. My inner voice was telling me I must be a real loony, something I had always been a little afraid may be the case. I had tried my best to suppress and out-will some of my mental health struggles I had in adolescence, and now I supposed it was all coming out in the wash.

Perhaps it was the calmness of his manner and the way he asked penetrating questions without seeming threatening, but at some point during our first session I felt deep in my being that here was someone who could help me, finally. I felt he "got me," almost from the first few minutes. My ego was definitely involved in making this assessment. I often believed I was smarter than many, including some former therapists I had seen, whom I felt couldn't fully understand someone with a superior intellect such as mine. This attitude demonstrated the kind of pedestal on which I had placed myself and the isolation trap it had reinforced. Not only could Dr. Y. keep up intellectually but he could and did stay way ahead of me. Also, I discovered in that very first session that I could not lie or mischaracterize or avoid or evade the truth. When he asked me if I had had anything to drink that day, my standard denial response was replaced with "yes." I was shocked and relieved at how easily the truth came pouring out.

Yes, here was someone I could talk to. Here was someone who could help me. But first, rehab.

First Meeting (Dr. Y.'s Perspective)

Initial Impression of Lynda Jensen

Like a meticulous daffodil that had braved forth during the final frost of winter, Lynda's delicate, fragile, vulnerable appearance belied the strength, stubbornness, and persistence of a perennial. Her carefully appointed attire; her well-tended hair, makeup, and figure; and her professionally cropped words were betrayed subtly by a fine manual tremor, the waft of alcohol, and more than a trace of shame. I could not foretell whether her crystalline encasement of perfection would serve to protect or to entomb her. But slipping through the splinters in her icy illusion of flawlessness were the fineness and firmness of high intelligence blended with deep humanism, a mix that I hoped would, in time, concretize into the bedrock of our treatment.

I sensed that if Lynda feared anything from our budding venture, it was to be discovered as deficient and undeserving. And if Mrs. Jensen expected anything from our nascent enterprise, it was to be disappointed—just as she had been disappointed with previous therapists and just as she had disappointed herself by returning to drinking, yet again. A different doctor, a different setting, but the same disappointing result. The winters of rimes and thaws had worn down the hopefulness of this weary perennial.

"My Name Is Lynda. I Am an Alcoholic"

In our first meeting, Lynda repeatedly referred to herself as "an alcoholic," to which I eventually raised exception:

> **Dr. Y.:** Although I understand and accept fully your point about the dangers and destructiveness of alcohol to your health and to all that you hold dear, I have a problem with your calling yourself an alcoholic.

Mrs. Lynda Jensen: But that's what I *am*, Dr. Y. Up until now my problem has been that I just won't accept that fact. *My* not accepting that I *am* an alcoholic will be the ruin of me. *Your* not accepting that I'm an alcoholic will not be helpful to me.

Dr. Y.: I totally accept that you should never again drink. I also accept that your inability to resist drinking could lead to unthinkable consequences, even to the point of being fatal to you and others. However, I also believe that calling yourself an "alcoholic" has several major downsides. One limitation is the implication that "everything will be OK" if *only* you would stop drinking. I am certain that you would be far, far better off if you become abstinent, but I doubt that everything would be OK with you and in your life.

Lynda: At this point, I will settle for being "far, far better off." I just don't seem to be able to stop.

Dr. Y.: That touches on the second point that I am getting at. You *have* stopped drinking several times in the past, but you always go back to the bottle. If you stop drinking but don't feel that much better about yourself and your life, you will become demoralized. If you don't discover and address the psychological issues that underlie your abuse of alcohol, your chances of remaining sober are poor. If you have an untreated psychiatric disorder, such as depression or anxiety, that may not go away if you stop drinking—although alcohol always makes it much worse—so you have a risk of returning to alcohol as you try to drown your pain and hopelessness. By calling yourself an alcoholic, there is the incorrect implication that alcohol is *the* problem.

Lynda: Why else shouldn't I consider myself an alcoholic?

Dr. Y.: Because you are so much more than "a problem," or an illness, or a simple chemical compound, or a pejorative label. I believe that labeling you an alcoholic is a prejudice, with all of the limitations of any prejudice. It narrows understanding, discovery, and the potential for change and growth.

Lynda: So what would you like to call me and how should I think of myself?

Dr. Y.: I am just getting to know you, but I do know that you are a wife, mother of four children, and an engineer. You are also a person who suffers from the illness alcoholism.

Lynda: Because I am an alcoholic, I haven't been functioning well as wife, mother, or engineer. I don't feel much like a person, either.

Dr. Y.: Without question your alcoholism can undermine all that you hold dear in your life and all that you value in yourself. Other illnesses, left untreated, can do that, as well. For example, any person with an acutely inflamed appendix or who has just experienced a heart attack must immediately address their conditions. If they don't do so, they can't function. They might die. Nonetheless, we don't call them "an appendicitis" or "a myocardial infarction." Physicians refer to them and they refer to themselves, quite appropriately, as a person with appendicitis or a person who has just experienced a myocardial infarction. The person should never be excluded from this discussion and should never be upstaged by the illness.

I view you and believe that you should regard yourself as a person who suffers from an illness called alcoholism. Throughout your treatment with me, we will review together the scientific literature—the epidemiology, genetics, neurobiology, and pathology—that leads me to believe that alcoholism warrants being conceptualized as a medical illness. It is important that we recognize the dangers of alcoholism in the context of *both* your strengths and your weaknesses. In this way we will learn why you are vulnerable to this illness and how you will wield your many, many strengths and abilities to overcome these vulnerabilities.

Finally, I believe that AA, which I admire greatly, to which I refer many patients, and which I believe has saved the lives of countless individuals, would better serve its members to change its name to "Alcoholism Anonymous." I believe it is imperative that you continue to attend AA meetings regularly, but someday I hope that you will consider introducing yourself like this: "Hello, my name is Lynda. I am a person who suffers from alcoholism."

"Special" Doctor

On rereading Lynda's written account of our first meeting, I became uneasy. The first time I read her description of our initial session I was flattered that such a fine and accomplished person would regard me as an exceptional professional with such special powers to understand her and to help her save her life. Even worse, I had to admit to myself that *I believed she was right!* One might have hoped that, after so many years of clinical experience, I would have been more alert and immune to the risks of idealization. No such luck. Without considering the inevitable consequences, I was standing right up there beside Mrs. Jensen on the "pedestal" where she said she had placed herself because of her "superior intellect." It's a long, long way to fall for a mortal psychiatrist. Mrs. Jensen also idealized her father, who let her down with his violent outbursts and by dying and abandoning her when she was 4 years old. Her feelings for her father, which are seminal to her psychodynamics and personality formation, would certainly be reflected in her transference to me and would be intensified should her idealization of me continue. Fortunately, the last sentence of her account revealed that she was more aware of the instability of that pedestal than was I: "Yes, here was someone I could talk to. Here was someone who could help me. But first, rehab." If I were such a hotshot doctor, why would she have had to hit bottom and enter rehabilitation shortly after our first session?

Now I get it…finally, and therefore I knew how to proceed with treatment. It was essential that I make special efforts to demystify our psychotherapy with openness, information, and interpretation each time Lynda elevated me. And I must be ever cognizant of my encouraging or accepting her belief that I have special powers, qualities, and abilities that I certainly do not possess. Since my three daughters, who always helped keep my ego in check, had grown up and departed to California, I decided to accept a few new adolescent patients into my practice. I could always count on adolescents to hold in check my vanity and sins of pride.

Hitting Bottom (Lynda Jensen's Perspective)

As I indicated previously, soon after entering the doors of this very fine rehab program, I was uttering mantras of change: "do or die," "now or never," "the time is now," "no matter what," and "who gives a shit."

But first, a few words about how I got to this place. Shortly after visiting Dr. Y. and a "quick" trip to Istanbul for a conference, I was in Los Angeles visiting with all four of my adult children to celebrate a host of milestones—my grandson's third birthday, the recent birth of my first granddaughter, and saying goodbye to my daughter, who was going to be leaving the country for an extended sabbatical.

I could write a whole chapter on this extended weekend visit because it represented my so-called "bottom," bringing unspeakable pain, hurt, worry, and fear to all my children and despair, remorse, isolation, and a sense of hopelessness to me. I drank on and off in secret over the course of the extended visit and hoped no one would notice. The opportunity to see all of my children together and to spend time with my grandkids, including my brand new baby granddaughter, were the things I held most precious in my heart. But I was not fully present or capable because I could not put aside my drive to drink. It was as if an alien monster had overtaken me.

I was staying in Los Angeles through Tuesday morning so I could attend an Obama fundraiser on Monday night at the home of Melanie Griffith and Antonio Banderas. This weekend illustrates how crazy and surrealistic my life had become—Istanbul the week before and now a Hollywood fundraiser, as I continued to spiral down. In between all this activity, I was looking to buy a house or condo in L.A. To cut to the chase, I was supposed to have a final dinner with all the kids on Sunday night, but I ended up canceling. I had been drinking in my hotel room to the point that I didn't think I could show up and act "normally." I made some sorry excuse that I was too tired. They all knew better. I continued to drink—pass out, wake up, drink some more, fall asleep or pass out, and so forth and so on, and on. I couldn't make it to the Obama fundraiser on Monday night. Instead of leaving for home Tuesday morning, I stayed on, having planned to leave Wednesday morning—after I could sober up enough to travel.

In the early evening on Tuesday, my hotel phone rang. I was told that my sons were downstairs and wanted to come up to my room. I reluctantly agreed. Racing around my room, I stuck empty wine and minibar bottles into my suitcase and barely managed to splash some water on my face.

Although I was afraid of what I knew was about to happen, I was also relieved. I wanted someone to come riding in on a white horse and announce that the jig was up. Earlier, in preparing to leave the next morning, I had put some money out as a tip for the housekeeper with a pathetic note: "Please pray for me." I was reaching out for help in my own inept way, not feeling I could pray for myself.

Now help was here in the form of my sons, fully backed by the support and agreement of my other children and my husband. My sons sat down with me and gently prodded me into seeing the merits of going to rehab "without passing go." At first I debated whether it would be better for me to go home and try AA and therapy first, but their consistent message was not to wait, to go for it now. They had already checked and learned I could get into a top 90-day program recommended for professionals and business executives, which they probably knew would appeal to my elitist side when I attempted to backpedal. Before agreeing to go into the program, I made the excuse that I couldn't just take a 90-day leave from my job without clearing up pending matters at work and that I might get fired. One of my sons replied, "Who gives a shit, Mom, this is your life!" That "who gives a shit" hit me like a ton of bricks. It cut through my fog by flagging how dire my situation was and that dealing with it *now* was more important than keeping my job or anything else. That comment sparked a moment of clarity and marked the beginning of a profound psychic change that would play out over the coming weeks and months.

As we drove to the facility that evening, I continued to struggle with the reality of my life—what I was leaving behind and what I was moving toward. Every time I questioned whether 90 days might be overdoing it and that perhaps I should sign up for 30 and see how it went, my sons held firm and kept convincing me that 90 was the way to go. "OK," I thought, "who gives a shit; this is my life."

As I walked through the doors to rehab, I promised myself I would not revisit the decision to stay 90 days. I would do the 90 days "no matter what," even if I might start to get restless or bored or feel the time was not being well spent. I would not question the decision. I would keep to it no matter what. I made a commitment to myself that I would not break. Likewise, my sons assured me they would alternate Sunday visits, a commitment that they faithfully kept.

I knew deep in my soul that this was my last chance. It was "now or never," "do or die" time. Learning to live a life of sobriety had to become and remain my highest priority, and I had to learn not to "give a shit" about anything real or imagined that got in the way of that.

Hitting Bottom (Dr. Y.'s Perspective)

Big Picture

The contrasts between two of Lynda's mantras, "do or die" and "I don't give a shit," are most revealing. Their surface meanings, of course, are quite clear. "Do or die" refers to the vital imperative that she stop drinking and how hard she must work in the residential rehabilitation program and in AA to learn how to stay sober. "I don't give a shit" refers to the necessity for her to prioritize her recovery from alcoholism over her all-consuming work demands and other responsibilities. I also sensed much deeper, psychological meanings in both mantras that impact her self-definition and reveal a fundamental conflict that led to her alcohol dependence. I inferred that if this conflict were not discovered and resolved, she would return to drinking—no matter how many mantras she repeated, how many recovery programs she completed, nor how many AA meetings she attended. I suspected that she believed that her very existence, value to others, and self-worth depended on her performance in all spheres of her life, and I further suspected that she resented it deeply. She felt not like a human *being*, but a human *doing*. If this theory proved to be correct with confirmatory evidence from her personal history—and in our ongoing therapeutic relationship—her *resentment* (a euphemism for deep-seated rage) for having to perform for acceptance would lead to a "catch-22" type of conflict in which she would find ways to undo her achievements—whether in work, in her personal life, or in her therapy with me.

The "I don't give a shit" mantra (which brings the polite, formal, and always-appropriate Mrs. Jensen to delighted laughter each time she recounts it) on the surface refers to prioritizing treatment and recovery over her perfectionistic work ethic. On the other hand, that mantra could just as easily be a toast before chugging down a drink that she knows she shouldn't have. Said more specifically, her toast would be, "I'm fed up with trying so hard to get everyone's approval to exist. Screw you! Screw work! Screw my family! Screw recovery! And, most of all, screw me! Now let's drink up!" The "proof" of this theory would come in Lynda's self-recriminations and feelings of guilt and shame *following* drinking, which would be the result not only of her failing to remain sober but also primarily, I believe, because of the unconscious aggression that she had directed toward herself and others *by* drinking.

Bigger Picture

In psychotherapy, as in nanotechnology and poetry, the large is revealed by the small. When Lynda returned for our second psychotherapy session after completing her work in the 90-day alcohol residential rehabilitation program, she recounted what she contributed above. In her account, she detailed leaving the "Please pray for me" note for the hotel housekeeper. Her primary point was to communicate how desperate and pathetic she felt at that time. I got that message but heard a much larger one.

> **Dr. Y.:** Do you usually leave a note for the housekeeper?
> **Mrs. Lynda Jensen:** Yes, along with their gratuity. They work hard, but they don't make much money.
> **Dr. Y.:** Do you believe that most people do that?
> **Lynda:** Yes, if they can afford it.
> **Dr. Y.:** It would be a better world if you were right.

What I learned from this interchange and what has been confirmed by numerous examples in subsequent treatment sessions is that Lynda always tries to do the "right thing." I wondered how she feels and deals with her feelings when, inevitably, *she* does the right things and *other people*—especially those on whom she depends—do not. From the earliest phase of her treatment, I harbored the suspicion that when people let her down Lynda denies her perceptions and buries her feelings. I suspected that her anxiety, depression, and alcohol abuse were directly related to denial, a psychological mechanism that would also have far-reaching implications and repercussions for her most important choices and intimate relationships.

Although not the point that she was trying to make (i.e., how desperate and pathetic she becomes in the grip of alcohol), the most important message that I received from her note to the housekeeper was that Lynda is a fine human being. She always tries to do what is right and to do so in the right way. Although I realized that a lot of work was ahead—in and outside of treatment—I was optimistic that her *fineness* would carry the day.

Lynda Jensen's Psychiatric History

Earliest Memories (Lynda Jensen's Perspective)

A good place to start in talking about earlier years is fearfulness. I have tried to pinpoint my earliest memory of being fearful. I believe it to be before I was 4, when my parents had huge, verbally and physically violent fights at the dinner table, sometimes ending with my father pulling the tablecloth off the table and sending all the china and silverware and glassware flying into the air and crashing to the ground. Sometimes it ended with my father hitting or choking my mother. At these times my two older brothers and I retreated to the front hallway and sat on the stairway, waiting for "it" to be over.

I also remember the fear and confusion I felt when after Sunday church services we would sometimes go to the Chalet restaurant for brunch, after which my mother, brothers, and I would wait in the car for my father to come out. He was at the restaurant bar drinking and socializing. Mom would valiantly go back into the restaurant to get him but return empty handed, repeating this process several times over before my father would finally emerge. I knew this wasn't right, that something was wrong with this picture, but not one of us talked about it, ever.

I also seem to remember times when my brothers would get in trouble and we'd all gone down to the basement where my father would administer the belt. It was ominous, dark, and scary down there. I was always spared.

I am not sure how many times these incidents occurred, I believe at least several times for each. I know I was not yet 4 because my father was hospitalized right around my fourth birthday. Looking back on these things I realize the entire house must have been permeated with a sense of fear bordering on terror, because my father was an alcoholic who became unpredictable and often violent when he drank.

I do have happy memories of times with my father before his early death. Like when we got our dog and he let me name him, much to my brothers' annoyance when I selected "Nixie" after the black cocker spaniel in my *Nixie, Trixie and Dixie* Golden Storybook. My father also let me stay up late with him, watching TV and hanging out, after making my brothers go to bed earlier. He also brought me gifts when he returned from business trips. I remember one in particular—a beautiful golden plastic trumpet that came in its own velvet-lined case that made Nixie howl when I played it and drove my brothers mad. I don't believe he brought gifts for my brothers. There are other fleeting memories—my father taking me to get my prized red tricycle that I named "Speedy" and visits to the local hardware store to buy dog food and various other items, a place with such a distinctive smell that I can still conjure it up today. I felt love, security, and the sense of being cared for in these brief times together.

Earliest Memories (Dr. Y.'s Perspective)

Lynda's earliest memories are colored by two powerful emotions: fear and love, in all of their many hues. Through the scabs, dressings, and bandages of her "conscious mind," she looks back on and recounts these feelings with the perspectives and cognitive vocabulary of an adult and with the detachment brought about by six decades' dilutions of time and distance. Her unconscious emotional memory, however, retains the unhealed wounds of the terror and powerlessness of her early childhood, and these feelings color and influence her *every* adult perception, conclusion, and decision. The predominant themes are powerlessness, impending peril, confusion, and the conflicted feelings associated with survival and being loved by and being *special* to a man who was dangerous and out of control. Lynda deeply loved her father, with whom she identified. Understandably, as an adult Mrs. Jensen would wish to be powerful and to be allied with potent people and institutions but, unlike her father, to maintain consistent control. Simultaneously, the power and "specialness" of success involved many dangers, including competitive retaliation by equivalents of her brothers and her mother and the sudden loss of the security, love, and specialness of the sources of power.

Alcohol is intimately involved with Mrs. Jensen's most vivid early memories and most profound feelings. Her father held all of the power in the family. All eyes were on Daddy, his moods at the time, and whether or not he had been drinking. The family's emotional status depended on Daddy's capricious disposition, as did their safety—except, perhaps, for Lynda, who was *special.*

My Father's Death (Lynda Jensen's Perspective)

What Happened to Daddy?

Right around the time I turned 4 my father became ill with what was ultimately diagnosed as acute leukemia. He died within 4 months. To the best of my memory I saw him only two times during this period of illness. Once was in the hospital when he came down to the lobby to say hello to me. (In those days children weren't permitted into patients' rooms.) The next and last time was shortly before his death, when his doctors let him come home for Christmas Eve. He lay on the couch and we had a very quiet holiday, quite different from other Christmases when all the relatives would come around. I remember getting the odd Christmas present of plastic dishes and a child-sized set of silverware, with none of the customary dolls, stuffed animals, or fancy dresses waiting for me under the tree. It was serious and scary, and Daddy was so quiet and not at all like Daddy.

Weeks later, when it dawned on me that we hadn't gone to the hospital in some time, I asked my brothers, "Why haven't we gone to see Daddy?" One of them hastily answered, "Oh, Daddy has been moved to a hospital far away and we can't go see him for a while." Possessing only the sensibility of a 4 year old, I somehow knew this answer didn't seem right. So I went to my mother and asked her where Daddy was. That is when she told me he had died. It was some time after the funeral, but I don't know how long, whether it was days or weeks.

In my mother's defense I am sure she was doing what she thought best, based on a belief that a 4 year old can't grasp death and so it is better to shelter her from the truth. She probably believed I wouldn't understand and therefore would not be all that affected, reflecting a 1950s philosophy that "children get over these things so easily." But for me it was like Daddy disappeared into the wild blue yonder, and now no one was supposed to talk about it. The sense I got was that everyone else in the family was a little relieved and almost glad he was gone. The reign of terror was over. For me, who treasured the good times with him and felt loved by him as flawed or as sick with alcoholism as he was, the fabric of my life had been ripped apart, exposing a gaping hole that could never be mended. I believe I internalized a message that I didn't matter or count because I was not supposed to be affected by my father's death.

Shortly after learning of my father's death I had a very vivid dream in which he appeared to me looking vibrant, healthy, happy, and calm. He explained that he was no longer sick and assured me that my life would be a good one and that I shouldn't worry or be afraid. I would be taken care of. This dream of my father coming to me was so real that throughout my childhood I continued to believe that it was real and that he had come back to say goodbye. My friends were never hesitant to ask about or let me talk about my father and what it was like to lose him at such a young age. When responding to their questions about the things I could remember, along with my stories of Nixie and Speedy, I would always recount the dream. My friends would be amazed and captivated and somewhat in awe, and I gained a few notches of respect and authority in their eyes as having had a peek into the great beyond by communing with my dead father, although I honestly don't believe that is why I held onto the truth of the dream.

Carrying On

The next few years were not unhappy times. My mother carried on, probably lonely and operating partly in a fog, but at least protected from the violence inflicted on her by my father. I enjoyed school and loved roller skating, ice skating, and wandering in the snowy woods by our house, playing with my friends, watching "The Mickey Mouse Club," and visiting the library with my mother. I also relished going with her to the beach in the summers. With my metal beach tag pinned to my bathing suit signifying our season pass, I felt official and like I belonged. I loved running in and out of the waves and the vanilla and raspberry ice cream Dixie cup she would buy for me at the end of our visit, which I ate slowly with my wooden spoon.

I did have little compulsions and fears. I was an inveterate thumb sucker. It took a huge effort and a lot of guidance and support from my mother for me to successfully quit in the spring of my kindergarten year. I was terrified when learning to ride a two-wheeler, with my patient brother taking the training wheels off and putting them back on numerous times until I finally felt secure about balancing. I would be thrown into angst if I got a spot on my dress, which necessitated an immediate change of outfits. I had to use a separate utensil for every item of food on my plate, with separate forks for meat, potatoes, corn, and whatever else was being served. I loved getting new shoes but hated it when the soles got scuffed, re-examining them after every few steps to see how well the smooth clean surfaces were holding up. I am not sure how many of or with how much more intensity these idiosyncrasies showed up after my father's death, but I do note I often heard about my father's demanding standards and eye for quality as demonstrated by things such as his insistence that my mother buy only leather-soled shoes.

The times I felt as if I didn't belong were few in those days and mostly revolved around some adult asking me about my father, such as what he did for a living. I dreaded answering, mainly because of the uncomfortable reaction I would detect in the questioner. I'd answer, "Oh, my father's dead." This would be followed either by a complete thud of silence or a quick change of subject, such as, "So, how do you like school?" Later I learned to respond to the question about my father in a more formal manner, explaining that he was "deceased." I thought this might present a more dignified statement of fact and thereby create a smoother landing after the grim news was delivered. The key point here is that I didn't want to be thought of as different, which in my world view meant lesser, but the universal reaction of adults to news of my father's death reinforced in me the belief that I was.

Changes

My life became more fear filled a few years later when I turned 7 and my mother pretty much ran out of the money that was left at my father's death, resulting in our having to sell our home and move to a smaller house in a less prestigious suburb. Shortly thereafter she went to work.

I really don't recall being upset by the move—either house or new school. It seemed like an adventure. When we got to our new neighborhood I remember being very excited about exploring it and learning to navigate the surrounding blocks and generally finding my way around. I seemed to make new friends in the neighborhood almost immediately and I liked my new school. I didn't really notice or care that our house was a lot smaller or that the town was more country bumpkin village than upper class suburb. All those details went right over my head. My middle brother was upset about these things. He was in seventh grade, and the disruption these changes posed in his life was, for him, major.

In the midst of this new sense of adventure, I didn't foresee the problems lurking just ahead despite the brewing warning signs. My middle brother was not at all happy, resisting the move tooth and nail and declaring he wasn't going to leave. As I recall, we had to pull him out physically the day of the move. Another dark sign came that day in the form of my mother's reaction to my excitement over what was perhaps the first snow of the season. I delighted in the snow and reacted instinctively by throwing myself onto the ground to make a snow angel. My mother became very angry, almost to the point of tears, asking what in God's name possessed me to get all snowy and wet just when we were busy trying to get ready to leave? It didn't seem like such a big trespass to me. It was only a snow angel. This wasn't the way my mother usually reacted to such things. This was a new and different side of Mom, one that kind of frightened me.

In fairly short order after the move things became very difficult for our family. Mom went to work and was less available for me. I missed her. In fourth grade I wore a house key on a chain around my neck so I could let myself in after school and waited patiently for my mother or brothers to come home. My dog was my companion. If Mom was late, I would stand by the front door window and watch for her car, afraid to think about what would happen to me if something terrible were to happen to her.

My sense of being different from other kids was exacerbated during this phase because now not only did I have an MIA father, I also had a working mother. This was not "normal" in suburbia in the fifties. Two parents—a working dad and stay at home mom—plus two or three kids and two cars in the garage were the gold standard of the times. My brothers made fun of the fathers in our neighborhood, exposing them as losers because of their tiny houses and tiny ambitions. We were much more intelligent and destined for bigger lives, they declared, like our father, whose brilliance and business success they were quick to claim as their own even though they hated his alcoholic ways. But I envied the families of those dads, whose lives may have been "small" but to me seemed normal, steady, predictable, and stable.

As my middle brother continued to flounder—trying to flunk out of high school when my mother would not let him quit and generally hanging around the wrong kids and getting into deeper trouble—my mother became in turns increasingly preoccupied and distraught. Meanwhile, our financial difficulties were mounting to the point that our home was nearly foreclosed on several times. I would overhear my oldest brother and aunts and uncles talking about my mother as if she were a child who couldn't take care of herself, and I felt sorry for her and mad at her all at the same time. I wanted her to be stronger and more capable, both in controlling my middle brother and in her ability to make a decent living, but I could see that both those challenges were beyond her. I wanted her to be a better housekeeper and make my brothers help out more. Our house was always the one with paint peeling, lawn overgrown, and in general disrepair, which heightened my sense of being different and not as good as others. In my assessment we stuck out like a sore thumb on every level.

My Desperate Drive to Control

I believe several of my key personality traits or habit patterns emerged from this period, including a desperate drive to control. I wanted to control my mother by somehow pumping her up to become more capable. That did not bear fruit, except around the edges of things. For instance, I remember going on a Christmas shopping outing with my Mom when I was in about fifth grade. She was a very generous person at heart and wanted to deliver the goods at Christmas. As she pulled out the charge card over and over, I became increasingly agitated and tried to remind her there would be big bills to pay later on. It was as if I were playing the role of her little accountant or financial planner, sporting pocket protector and horn-rimmed glasses, adding up the cost of goods purchased and trying to mitigate the damage being done.

I also took to cutting the lawn and weeding the flower beds when my brothers wouldn't and doing just about anything I could to make our house look better from the street. I used to take long walks, studying other people's neat and tidy exteriors, and longed to be part of that world that seemed so far out of my reach.

Most of all I increasingly looked at my Mom's life as the model for what I didn't want for mine. I didn't want to be the woman stuck with a husband who is mean and violent and then dies and leaves her high and dry to raise three kids on her own with only a high school education and whose life is just one struggle away from collapse.

This grade school me was very selfish. I wanted my Mom to be different from who she was because I wanted a different life. She couldn't give me what she didn't have. I often overlooked her many wonderful qualities, such as warmth, generosity, patience, a forgiving nature, dedication to raising us and making sure we received good educations, never being resentful or mean spirited, just to name a few. I zeroed in on those things I felt were the missings rather than the positives.

Of course, I was only a child and children tend to be selfish. But, I want to make a more fundamental point about selfishness and alcoholism, which is to say that many alcoholics exhibit deep levels of selfish, self-centered, and self-seeking behaviors even before they become problem drinkers. For a variety of reasons we are often scaredy-cats afraid of all manner of bad things happening, so we work very hard at controlling our environments, including the people within those environments, to try to get them to behave our way, which we of course believe to be the preferred one if anyone would just bother to listen. This is a subtle form of selfishness rooted in fear and the corresponding attempt to control. A great deal of recovery work focuses on untying this Gordian knot of fear, control, and self-centeredness.

Turning Point

Sixth grade was a pivotal time and turning point in my life. I had one of those once in a lifetime teachers, Miss Netto, who changes one's life, and she did mine. She was a new teacher with big ambitions for her students, and she set the bar high. She had us doing term papers with bibliographies and taking on interesting and challenging multidisciplinary research projects and reading novels. Altogether, this represented my first conscious experience in cultivating an intellectual curiosity that would last the rest of my life. Moreover, she helped me see I was a promising student, conveying her high hopes for my future. And I believed her.

I felt I had been given a key that would unlock a new and better future for me. If I were truly becoming a good student, I could see a future of college scholarships and a path much different than my mother's. I started praying before and after tests both to God and to my deceased father, who I thought might be "up there" keeping an eye out for my interests. The prayer was along the lines of "Please help me to do well on this test so that someday I can get a scholarship and go to college." When I received a good grade I would pray again: "Thank you for letting me do well on this test. This will really help."

Death of Lynda Jensen's Father (Dr. Y.'s Perspective)

There is a story, perhaps apocryphal, about the poet Robert Frost, who had just read aloud one of his poems to a live audience when a person in the audience asked him to explain the meaning of a particular verse. Frost responded by re-reciting the entire poem. His message was unambiguous: if he were able to articulate his meaning any more clearly than through this verse, he would have revised the poem accordingly. Even in my wildest dreams and aspirations, I know that I am no Robert Frost, and Lynda's perspective on the death of her father is a prosaic masterpiece of explication of the roles of family dynamics and tragedy in childhood in the development of personality and the formation of symptoms. Thus, I will keep my perspective on this formative period in Lynda's life relatively brief. Her poignant account says it all.

The predominant themes in this component of Lynda's history are *loss*, *damage*, and a young child's *imperfect attempts at repair*.

Loss

The terminal illness and death of her father was shrouded in silence and clouded by no attempts by adults to help 4-year-old Lynda and her brothers cope with this sudden loss. Although a young child, Lynda somehow understood that, even though he was unstable, her father had been the family's source of financial and social stability and was her primary ally and protector—both within and beyond the family. Through her vivid dream and imagination she sought to restabilize her life by bringing an idealized, all-powerful father back home to love and protect her. That worked…for a while…and at a dear cost.

Lynda's symptoms of thumb sucking and compulsions align not only with classic psychodynamic theories of critical stages of infant and childhood psychosocial development but also with symptom formation when children experience and respond to psychological trauma within these developmental periods. Such responses to trauma laid the foundations for the future adult problems for which Lynda sought treatment. According to these theories, Lynda's self-soothing thumb sucking would reflect a regression to her *oral stage* of development in order to experience reduced anxiety and security by remerging at the breast of her all-nurturing and protective mother. This theory would be corroborated by Lynda's acknowledging her mother's kind and supportive response to the embarrassing habit and by our understanding of what, as an adult, Lynda liked about and "got" from drinking alcohol—apart from all the problems it engendered. Alcohol use can be viewed as a reflection of Lynda's seeking orally engendered comfort, security, and pleasure when these were in painfully short supply in her daily life as an adult.

Lynda's obsessions—getting a spot on her dress, scuffing the soles of her new shoes—and compulsions—checking the soles every few steps—would be viewed theoretically as a fixation at her *anal stage* of development wherein she would receive approval from authority figures and a sense of personal mastery and gratification by controlling her bowel movements. Like her oral fixation, the symptomatic manifestations of anally based dynamics in her adult life become especially pronounced during times of stress and conflict. As an adult, her efforts to perform perfectly and to control herself and others were her attempt to be loved and accepted. However, she would resent having to perform for what seemed to be bestowed on others "for free." Lynda's resentment (i.e., disguised rage) would lead especially to frustration, self-directed anger, and passive-aggressive retaliation whenever others failed to appreciate her or her achievements sufficiently or when they let her down by not reciprocating in kind. Destroying oneself and one's life through alcohol is, among many other things, a form of passive aggression directed toward self and toward others who care about and depend on that person.

Damage

Magical Thinking

Even before Lynda's father died, there was no communication about the critically important family issues—such as the physical and emotional effects of her father's alcohol-related rages and violence on her family. Her *not* being informed of the seriousness and long-term implications of her father's illness coupled with the suddenness of his death delivered a clear and terrifying message to young Lynda: "What you don't know *can* hurt you!" Her response was to try to know about and to control whatever she could—from keeping her dresses unspotted and the soles of her shoes unscuffed to using separate forks for meat, potatoes, corn, etc. She sustained a *magical belief* that, through this omniscience and total control, she could prevent another rug from being pulled out from under her and leading to her cascade into a dangerous, dark abyss of uncertainty.

Directly related to young Lynda's "need" for control is the self-centered way in which 4 year olds view the world. Devoted parents sternly warn their young children, "Don't touch the burner on the stove, or you'll burn your finger" or "Don't play with Mommy's scissors, or you will cut yourself" or, in fear-borne anger, "Don't run into the street or you'll get hit by a car" or the like. There are occasions when children do not listen to their parents, only to suffer the untoward consequences about which their guardians warned. In such circumstances they are reminded, "you were punished because you didn't listen to us," which, when translated into a 4 year old's black and white vernacular, becomes "I got hurt *because* I was bad." As an extension of this form of logic, a child believes that "good things happen when I am good, and bad things happen when I am bad." Thus, when her father died, young Lynda concluded, unconsciously, that this tragedy occurred "because she had been a bad girl." One psychological "benefit" of such a conclusion—bestowed at an enormous toll—was that her "responsibility" for her father's death lent some degree of predictability and control to what otherwise would be an arbitrary, dangerous world: "If I am a good little girl—even better, if I am a perfect little girl—nothing so terrifying will ever again happen to me or to anyone I love." This bargain came at the expense of Lynda's unconscious belief that she was *responsible* for and thus *culpable* for the death of her father.

Electra Complex and "Damaged Goods"

A second source of both experiential and psychological damage was associated with young Lynda's gaining a more realistic view of her mother. Incrementally, she was compelled to accept that her mother, although loving and well-intended, was severely limited in providing for the family's ongoing needs. This painful reality was evidenced in Lynda's brief anecdote about the Christmas shopping episode with her mother when she was in the fifth grade. While her warm-hearted and well-intentioned mother was blithely using a credit card to pay for an abundance of Christmas presents, 10-year-old Lynda was becoming increasingly upset and agitated over her mother's obliviousness to the reality that, at some point, these gifts had to be paid for. Most children of Lynda's age would have been focused on the gifts, not on the long-term implications of their being bought on credit. Lynda's eventual response to her mother's lack of what is called *executive functioning*, or the ability to anticipate and respond rationally and sequentially to future needs (e.g., have the money *before* you splurge on gifts), was to become *her mother's mother.* She placed herself in charge of planning and doing what was needed for herself as well as, to a lesser extent, for her mother and her brothers.

Lynda's 1) belief that she was *favored* by her father, 2) feeling *responsible* and *to blame* for her father's death, and 3) *displacing* the role of her mother are the classic ingredients for Oedipal, or in the case of women, Electral psychodynamics, as was presented in Chapter 4, "Stuck in My Job," with regard to Clarke Myerson's relationship with his father, Nathan. Lynda's unconscious psychological response to the competitive envy and retaliation of her mother and brothers was to begin to regard herself as "damaged goods," which would be interpreted by psychoanalysts as a *castration equivalent*. Beyond maintaining a smaller, less potent target by being damaged, she also could claim that she had been duly *punished* for her ambitious transgressions. Therefore, there was no need for her to be attacked further by her rivals. Lynda felt exposed and shamed when asked about her father by peers and their parents. She was also sensitive to being different from her friends and their families by having a working mother and an inferior, deteriorating home, which also reflected her being different and *not belonging* by virtue of her being "a bad girl" and "damaged goods."

Repair

Let us engage in a healthful, justifiable "pause" in appreciation of, and in respect and praise for, gifted teachers. Among the many treasures that they bestow is the rescue of troubled young souls by helping them recognize, accept, and actualize their worth and, as Lynda described, to offer them a key to "unlock a new and better future." For young Lynda the golden key was the discovery of her passion for learning and her aptitude for excelling intellectually, which she has done since junior high school.

Because Lynda would bring with her adulthood successes the vestiges of her psychological responses to her early life trauma, her repair is incomplete. Without her having had the opportunity to address the psychological implications of her early childhood, one could anticipate that whereas Lynda's future was likely to be better, it would not, entirely, be new. For example, there are two important, fundamental, and persisting adult manifestations of her perceiving herself as "damaged goods": 1) she believes that she must *be perfect, perform with perfection,* and *be in total control* in order not to be exposed as being deficient and broken, and 2) she engages in and puts up with devaluing, exploitative relationships—until she can't stand it anymore. And then she is vulnerable to drinking. My job as her psychotherapist, therefore, is to become Lynda's objective and trusted guide as she revisits, reevaluates, and reformulates the events of her childhood and the conclusions that she reaches about herself and others.

Growing Up (Lynda Jensen's Perspective)

High School

I am strongly tempted to fast-forward my account to adulthood because I feel self-conscious about going into such depths about my life. I don't want to be perceived as a whiner, and I hear a critical voice whispering in my ear to "just get on with life, for God's sake. Stop wallowing in the past." My response to that voice is Dr. Y., who tells me that it is not always best to bury my thoughts and feelings and that to perceive myself as an undeserving, self-absorbed whiner might be a defense against facing, for the first time, frightening memories and feelings. So on through adolescence to adulthood.

Adolescence presented the same family challenges but with some important distinctions. School became an increasingly positive force in my life. I continued to do well and loved learning and putting time and energy into my studies. Starting in seventh grade, however, I began to experience bouts of out-of-body sensations. It was as if I were a talking and thinking mind dismembered from my body. I'd be speaking with someone, and all of a sudden this sensation of being detached from my body would wash over me. I'd see my hand as if it didn't belong to me, as if it were a separate object or belonged to someone else. Needless to say, this was very frightening. I'd try to stay calm and never succumbed to an out and out panic attack, but it was terrifying.

After a few of these episodes, I talked to my mother and tried to describe what I was experiencing and my accompanying terror over not being able to control what was happening to me. Her response, which was beautifully simple but not at all helpful to me at the time, was "just don't think about those things if they bother you so much." Ultimately, I kind of trained myself to handle these episodes calmly, continuing to talk and present an outward appearance of normalcy while inwardly noting the out-of-body experience and reminding myself it would pass, which it always did…eventually.

College

Because of my family's financial situation, I never was sure I'd be able to go to college until close to the actual time for leaving. I wasn't 100% certain that my scholarship money, together with what

I had saved from the many jobs I had since I was 11 years old, would add up to what was needed. A couple of last-minute windfalls pushed me over the line: these included a scholarship from the Benevolent and Protective Order of the Elks and an additional academic scholarship from the Mothers' Club at the University of California, Berkeley, where I attended. My mother said she would try to help by providing some money from her Social Security benefits and my father's veterans benefits, and I would work almost full time throughout the academic year and summers. All in all, I could hardly believe I was actually college-bound. It had been an almost mythical dream for all of those years starting in sixth grade, and now it was becoming a reality.

I decided to major in math, with the goal of being a secondary education teacher, and I minored in French and English. I was on my way to a new and better world! Slowly, I became in tune with the rhythm of college life. I really enjoyed my classes, particularly my mathematics, English lit, and French classes. I was taking third-year French, having tested out of 2 years, and the classes were small and held entirely in French. I got straight A's, joined a sorority, and started developing a closer knit social life, although I was still haunted by a sense that I didn't quite fit in. And then, when I was a sophomore, I met Laurence.

Laurence

Laurence seemed different from the very few other guys whom I had dated in college. Until his junior year he had been on the varsity lacrosse team, but he had become disillusioned with the coach and program. He also felt that lacrosse was interfering with his ability to earn the GPA he needed to get into med school. I thought he was both fun and serious, and I really liked that he came from a large, close, and wealthy family in Southern California. I thought that, like me, he was someone who was serious and wanted to do something meaningful with his life. Most important, he came from a solid base and was striving for a secure future.

We continued to be a couple over the remaining school year. That summer I learned to taste life as he knew it, through many La Jolla, California, parties and social events. I was experienced in how to buy nice clothes on sale with my earnings from my part-time jobs and knew how to present myself with a certain modicum of refinement, so I fit in with his family. I felt that I was regaining the alpha dog station I had lost when my father died, although I didn't understand it that way at the time. I was gravitating more and more toward the bosom of Laurence's family and further away from mine.

On one occasion, however, we had a big argument when I casually mentioned that I worried about his eating so much junk food. Upon his questioning me, I admitted that I had noticed that he was getting a bit overweight now that he was no longer playing lacrosse so intensively. I quickly learned this was not a permissible topic. He exploded and broke off our relationship. I was shocked and crushed because I hadn't expected such an extreme reaction. I felt abandoned and desperate to get back into his good graces. I was vulnerable and felt terribly wounded. I'm not sure why I fell to such emotional depths. As I recall, I finally groveled my way back into his life and good graces, and we became a couple again.

In December Laurence had completed college and was living back at home while waiting to hear about whether or not he was accepted to medical school. One night he surprised me with an unplanned visit to campus to tell me that he had been accepted to Loma Linda Medical School near Los Angeles. I was the first person he told. We celebrated by driving back to La Jolla to tell his parents. Soon thereafter he surprised me again, but this time less favorably. He had decided to go to Argentina and study Spanish for a semester before entering med school. He also talked me into the "wisdom" of our dating others while he was away. Again, I was crushed and felt totally abandoned.

I did not hear very much from Laurence for several months and, glumly, went about planning my future. One afternoon, just as I was going into my abstract geometry class, Laurence showed up unexpectedly outside the math building. I thought he was still in Argentina, but here he was back on campus and standing right in front of me. He asked me to marry him. I was shocked and swept off my feet. In an instant I forgave his abandonment of me and said yes. We married that June. I was just shy of my 21st birthday, and he was not quite 22.

I decided to apply to the Computing and Mathematical Sciences section of the Engineering and Applied Sciences Division of Cal Tech, which is located not too far from Loma Linda Medical School. Cal Tech is an absolutely outstanding university in my area of interest. It is a small school with incredible standards and is notoriously difficult to gain admission to. Still, I thought it was worth a shot so that I could be near Laurence. About 6 months later, just after I was notified that I was to be graduated at the very top of my class at Berkeley, I also learned that I was admitted with a full scholarship to Cal Tech. I was ecstatic and couldn't wait to tell Laurence. I was dismayed that Laurence was far less enthusiastic about my acceptance to Cal Tech than we both had been when he got into Loma Linda Medical School. Finally, I decided it was best to put his tepid response out of my mind; he probably was just overworked from his first year of medical school.

Newlyweds

We were just kids, masquerading as grown-ups. Looking back, I had
thought at the time that my enthusiasm was fueled by some sort of
romantic love, but now I realize it probably came more from a desire, perhaps even need, to be taken care of and to become absorbed
into what I saw as his secure, successful, and lively family. To be part
of a family system that didn't sit around waiting for bad things to
happen but, rather, charted its own course of happy destiny was
more than I had previously dared to imagine for myself.

When I said yes to Laurence's proposal, I certainly didn't stop to
think through all the implications, such as what it would be like to
be pursuing a Ph.D. in engineering and computer sciences with
brilliant peers and demanding professors while married to a medical
student whom I would rarely get to see, or to be living in a tiny basement apartment in a place where I did not know anyone.

As expected, Cal Tech was a challenge, and it took me some time
to ease into this new way of thinking, analyzing, and verbalizing basic and applied science. Also, it took me a while to believe I could be
successful at it. All of my classmates were brilliant, with most coming from Stanford, Cal Tech, MIT, and prestigious Ivy League
schools. The professors were world class and demanding, and they
expected a lot of us. The long and short of it was that I felt insecure
about whether I could hack it. Also, this was at a time when only
about 5% or 10% of the class was made up of women. To my surprise, once I settled in with the culture of Cal Tech and understood
the beauty of applied basic sciences, I did very well. I had found an
academic home.

As I was becoming more acclimated into the ways of graduate
school in engineering and computational sciences, my marriage began showing signs of deep cracks below the surface of things. At the
start of my second year, Laurence began volunteering at a free
health clinic. He worked alongside a nurse with whom he began to
hang out after clinic hours. When I protested that it didn't seem appropriate, he'd respond with "Lynda, you're just too insecure and
jealous." He'd make it seem as if I were trying to smother him by
being unreasonably possessive. He'd also point out how I couldn't
possibly understand what medicine was all about and that he needed
friends and colleagues with whom he could talk. I'd walk away telling myself that I must be the one with the problem, admitting that
yes, indeed, I was insecure and that it was reasonable for him to have
female friends other than me.

But things got worse. She began calling him in the middle of the
night wanting to talk. He was now suggesting that we socialize with
her and her husband. It was dreadful and I felt total emotional, psy-

chic, and even physical pain. He kept telling me she was just a friend and I kept trying to accept that at face value. I needed to keep up my studies and would force myself to concentrate, but all the while I felt my insides were being ripped up into pieces.

One day I had an epiphany when walking to class. My inner voice said perhaps she is just a friend; I really don't know, but that doesn't matter. What matters is that I can't live with my husband having this kind of friendship with another woman. It may be OK for another wife, but it wasn't OK for me. I worked up the courage to tell him this and to say that he'd have to make a choice. He could have these kinds of friendships or he could have me, but he couldn't have both.

That took care of things, at least for then. He broke off the friendship and recommitted to me. I believed I had dodged a bullet and that I could get over what I hoped would be an isolated experience. I let go of asking more about the full extent of their relationship and tried to put it into the past and hoped it wouldn't bleed into my future.

Quite unexpectedly, I became pregnant in the spring of my second year at Cal Tech; Laurence was a third-year medical student. This was quite unexpected because I had not had a period in over 10 months or so and my doctor had been concerned I might have fertility issues. I wasn't feeling very well for a few weeks, and we were surprised but excited when the random pregnancy test came back positive. I gave birth to our son, Matthew, the following December, a few days after my finals, and went back to school when he was 10 days old. We found a wonderful babysitter, and it was still hard going but also a magical time. My baby son helped me gain a new perspective about what was truly important, which sharpened and informed my priorities. I used my time as efficiently as possible, going to the library between classes to study rather than socializing with classmates and returning home to our apartment as soon as classes were over for the day. I'd study whenever Matthew was sleeping. Because Laurence was on his clinical rotations in medical school, he was always away or needed his sleep when he was at home. He did not participate in caring for Matthew.

As that semester continued, the effects of sleep deprivation began taking a toll. I started experiencing severe insomnia, unable to fall asleep even after Matthew was safely tucked in and fast asleep in his crib. It was as if my system were on high alert 24/7 as I lay in bed, my mind darting back and forth between listening for Matthew to wake up and thinking about how much more reading I had to complete for my classes and independent research. There were nights I would get up, go into the kitchen, and reach for a bottle of alcohol. I'd pour a glass and try to silence my mind so that I could sleep. This is my first recollection of using alcohol as medicine. I remember thinking that this was a little weird and creepy, as memories of my father flashed into my head, but I felt desperate and I counted on alcohol's effects to work for me.

As I entered my third year of graduate school, I became pregnant with Dennis. Laurence graduated from medical school a few weeks earlier and decided to take a trip to see some old friends on the East Coast. I was in the midst of midterms, newly pregnant, and caring for a 1 year old. Having hoped that Laurence would use his rare free time to be with me and help me care for Matthew, I felt a little abandoned in having to wrap up my year alone and without help. But he wanted to have some time "just having fun" before starting his internship and was undeterred in his decision to go. I was not happy about this and did my best to understand and put a positive spin on it. I didn't want to let what both he and I agreed were "my selfish feelings" get in the way of his career. Somehow, I managed to finish out my year well and was absolutely surprised when told that I had the top grade in my entire year.

When contemplating what came next in our marriage, I am finding it very difficult to think about it, much less write about it. I can now see and feel my past self barreling ahead so innocently and naively, and so very ill equipped, toward a precipice of loss, heartache, and hardening of spirit and soul from which I am only now beginning to recover. It was one of those singular turning points that I see now but didn't then, and I feel a deep sadness for my former self.

Growing Up (Dr. Y.'s Perspective)

High School

Lynda began her discussion of adolescence with an apology:

> I am strongly tempted to fast-forward my account to adulthood because I feel self-conscious about going into such depths about my life. I don't want to be perceived as a whiner, and I hear a critical voice whispering in my ear to "just get on with life, for God's sake. Stop wallowing in the past."

I interpret her qualms as her understandable resistance to revisiting her painful past. Other patients with similar misgivings are less polite and accurate:

> All psychiatry wants their patients to do is to wallow around in the past and to blame *others* for their problems. I prefer to deal with the here and now and to leave the past where it belongs—in the past.

People who make this assertion are often fearful of facing and dealing with the painful realities of their pasts, and they usually learn that there is no way around the pain—only through it.

Lynda next discusses her feelings of depersonalization and derealization and her mother's advice about how to deal with them:

> Starting in seventh grade, however, I began to experience bouts of out-of-body sensations. It was as if I were a talking and thinking mind dismembered from my body.

Feelings such as those described above by Lynda occur frequently with people with significant anxiety disorders, including panic disorder and generalized anxiety disorder. In addition, they commonly occur in people who have suffered from severe life stresses that overwhelm the psychological and biological coping systems, such as posttraumatic stress disorder. Anxiety disorders—particularly panic disorder—have a strong hereditary component and a powerful comorbidity with alcohol use disorder. Not only did Lynda suffer from alcohol dependence but so did her father and many other members of her family. Very likely, to some extent, both she and her family members were endeavoring to "treat" these psychiatric conditions with ethanol—which is akin to trying to put out a fire with jet fuel. Not only does it not help, it makes the psychological problems dangerously worse.

Another pathological way of "dealing" with depersonalization is to *not* deal with these symptoms. This is exactly what was proposed by Lynda's warm, well-intentioned, yet ineffectual mother:

> After a few of these episodes, I talked to my mother and tried to describe what I was experiencing and my accompanying terror over not being able to control what was happening to me. Her response, which was beautifully simple but not at all helpful to me at the time, was "just don't think about those things if they bother you so much."

Not dealing with psychological symptoms, technically termed in psychiatry *compartmentalization*, is often as dangerous and disabling over the long run as using alcohol. Patterns of avoidance of key problems sow the seeds of poor choices and decision making that, over time, reap a bitter, hurtful harvest. In the next sections, we will trace how this dysfunctional approach is tragically manifested in Mrs. Jensen's life.

College

During college, Lynda gained the confidence that her game plan of combining her superior intelligence with hard work was paying off. Although she worked nearly full time to pay for her education and although she was taking the most challenging mathematics and humanities courses at a fine and competitive university, she was an academic superstar. She also was coming into her own socially. Would her formula for success be sufficient to overcome the trauma of her childhood, the effects of which she did not have the opportunity to address directly?

Laurence

As a college sophomore, Lynda was coming into her own when she met Laurence. She was excelling academically and had an active social life. One can understand how she would be swept off her feet by a handsome athlete who came from a large, close, and affluent family and who seemed to be serious about his future as a professional. Lynda believed that she had been bestowed with these assets until the death of her father and that all of these assets could be reinstated with a relationship with Laurence and his family. With the clarity of hindsight, however, Lynda was too young and inexperienced to comprehend the great risk of hitching her future so completely to someone else's star. Lynda had idealized the part of her early childhood prior to the death of her father and was vulnerable to "losing herself" to regain a fantasy:

> I felt that I was regaining the alpha dog station I had lost when my father died, although I didn't understand it that way at the time. I was gravitating more and more toward the bosom of Laurence's family and further away from mine.

I don't regard it as a coincidence when a person abrogates her power and personal agency to another person, because "it takes two to tango." Like radar, people with high levels of narcissism detect others who are particularly vulnerable to putting up with their machinations. And the evidence of Laurence's pathological narcissism was apparent in the earliest phases of their relationship. Examples include his overreaction to Lynda's observation about his eating habits, his sudden abandonment of Lynda when he went to Argentina and his theatrical return to her with a proposal of marriage, and their antipodal responses to the other's acceptance to graduate school. People should pay more attention to being on emotional roller coasters early in a relationship. Ignoring the implications of these feelings is inviting a ride that is more painful than exciting. And, as she indicated, Lynda had learned to "deal" with unsavory feelings by rationalizing and burying them:

> I was dismayed that Laurence was far less enthusiastic about my acceptance to Cal Tech than we both had been when he got into Loma Linda Medical School. Finally, I decided it was best to put his tepid response out of my mind; he probably was just overworked from his first year of medical school.

Newlyweds

Lynda's pattern of not acknowledging the implications of painful realities that she was perceiving was becoming increasingly more difficult to sustain. Her inability to stand up for herself had at least three distressing consequences: 1) Laurence continued to violate her trust while disavowing doing so, 2) Lynda's denial of what was going on in her marriage was affecting her mental stability, and 3) Lynda's dependence on alcohol began. There is only so much than one can swallow and keep down without a lubricant and depressant. Unfortunately, alcohol is both.

> As that semester continued, the effects of sleep deprivation began taking a toll. I started experiencing severe insomnia, unable to fall asleep even after Matthew was safely tucked in and fast asleep in his crib. It was as if my system were on high alert 24/7 as I lay in bed, my mind darting back and forth between listening for Matthew to wake up and thinking about how much more reading I had to complete for my classes and independent research. There were nights I would get up, go into the kitchen, and reach for a bottle of alcohol. I'd pour a glass and try to silence my mind so that I could sleep. This is my first recollection of using alcohol as medicine.

Infidelities and Losses (Lynda Jensen's Perspective)

> Laurence completed medical school and decided to specialize in general surgery. It soon became apparent that his relationship with the nurse back when I was a first-year graduate student was not to be

an isolated incident. I discovered he reconnected with a former girl-friend when he visited L.A. Then, as he rolled through his intern-ship year, a number of other new women friends popped in and out of the scene. I confronted him but didn't lay down a clear ultimatum as I had previously. I felt trapped now with two babies. I lost the clar-ity of mind and voice that I was able to muster up the first time around. I was devastated by the realization that it was all happening again and yet not really wanting to admit it. Walking away from my marriage did not seem like an option; I needed for it to be OK. At one point when I pleaded to know what was really going on, he shot back with something along the lines of "You don't really believe I ha-ven't had sex with anyone else, do you?" I felt humiliated and crushed. After a while I asked for a separation. He protested but then moved out of the house for a short period of time. In quick succes-sion his father underwent a heart bypass operation and my mother was diagnosed with terminal cancer. We put our marriage difficulties on hold for the time being. I was very involved in caring for my mother through her treatment and last months of life. I didn't ask what Laurence was doing when he wasn't with me, and I tried to block it out the best I could because I needed every inch of emo-tional bandwidth I had to deal with the fact my mother was dying.

When my mother died, I was 26 years old and at sea. I was doing well on the job, but my marriage was so far from what I had pictured for myself that I began to lose sight of what that original picture looked like as it continued to fade away. We moved to the San Fran-cisco Bay area, where Laurence began a practice and I was hired as a software engineer by a major computer firm in Silicon Valley. Lau-rence made a plea to renew our marriage. He said things would be much better now that he had completed his training. He was joining a big group of surgeons, so his call schedule would be manageable, he'd be happier, we'd be financially secure, and life would be good. I decided to give it another try.

A number of factors propelled this decision to try again. I con-tinued to worry about the kids, particularly Matthew. I told myself they would be better off if Laurence and I stayed together. I con-cluded that he must have loved me because I had given him every opportunity to fly the coop and he still wanted to stay married to me. I believed, or was at least making the attempt to believe, that I could permit him his sexual waywardness as long as I understood that he loved me and didn't want to leave. I'd tolerate what he may or may not be doing on the side. I would simply not allow myself to think too much about it. We had two more children, daughters, and he continued to be unfaithful on a regular basis.

My career progressed in tandem with the explosive growth of the field—from personal computers to laptops to mobile devices. As one of the first women with training and experience in computational science and engineering, I had developed an international reputation as a pioneer in this area. Much of the responsibilities at home in the raising of four young children and coordinating our household were in my court, as well. I was becoming tired and resentful. Eventually, I could take no more and insisted on a formal divorce from Laurence. Although he had insisted on joint custody legally, he was not dependable in providing for our children's needs or helping me out in disciplining them or managing their lives. I would arrange for all of their appointments, activities, and school supplies and would be responsible for carpooling duties, getting them to practices, attending their school functions and games, and whatever else needed organizing. Sometimes when I'd return home after a long day at work, when the kids were with Laurence, I'd pull the car into the garage and just sit there for a while, thinking to myself how easy it would be to let the car keep running and just kind of fade away. I also began to drink heavily during this time.

Infidelities and Losses (Dr. Y.'s Perspective)

There is little to add to this section beyond what Lynda describes and what I have written previously. The seeds of the distress and dissolution of Laurence and Lynda's relationship were sown and were evident long before its dry harvest. *Laurence was unfaithful to Lynda, and Lynda was unfaithful to herself.* As time moved on, the gaping chasm between how she functioned in her work and in her maternal roles and what she put up with in her relationship with her husband became more than even she could tolerate or traverse.

In the next section we will focus on Lynda's soul-depleting struggles against the relentless currents and tides of alcohol. As one might anticipate, the same unaddressed psychological conflicts that set the stage for her dysfunctional marriage would also undermine her attempts to conquer alcohol dependence.

"Downing and Drowning": My Struggles with Alcohol (Lynda Jensen's Perspective)

From my mid to late twenties, drinking had become ritualized into almost all of my job and social functions. We'd have wine at parties, brunches, dinners out, ski trips, and other outings. I had a group of young engineering friends, and drinking just seemed to be a part of having fun. Drinking was also involved in every corporate party and even at lunch when there was something to celebrate. I always liked the way it made me feel—relaxed, confident, open and friendly, and comfortable in my own skin, like I fully belonged. I sometimes drank too much but for the most part controlled my intake and didn't stand out from others. I frequently had wine with dinner at home. My best friend, Susan, and I talked about opening up a wine bar in a cool area of the city, setting ourselves up to eventually leave the computer industry. (We both went on to become senior vice presidents in our respective firms, and the wine bar idea fell by the wayside.)

During these years my drinking continued pretty much at the same pace as before, with wine every night at dinner, typically about two glasses, and another glass later in the evening with my bath. The wine was my medicine, helping me to let go of work and all the challenges of the day and sink into being at home, smoothing the transition, which I generally found difficult. Every so often I would quit for a month or so to prove I could, but I'd always return to my daily evening wine routine. I wouldn't want to go out to eat unless it was a restaurant that served wine, reflecting how important it was for me to get my daily fix.

Right around the time I turned 50, my drinking took a critical turn. I found that instead of two glasses of wine at dinner, I was downing three, four, or more. Afterward I'd look at the nearly empty bottle and it was as if the wine had just disappeared into the ether, and I'd be surprised to see how much I had drunk. One Friday night I came home from a business trip and we ordered Vietnamese takeout. Naomi and Eloise, my two youngest, had a bunch of their high school friends in for dinner. After dinner Eloise and her group were leaving for an evening of fun, the plans of which were too vague for my liking. We had an argument, and I said she couldn't leave without telling me where they were going and when they'd be home. She blew me off, probably because I may have been showing the effects of my early evening wine, and she just left with her friends. I was so angry that I double-locked the doors of the house with the rationale that she would have to ring the doorbell and face me when she returned home. When she got home she rang the doorbell, but I was passed out in bed from too much wine and didn't hear her. She thought that I had intentionally locked her out. This was January in Northern California, and the weather was particularly cold. She called her sister, and the two of them went to their dad's to sleep. The next morning when I awoke I was shocked to see I had gone through one and a half bottles of wine the night before. When I learned about what I had done to my two daughters, I was horrified and remorseful at the deepest level of my being. I felt I had pulled the world down on my beautiful, innocent daughters, two beings for whom I'd go to the ends of the Earth to love, cherish, and protect. When we sat down the next morning I told them I had wanted only to talk, not lock them out. I also admitted for the first time to people who mattered to me that I had a problem with alcohol, which I could now plainly see, and that I was going to quit drinking. And I really meant it.

Trying to Stop (Lynda Jensen's Perspective)

In the ensuing months I went to AA, although I quickly concluded it wasn't for me. The people there seemed too obsessed with alcohol and in my view hadn't really put it behind them, as evidenced by their relentless storytelling about their past use. There was also a little too much of the God thing for my liking. On my own, I'd go for weeks not drinking then declare I was going to try moderation rather than total abstinence. Then when that didn't work I'd go back to abstaining. I tried meditation, a weekend "how to quit drinking without AA" retreat and one-on-one therapy sessions with a chemical dependency counselor, among other things. I wandered in this fashion for about 8 years—back and forth between trying to moderate, failing at that quest, then abstaining for some period, then repeating the above. I would vow to quit and make the attempt but then could not stay quit. A voice would pop into my head and tell me that I could get this thing under control and drink moderately if I just worked harder at it. Or it would argue that by periodically abstaining, I might perhaps eventually lose my taste for it so that quitting would sort of just evolve over time. (This was the way it had worked for me when I quit eating beef.) Basically, alcohol's siren call and its promised relief proved too much for me, and I'd continue to succumb despite my resolve.

I lied to my family, telling them I was not drinking when I actually was, and rationalizing the lie by my continued attempts at quitting. Like an eternal optimist, which I am not, I told myself I'd eventually grow out of the need for wine if I just kept trying. This entire process was very hurtful to my family members and greatly damaged their faith and trust in me. I felt increasingly guilty and ashamed about my behavior, which strengthened my desire to drink. I began to think of myself as a pitiful failure when it came to alcohol. All my achieving ways were not up to this match.

Bernard (Lynda Jensen's Perspective)

Several years after my separation from Laurence, I met Bernard, who, at the time, was an attorney in a large law firm in New York City. At the time we first met, I thought he was energetic and attrac-

tive, and I admired his intellect and legal talents. He was divorced
and had several teenage children, and mine were much younger. I
didn't see him again for another year but became reacquainted with
him at a business meeting on the East Coast. We began to date and
were married about two and a half years later. Laurence had already
remarried by that time subsequent to getting an annulment, which
he claimed he did to keep his parents happy by remarrying in the
Catholic Church. This hurt, but I acquiesced. Nonetheless, I tore
up the annulment papers when I received them in the mail and
promptly threw the scraps in the wastebasket.

In the early years of our marriage, Bernard lived and worked in
New York City, while I continued to work and live in the Silicon
Valley region of California. We dedicated ourselves to carrying on
a long-distance marriage, seeing each other mainly on weekends—
when possible. When I was married to Laurence, I was able to work
for my company on a flexible basis so that I could be home with the
kids most afternoons and manage the household. The amount of
money I earned was of secondary concern, with Laurence also being
a strong financial breadwinner at that point. My life with Bernard
would be different. He quickly suggested that I was going to have to
increase my time at work because he had lots of financial commitments: alimony payments to what were now two ex-wives, child
support for his youngest child, plus all the added expenses we would
have by way of maintaining two homes and traveling back and forth
to see each other. He was also carrying the mortgage on a beach
house and a lot of college and graduate school debt.

I thought I could make our marriage work by squeezing my
travel and late evening work into the times the kids were with Laurence and by having a full-time, live-in nanny. I did make it work,
but I was never as happy with that configuration. I was now working
all the time and worrying so much about money. Thus, I went into
this marriage with my eyes only partially open. It was as if I were on
a one-way track to get married and ignored the obvious signs of
trouble ahead. I lived in a fantasy zone, believing Bernard would
find a way to move to San Francisco eventually, even though he
never indicated he could or would. I thought he wouldn't be able to
stand being apart from me and would compromise on his stance on
staying in New York. That never happened. We continued to do the
long-distance thing through 13 years of marriage.

As I write this chronicle of my life, I see more clearly how I continued to place myself in a victim role in my marriages. With Laurence, I stayed way too long in a marriage bereft of intimacy and
honesty. I felt lonely and sorry for myself, and I compensated
through overachievement in the office and home. With Bernard, I
settled for a marriage where my husband couldn't be consistently

physically present, and I felt lonely and sorry for myself that I had to do so much on my own. And I resented having to work so hard to make ends meet. I acted as if it were written somewhere that this was the way it was to be and that I didn't have the power to make other choices. This was to be my lot in life, or so it seemed.

In the early 2000s Bernard and I decided to leave our respective firms, he to retire and I to take on a senior research and development position in a new start-up company in Silicon Valley. I imagined that we'd both travel less and be home more. My sons had already completed college and had begun their careers, and my daughters were in college. My priorities included having more free time for family and leisure and to take better care of my health issues. Bernard was going to manage our investments, which we then believed were sufficient to allow us to cut back in this way. Within a year, however, Bernard had lost most of our liquid assets in the tech stock bubble crash. I encouraged him to go back to working in a law firm in San Francisco, but he did not like the idea of having to work so hard once more.

Meanwhile, my new company took off like a rocket, and I, as one of the earliest employees, was a major executive in its management and development. Soon, I became one of three managing directors of a top high-tech firm. However, I was working harder than ever, and Bernard was not working at all.

I turned my mind to viewing this change as a new challenge that would demand the best from me and would therefore reenergize my focus and priorities. I threw myself into bringing innovation and value into my role and all the associated duties and had to stretch myself to cover a broader range of activities than I had managed in previous jobs. Going back to drinking wine at night with dinners, albeit more than two glasses, with occasional times of total abstinence, I limited my drinking to a more controlled and moderate pattern.

Bernard (Dr. Y.'s Perspective)

Tearing up and discarding the notification by the Catholic Church of the annulment of her marriage to Laurence did not erase the years of heartbreak and disappointment that Lynda had suffered in a marriage to a man whom she could not trust and who prioritized his needs over hers and those of their four children. Nor did it expunge Lynda's unconscious conflicts and psychodynamics that would lead her to attract and be attracted to other men with this personality profile.

Although Bernard does not have affairs nor does he lie to Lynda, many of the basic elements of his behavior and their marriage are analogous to those of her first husband and marriage. Examples of the parallels are numerous: 1) Lynda believes that she and her husband are not a team in sharing the economic burdens and household responsibilities—i.e., she feels alone and exploited; 2) like Laurence, Bernard takes very good care of Bernard in that he is quite comfortable with an affluent lifestyle without making the personal sacrifices required to advance the needs of Lynda or their marriage; 3) there is poor communication in the marriage about sensitive but important issues in their relationship—with both parties sharing equal responsibility for this deficit; and 4) while accepting the material and organizational benefits of Lynda's talents, hard work, and career success, both Laurence and Bernard failed to confront her meaningfully about her alcohol abuse or to participate actively in the treatment thereof.

I would postulate that if Lynda were to overcome her alcohol dependence—much of it related to her low self-esteem and rage over allowing herself to be exploited in her marriage—the power structure in the marriage and Lynda's demands for improved marital participation and intimacy from her husbands would have changed accordingly. Marriage is not so different from other complex human systems and arrangements, such as politics, business, and professions—when there are problems with promises, expectations, contracts, and relationships, just follow the power and money to determine where these faults lie hiding. In both marriages, the financial and family functional *responsibilities* but none of the *power* were Lynda's domain, and she did not know why. Inevitably, she returned to alcohol to "dis-solve" the problem, with the predictable results.

Going Under (Lynda Jensen's Perspective)

> Five years into this new life my drinking started to escalate. It came to a head when Bernard suggested we both stop drinking to get ready for a trip to Africa to climb Mount Kilimanjaro. I agreed, thinking this would be the perfect opportunity to quit for good. I found out, however, that this attempt to totally quit "for good" exacerbated the situation for me. I discovered that I couldn't quit. The mental obsession to drink was overpowering and seemed to get stronger. What's worse, because Bernard was doing just fine and keeping to his part of our pact, I felt terribly guilty and was now drinking here and there in secret.

After a few months of this pattern, I reached out to family members and friends and admitted to them that I was an alcoholic, that I knew I needed to quit, that I was going to try doing so through AA. For the first time, I also said I was willing to consider going into a treatment program if necessary. Meanwhile, I was wrapping up a huge project for work that was taking up pretty much all of my waking time, leaving little time for AA. This led to a cycle of working very hard, then drinking, then recovering from the effects, then doing it all over again. I didn't make time for AA and decided that once the project was complete I'd clear away all commitments and focus on getting sober. I spoke with my boss and confessed that I had a problem with alcohol, that I wanted to quit but had not been able to do so on my own, and that I planned to go to a 28-day treatment program. He was extremely, genuinely supportive.

I finished up my project and left for rehab the next day. I didn't go to Africa, over Bernard's great objections and disappointment. I encouraged him to go, which he did. This was late 2007. I completed the program and reentered life as a newly minted sober woman. On return I was most worried about my marriage and work. Would Bernard understand and accept what a life change this would be for me and us? Would I be able to handle the time demands and stresses of work without caving in to the lure of alcohol's relief? I was told in my rehab program that I needed to make ongoing recovery my highest priority if I were to stay sober. I worried about how to do that in the midst of so many job demands.

I started off doing what I had been told to do. I attended AA meetings, got a temporary sponsor and started working the steps with her, and picked up my 60- and 90-day sobriety chips. Then summer came and I spent some extended time on vacation with Bernard and other family members. I started feeling like I kind of had this recovery thing nailed. I wasn't actively thinking about drinking. I believed I really didn't need AA much anymore. I was working my own program of recovery, and I honestly felt pretty good.

Then the financial meltdown of the fall of 2008 hit. Bernard was now investing the large amount of funds we had accumulated from my new job—after his having lost everything in 2001. Again, he had taken positions in highly risky investments and had invested the entirety. Again, he lost the enormous amount I had worked so hard over the past 5 years to earn and accumulate. I felt like I was back in 2001 starting all over again. It was like a recurring nightmare. What made it worse, Bernard did not have an explanation as to how this happened again, nor a suggestion about what he might do to help us recover. Neither did he seem to feel that responsible or distressed. He was quite satisfied being retired and letting me go on slaving like a mule. I felt like a fool for having trusted him to continue to invest a substantial amount of our net worth. I felt like it was all up to me again to swoop in and fix the situation. My resentment was enormous, and once more I returned to drinking heavily.

My children almost immediately caught on that I had started drinking again, even though they all lived states away. They could hear it in my voice and detect it in my patterns—like calling them at untoward hours of the night and early morning. They were hurt, angry, and let down. I said I would pick myself up, get back on the wagon, and use the relapse as a learning experience, which I truly intended to do.

Over the next few months I moved through the cycles of not drinking, then falling to the mental obsession and drinking again (always secretly as I was desperately trying to get control of things without letting on how much I was struggling), then not drinking for the next 2 weeks or so, and so forth. On a business trip later that spring, I started drinking after my meetings were over and stayed in my hotel room drinking through the next day. After I sobered up I spoke with my boss and offered to resign. He refused to accept my resignation, instead encouraging me to consider what I needed to do to get firmly back on track. I ended up attending a 6-week evening outpatient relapse prevention program and committed to AA again. I found a sponsor and threw myself into recovery. I asked Bernard to stay at our vacation home so that I could focus on putting recovery first. During that time, I consulted divorce attorneys, not sure about whether I could stay married and sober. I believed our relationship presented triggers for me.

This time I stayed sober for 11 months before falling off the wagon again, setting into motion the cycle of abstaining, drinking in secret, abstaining. I was distraught as I realized I was again being swallowed up by a force that seemed out of my control. I decided that AA must not work for me and started seeing a cognitive-behavioral psychologist with whom I was not fully honest about my repeated drinking slips, which only increased my sense of shame and guilt. The only progress I could see was that when I added up all my abstinent time from my first rehab until then, I had racked up a few more sober months than drinking months. That observation provided some ray of hope and a sense of progress, however distorted. But I fell back to old, sick ways of thinking, such as hoping I'd eventually just lose the taste for wine as I had for beef, or that if I drank like crazy just one more time it might fill me up in a way that I would never need to drink again. This was obviously deluded, sick thinking.

This pretty much sums up the last months of my drinking career, until I made my way to Dr. Y., that hotel room in L.A., and the Betty Ford Center, and then back around to Dr. Y. and AA, as described at the beginning of this chapter.

Going Under (Dr. Y.'s Perspective): Diagnosis and Discussion

Psychiatric Diagnosis

I diagnosed Lynda to have alcohol use disorder, severe (303.90) [F10.20]) and generalized anxiety disorder (300.02 [F41.1]) (American Psychiatric Association 2013).

Discussion

The painful litany of the process and consequences of Lynda's heroic but doomed battle with alcohol is repeated tens of millions of times each year. In its wake, countless people destroy their own lives, the lives of their loved ones, and even the lives of those whom they don't know—such as the legion of sober, innocent victims of fatal automobile accidents.

Notwithstanding Lynda's remarkable assets, the deck of alcohol dependence was stacked against her. Lynda always had these four losing cards in her hand:

1. Her strong genetic/hereditary vulnerability to anxiety disorder and alcohol use disorder
2. Her unaddressed and unresolved conflicts stemming from her traumatic childhood experience
3. The power of alcohol to hijack her brain and, hence, her will to address meaningfully important issues in herself and her marriage
4. Her lack of understanding of how to go about gaining this understanding and help (which, when generalized to the many facets of being stuck, is why I wrote this book)

Even if she were able to discard one, two, or even three of these cards, she still would lose her battle with alcohol. All had to be addressed and discarded simultaneously, which she had not done previously. Thus, Lynda was stuck in a painful, ruinous pause. In Chapter 9, "Stuck in a Bottle, Part II (Decide and Discipline)," the Fatal Pauses approach to helping Lynda overcome her alcohol use disorder using the 3-D Method and the Power of No and the Power of Go will be presented.

Reference

American Psychiatric Association: Diagnostic and Statistical Manual of Mental Disorders, 5th Edition. Washington, DC, American Psychiatric Association, 2013

9

Stuck in a Bottle, Part II (Decide and Discipline): The Case of Mrs. Lynda Jensen

O God, that men should put an enemy in their mouths
To steal away their brains!
Every inordinate cup is unblessed
And the ingredient is a devil.
—*William Shakespeare*, The Tragedy of Othello,
Moor of Venice, *Act II, Scene 3*

We know, too, that psychiatry can often release the
big neurotic overhang from which many of us suffer
after A.A. has sobered us.
—*Bill Wilson, Cofounder, Alcoholics Anonymous*

"I found my past was cast with a sticky substance from
which there was no easy escape and to which I was
pulled again and again."

Overview

In Chapter 8, "Stuck in a Bottle, Part I (Discover)," we were presented with a mystery: Why should a brilliant, self-made, successful professional who has been goal directed, hardworking, and dependable in all aspects of her life be *stuck* in a life-destroying problem with such a seemingly simple resolution? "All" she has to do to stop drinking is "Just say no!" *Just*. Prior to her consulting me, Mrs. Lynda Jensen had attended two excellent residential 12-step alcohol rehabilitation programs and, thereafter, had gone religiously to Alcoholics Anonymous (AA) meetings. Still she could not stay sober. What was missing?

In Chapter 8 we learned that Lynda's early childhood was challenging and confusing. She adored her father, who favored her while terrorizing her mother and her brothers. At age 4, Lynda was uninformed about and unprepared for her father's sudden death, and she was unsupported emotionally and materially in its aftermath. Nearly destitute, her mother was unable to provide mature, consistent leadership or support for her fledgling family. With a warm but unworldly and ineffective mother, young Lynda had no choice but to become her mother's mother, as well as her own—at many hidden costs. Why, despite consistent attendance at AA and focused determination, was Lynda unable to sustain sobriety? A clue to solving this mystery can be found in the following insight:

> **Mrs. Lynda Jensen:** In looking to my past for insights as to who I have become, I am struck with a certain irony as to how the bookends of my life are tethered together. In my youth I gazed longingly toward the future, and I strived to set things up so that my future world would be an all-around better place than what I was then experiencing at that point in my life. I imagined my future as one of fulfilled hopes, of attainment, and of earning my full acceptance in the world. But as my imagined future unfolded in real life, I found my past was cast with a sticky substance from which there was no easy escape and to which I was pulled again and again, like a swimmer unable to outswim a strong current no matter how furiously she paddles and kicks. Although I was now well settled into my formerly imagined future, I am not able to understand or let go of the patterns from the past that continue to hold sway over my present-day life.

In psychiatric medicine, no clear line can be drawn between psychiatric assessment and treatment. The very process of taking a psychiatric history is highly therapeutic. A patient secures comfort and relief in telling her story to a compassionate, impartial, nonjudgmental professional—even before causalities are identified, prior to a treatment plan being devised, and in advance of the implementation of therapy. Within this process it is critical to understand why previous interventions have been unsuccessful because they will provide fruitful clues as to what further treatment approaches should be tried and which must be avoided.

In my taking a psychiatric history from Lynda, four principal questions leaped to the fore regarding her alcohol use disorder. And she must have answers to these questions in order to decide to stop drinking.

1. "What is there about alcohol that draws me to that particular drug?"

The same question could be broken down into two separate but related questions: "What do I like about alcohol?" and "What does alcohol do for me?"

2. "If I like drinking, why should I stop?"
3. "Why hasn't AA worked for me?"
4. "What other than AA do I need to do to become unstuck—to become and remain sober?"

These questions will be addressed in the remainder of this chapter. People who are stuck in alcohol dependence and their therapists require accurate information about the nature of alcohol use disorder and its treatments. Because there is so much misinformation and confusion about these issues, in this chapter I will provide a review of the neurobiology of addiction, the medical aspects and implications of this disorder, and the roles of AA, psychiatry, and other mental health professionals in the treatment of people with alcohol use disorder.

What Does Lynda Like About Alcohol, and Why Should She Stop Drinking? (Dr. Y.'s Perspective)

Overview

Trying to intervene in an epidemic is inherently complex. Even when a great deal is understood about the causal agent—such as the bacteria involved in malaria or cholera—knowledge is also required to understand a plethora of other factors—environmental, epidemiological, political, social, psychological, economic, etc.—in order to deal effectively with the problem, both preventatively and therapeutically. I believe that a public health and public policy model for infectious disease applies usefully to substance use disorders, including alcohol use disorder. According to the Centers for Disease Control and Prevention, there are nearly 88,000 deaths attributable to excessive alcohol use each year in the United States (Centers for Disease Control and Prevention 2014). Alcohol abuse affects approximately 30% of all Americans and is the third leading cause of preventable deaths in the United States (Mokdad et al. 2004).

Brief History of Humankind's Use of Alcohol

Quite likely, on rare occasions our ancient ancestors serendipitously ingested small quantities of alcohol from a rotting piece of fruit—its sugars having been fermented by yeast fungi. No doubt, some probably liked what they had just sampled, whereas others found it unpleasant. However, the quantities of naturally occurring alcohol would have been so small that the infrequent samplings would not have affected our evolution or our brain or other biological systems.

Fermented drinks that have been intentionally produced by humans have been documented as first occurring in the Neolithic period, about 10,000 years ago. The use of wine and beer for religious, ritual, ceremonial, nutritional, medicinal, and recreational purposes has been recorded to have taken place in the Middle East and in the Mediterranean basin more than 4,000 years ago, and alcoholic drinks from honey and water (mead) also had widespread use around the western world at about the same time.

As farming and industrialization increased during and after the seventeenth century, access to and consumption of copious amounts of inexpensive alcoholic beverages became commonplace in most of the "developing" world. In tandem with increased access to alcohol by the general masses emerged all of the contemporary problems associated with the abuse of alcohol, in both acute (e.g., public drunkenness) and chronic (e.g., cirrhosis and dementias) states.

Of Alcohol Chemistry and Evolution

Ethyl alcohol, or ethanol, is the intoxicating ingredient found in all alcoholic beverages. With the linear chemical structure of only 2 carbon atoms, 6 hydrogen atoms, and 1 oxygen atom, alcohol is among the simplest of all biochemical and bioactive molecules that humans regularly intake. For comparison, cholesterol, which has 27 carbon atoms, 46 hydrogen atoms, and a single oxygen atom and a far more complex structure including 4 hydrocarbon rings, is produced in our livers and is present in nearly every cell of our body. Clearly, if alcohol were to enhance our survival, the human organism is more than capable of producing this simple molecule.

As reviewed in Chapter 5, "Stuck in My Body, Part I (Discover)" as related to obesity, the 10,000 years wherein human beings have been ingesting large quantities of alcohol comprise only a brief instant in humankind's 25 million years of biological evolution. Our bodies have not had sufficient time to adapt to or develop the protective elements to deal with the nearly universal regular consumption of alcohol-containing beverages in significant amounts. Alcoholic beverages range from about 5% alcohol content in beer to 12% in most table wines to 50% in the strongest (100 proof) liquor. The standard drink contains slightly more than half an ounce of ethyl alcohol, which translates into 5 ounces of wine; 12 ounces of beer; and 1.5 ounces, or a shot glass, of 80 proof (i.e., 40% alcohol) distilled spirits including whiskey, vodka, and gin. The quantity, frequency, and duration of the use of alcohol-containing beverages govern their effects in and on our bodies and, consequently, on our thinking and behavior.

Why Is Alcohol Dependence So Common and Dangerous?

Why would alcohol, which is actually safe and healthful for most people when used in limited quantities, be far more destructive and deadly to humans than all other organic, naturally occurring substances? For example, ricin (a toxin from the castor bean), cyanide (a poison from certain bacteria or fungi), and botulinum (a toxin from the *Clostridium* bacterium) are lethal to humans within hours to days after ingestion in minute quantities. It is estimated that 1 kg of *Clostridium* botulinum could kill every human being on the planet.

So why is alcohol dependence so common and dangerous to human beings? One paradoxical clue as to why alcohol dependence is so common is that in *moderate quantities* it is safe and pleasing to ingest. Second, alcohol is also relatively inexpensive, widely available, and culturally accepted in nearly every society. Third, as opposed to many biological toxins, we don't become violently sick soon after ingesting alcohol in moderate quantities. Similar to tobacco, the most serious and destructive effects of this substance do not usually occur until after prolonged, heavy use. Fourth, despite abundant evidence to the contrary, legions of people who drink large quantities of alcohol for long periods of time believe that they "can handle alcohol" without grave consequences. Invariably, they are tragically mistaken.

Fifth, a key biological clue in understanding the danger and lethality of alcohol is how it works in the body. Through biologically mediated positive and negative reinforcement systems, alcohol hijacks the reward systems and the decision-making apparatuses of our brains to encourage and increase its own use. In other words, alcohol interferes with our brain biology to drive us to drink more alcohol and to discourage us from stopping. We get high and feel pleasingly disinhibited when we drink sufficient quantities of alcohol, and we can become uncomfortable and sick (e.g., hangovers, delirium tremens) if we stop. Thus, alcohol falls into a classic model for all substance dependencies:

1. Compulsion to seek out and take the substance
2. Substance-induced diminution in control over resisting its further use
3. Negative physical and/or emotional response when drug is discontinued abruptly

Is Alcohol Dependency a Medical Illness?

Throughout recorded history—depending on the era, locality, political/religious environment, culture, subculture, and familial/individual attitudes—heavy alcohol use and abuse have been conceptualized in broad and diverse ways. The spectrum ranges from normative, expected behavior to the evil work of the devil. Many people, including professionals, believe that alcohol dependency is best viewed as a problem of willpower and poor decision making. Alcoholism, many argue, is a choice, not a disease. After all, they argue, people can choose not to have another drink as long as they live, but they can't choose not to have cancer. These critics of a disease model of alcohol dependence express understandable concern that by calling alcoholism a disease, individual responsibility for stopping drinking and legal culpability for any resultant damage—such as from drunk driving—is weakened. Others express concern that conceptualizing alcohol abuse as a medical problem is supported by the medical profession primarily in order to advance its own guild-like interests in power, control, and enrichment.

Although manifestly subject to biases as a physician, I believe that alcoholism meets all the requirements of a chronic medical disorder. I also believe that, just as with other conditions such as schizophrenia and autism, a medical model reduces stigma, prejudice, and self and public blaming and punishment. The medical model also offers realistic, hopeful avenues for prevention and respectful, effective treatment through positive public attitudes and scientific research. The following are the five principal reasons that I believe that alcohol dependence should be conceptualized as a medical illness, termed *alcohol use disorder* by the current *Diagnostic and Statistical Manual of Mental Disorders* (DSM-5; American Psychiatric Association 2013).

Rational, Realistic Diagnostic Criteria Exist for Alcohol Use Disorder

Evidence-based arguments for conceptualizing any condition as a medical illness or disorder require, initially, an agreed-on definition or classification. Since 1956, the American Medical Association has officially regarded alcohol abuse as an illness, and since 1991, alcoholism has been classified as both a physical and a mental disease in the International Classification of Diseases of the World Health Organization and in the *Diagnostic and Statistical Manual of Mental Disorders* of the American Psychiatric Association. Most public health and medically related organizations worldwide accept these official designations and diagnostic criteria. As you will see, the classification system and diagnostic criteria, as I have abstracted them in Table 9–1, are compelling and also make good empirical sense.

Genetics and Heritability Are a Significant Factor

A wide array of epidemiological and genetic studies has overwhelmingly demonstrated that, like many medical conditions, alcohol dependence is a combination of genetic, experiential, and environmental factors. In fact, at 50%–60% of the variance, genetics and heredity are most likely the single most important factor (Kendler et al. 1997). In many cases, the interaction of genetic predispositions and environmental influences are required for the expression of vulnerability to alcohol. For example, an individual who has a genetic predisposition for alcoholism will be more likely to develop the condition if he or she grows up in a household of alcohol abuse, whereas those without

TABLE 9–1. World Health Organization and American Psychiatric Association diagnostic criteria for alcohol dependence

A maladaptive pattern of drinking that leads to at least two of the following problems or impairments occurring within a 12-month time period:

A. *Tolerance*—Need for increasingly larger amounts of alcohol to reach desired effects and/or diminished effect when using the same amount

B. *Withdrawal*—Uncomfortable and, possibly, dangerous physiological and psychological effects when trying to stop drinking abruptly; alcohol (or a closely related substance, such as a benzodiazepine) is taken to relieve or avoid withdrawal symptoms

C. *Impaired control*—Inability to resist temptation to drink or to limit quantities of alcohol when drinking

D. *Neglect of activities*—Important occupational, family, social, and recreational activities limited or avoided because of drinking

E. *Wasted time*—A significant amount of time devoted to obtaining, using, or recovering from the effects of alcohol

F. *Hazardous use*—Drinking to the point that self and others are endangered

G. *Continued use despite prior problems*—Persistent use of alcohol despite significant problems or getting into trouble when using in the past

H. *Compulsion*—Craving alcohol when not drinking

Source. Adapted from American Psychiatric Association: *Diagnostic and Statistical Manual of Mental Disorders*, 5th Edition. Washington, DC, American Psychiatric Association, 2013 and World Health Organization: *International Statistical Classification of Diseases and Related Health Problems*, 10th Revision. Geneva, World Health Organization, 1992.

the genetic predisposition will be far less likely, even if they grow up in the same family environment. Genes have been identified that either increase the likelihood that an individual will develop alcohol dependence or are protective against alcohol dependence. An excellent example is a genetic variant that reduces the function of acetaldehyde dehydrogenase, an enzyme required for the metabolism of alcohol. The net result is the buildup of acetaldehyde, which makes a person extremely sick in elevated doses. Thus, individuals with this gene variant rarely abuse alcohol.

I find alcohol dependence to be conceptually similar to familial hyperlipidemia, a hereditary condition in which people are prone to producing abnormally high amounts of blood fats. Individuals with familial hyperlipidemia are highly prone to developing coronary artery disease, whether or not they ingest foods that are high in saturated fats, such as red meats, egg yolks, palm oil, and dairy products. If they do ingest foods that are high in saturated fats, do not take cholesterol-reducing medications, and do not exercise, they are far more prone to develop more severe cases of coronary artery disease that occur at much younger ages. If a person does not alter his or her diet, does not exercise, and does not take lipid-lowering medications—*all of which are choices and decisions*—and has a severe myocardial infarction at a very young age, would we still consider that person to be suffering from a medical illness and treat the person in a hospital with medical interventions? I believe so. Similarly, people with strong family histories of alcoholism should be encouraged to monitor and restrict their intake of alcohol and perhaps even abstain from alcohol-containing beverages. If they do not heed this advice and become dependent on alcohol, I do not believe that their poor decision making and choices rule out having the full benefits of a medical conceptualization of their condition and medical interventions. Nor do I believe that a medical diagnosis of alcohol use disorder absolves a person from having full responsibility for the consequences of drinking.

A Body Organ Is Prominently Involved in Its Cause: The Brain

Alcohol is affected by and interferes with our brain biology to bring about the aforementioned conditions of substance dependence. Because the ethanol molecule is so small and so broadly distributed into so many organs and organ systems within the brain and the rest of the body, its effects on our brain and the rest of our body are multiple and complex. Conservatively, nine separate neurotransmitter and neuromodulating systems have been identified thus far as being important in the reinforcement of alcohol dependence. Among the most prominent of these neurotransmitters are dopamine, serotonin, γ-aminobutyric acid (GABA), and glutamine. Among the prominent receptors involved in alcoholism are the N-methyl-D-aspartate (NMDA), nicotinic, and cannabinoid receptors (Knapp et al. 2008).

These neurotransmitters, neuromodulators, and receptors interact in complex ways among each other in many regions and systems in the central nervous system. As many readers will readily recognize, these neurotransmitters and systems are also important in key brain functions such as mood regulation, impulse control, attention, consciousness, reality testing, motor regulation, and balance. Concurrently, in dysfunction, they lead to serious neuropsychiatric disorders, including depression, anxiety, panic, aggression, violence, attention-deficit/hyperactivity disorder, Parkinson's disease, delirium, dementia, seizures, and schizophrenia. We term the concurrence of alcohol use disorder and other psychiatric disorders comorbidity. Thus, the plot thickens as such questions are raised as "Does alcohol cause depression by its actions in the brain?" "Does depression lead people to self-treatment with alcohol, which results in a vicious cycle of people becoming ever more depressed and ever more dependent on alcohol?" Or is the vulnerability to alcoholism and depression linked by common genes? Whatever the case, the shorthand that *alcohol hijacks the brain* is, if anything, an understatement.

Pharmacological Treatments Can Be Effective for People With Alcohol Use Disorder

I strongly believe that people who suffer from alcohol use disorder should be offered, as indicated, a wide range of treatments, including medical detoxification, comprehensive medical evaluation to rule out co-occurring medical and psychiatric disorders, dietary counseling, psychotherapy, family counseling, couples counseling, spiritual counseling, peer support—including Alcoholics Anonymous and peer family support, including Al-Anon—and medications. It would be highly unusual that all of these categories of treatment are indicated for a single individual with alcohol use disorder; rather, it is important to match the specific clinical intervention with the particular needs of the person.

Several medications have been proven to be effective and are approved by the U.S. Food and Drug Administration (FDA) in the treatment of people with alcohol use disorder. Disulfiram (Antabuse) interferes with the metabolism of alcohol by blocking the action of aldehyde dehydrogenase, which leads to buildup of the chemical acetaldehyde. If someone who is taking disulfiram were to ingest alcohol, he or she would become nauseated, would vomit, and usually would develop a severe headache along with elevated blood pressure. It is a terribly uncomfortable and upsetting clinical state. Disulfiram, which has been in use for more than 50 years, can help people who have stopped drinking resist the temptation to take another drink (Jørgensen et al. 2011). However, it will help only those people who are compliant in taking the medication, and many are not compliant. I follow many patients who take this medication and they tell me, "It makes my life so much easier. I know if I take Antabuse that I will get violently sick if I drink. Therefore, I am far less tempted to drink. Also, I don't obsess about alcohol all day, and I don't crave it as much."

Naltrexone has been documented to decrease craving and the reinforcing effects of alcohol when imbibed (Sinclair 2001). This medication is FDA approved to be used to reduce drinking frequency, the amounts of alcohol consumed when drinking, and the likelihood of relapsing to heavy alcohol consumption. Naltrexone is an opiate receptor antagonist that is thought to block the release of dopamine, a transmitter that reinforces alcohol use. Naltrexone also blocks the reinforcing effects of alcohol on opiate receptors and systems.

Acamprosate is a third, more recently approved (2004) medication to treat alcohol use disorder (Maisel et al. 2013). This medication chemically resembles GABA, the principal inhibitory neurotransmitter in the brain. Acamprosate works by decreasing alcohol withdrawal–related symptoms. Withdrawal symptoms are sufficiently uncomfortable and upsetting to spur people to return to drinking in order to decrease this uncomfortable and unsettling state.

I believe that the use of effective, FDA-approved prescription medications to treat alcohol use disorder is another reason that alcoholism can be conceptualized as a medical illness.

Alcohol Abuse Is Associated With a Vast Array of Other Medical Illnesses

Although the myriad of severe psychiatric and other medical disorders caused by alcohol use disorder does not, necessarily, argue for conceptualizing alcoholism as a medical condition, most medical conditions are causally associated with other medical illnesses. Importantly, many life-threatening illnesses are first diagnosed by the recognition of a co-occurring condition, as represented in the following examples: 1) Not uncommonly, the presence of a pulmonary infection is the first sign of lung cancer; 2) the blood cancer multiple myeloma often first presents with back pain or even fractures of vertebrae; and 3) psychiatric symptoms—including depression, behavioral changes, and psychosis—are often the first indications of several neurological illnesses, including Parkinson's disease, multiple sclerosis, and brain tumors. Similarly, alcohol use disorder—including the most severe and longstanding cases—is frequently first diagnosed by physicians who are evaluating the patient for a related medical disorder such as pancreatitis, cirrhosis, gall bladder disease, hepatitis, or depression.

I strongly believe that because of the high prevalence of undiagnosed alcohol use disorder and because of the severe morbidity, mortality, and social disruption associated with alcohol use disorder, it is a physician's responsibility to be ever alert for its presence in patients. I also believe that conceptualizing alcohol use disorder as a medical disorder strengthens the mandate that physicians screen all of our patients for this condition. Additionally, I consider that the failure to diagnose alcohol use disorder in our patients or to ascertain that people with this illness receive effective treatment should constitute medical negligence—no different from failing to diagnosis and assure effective care for patients with life-threatening cancer or heart disease.

The number of serious medical illnesses causally associated with alcohol use disorder is legion, and a comprehensive presentation and discussion of these illnesses would exceed the page limitations and distract from the focus of this book. Rather, I will merely categorize and list a few of the most common disabling disorders that have *strong and clear causal associations* with alcohol abuse.

1. *Neuropsychiatric disorders:* epilepsy, dementias, polyneuropathy, essential tremor, fetal alcohol syndrome, depression/suicide, psychotic illnesses, panic disorder, sleep disorders, traumatic brain injury, violent behaviors
2. *Cardiovascular and blood-related disorders:* myocardial infarction, arrhythmias, hypertension, cardiomyopathy, anemia, pulmonary embolus, stroke
3. *Gastrointestinal disorders:* pancreatitis, cirrhosis, hepatitis, gallstones, gastritis, stomach ulcer, duodenal ulcer
4. *Cancer:* oral, tongue, pharyngeal, laryngeal, esophageal, stomach, duodenal, breast, colon, and rectal cancers
5. *Metabolic and hormonal disorders:* diabetes, gout, sexual dysfunctions, testicular atrophy, gynecomastia (in men), osteoporosis

6. *Skin disorders:* seborrheic dermatitis, urticaria, psoriasis, premature aging
7. *Infectious and inflammatory disorders:* a vast array of bacterial and viral infections—including sexually communicated diseases—and rheumatoid arthritis

A small sampling of the strength of the *causal* connections of these conditions is that alcohol use disorder is associated with a 50% increase in stroke and tenfold increase in suicide rate and is the primary causal factor for approximately 50% of people with pancreatitis and for 50% of people with cirrhosis. According to the U.S. Department of Transportation, in 2010, 10,228 people in America were killed in motor vehicle crashes involving alcohol-impaired drivers, and these comprise approximately one-third of all traffic-related deaths in the United States (National Highway Traffic Safety Administration 2013). According to the American Foundation for Suicide Prevention, alcoholism is a factor in about one-third of all completed suicides in the United States, of which there were more than 38,000 (total) in 2010 (American Foundation for Suicide Prevention 2014).

Alcoholics Anonymous and Psychiatry (Lynda Jensen's Perspective)

In both AA and my 12-step rehab program, we are taught that fear is one of the key drivers underlying our drinking and that we have used alcohol for relief. I believed for a long time that it worked well for me in that respect. These fears are generally the stuff of the so-called primitive brain, such as fear of not being loved, fear of abandonment, fear of not being "normal" or accepted, fear of failing, fear of financial ruin, and the like. Along with fear come attempts at control. Alcoholics often struggle with trying to control the uncontrollable. The serenity prayer recited at many AA meetings captures this well: "God, grant me the serenity to accept the things I cannot change, courage to change the things I can, and wisdom to know the difference." For many of us the need to control orders the activities of our daily life, and a big part of recovery is learning how to let go and trust in the process once you are right with your motives and your Higher Power. In recovery we begin to understand that things we try to control eventually dominate us.

At heart a lot of us in "the Program," as we refer to the 12-step program of recovery outlined in the book *Alcoholics Anonymous,* are scaredy-cats just trying to control things the best we know how. Taking a few drinks gives us the illusion that everything is finally OK and right with the world and that we can let go for a little while. It presents an easy solution for how to turn off our 24/7 on switches, not requiring self-examination or change that is difficult. In my view recovery requires a great deal of courage and persistence and a bold leap of faith born out of desperation in finally facing up to the demons that we have long avoided.

Alcoholics Anonymous and Psychiatry (Dr. Y.'s Perspective)

"Ancient" History, Part I: AA Perspective—"Alcohol in a Pill!"

Like different species of twisting vines about a wind-tossed bough, AA and psychiatry have both stabilized and strangled people who suffer from alcohol use disorder. Although both organizations purport to have the same goals, nonetheless, many psychiatrists and AA members have had a long, troubled history in working together to help people with alcohol use disorder. At times an unholy war has raged between AA and psychiatry, with the usual first casualty of every war: truth. And, in this case, the second casualty of the struggle between AA and psychiatry has been the people with alcohol use disorder who are supposed to be helped by both entities, ideally through their working together toward that purpose.

Since AA's founding in 1935, many AA members have accused psychiatrists of "drugging" people who suffer from alcohol use disorder with medications that amount to little more than "alcohol in a pill." In far too many circumstances there was and remains today much more than a grain of truth to this accusation. People with alcohol and other substance use disorders have and continue to be misprescribed medications in the sedative/hypnotic, antianxiety, and analgesic (i.e., pain) categories that are not only ineffective in their individual cases but also highly addictive. The following are several— certainly not all—of the most commonly prescribed addictive drugs.

(**Warning:** The following list is by no means complete or inclusive of prescribed medications that are highly addictive and broadly abused. Additionally, many of these medications can be medically indicated for and useful to people with histories of alcohol and other substance use disorders. However, such use must be under the on-going guidance and monitoring of a physician knowledgeable in the safe use of these medications for persons with histories of alcohol and other substance use disorders.)

- *Barbiturates:* amobarbital (Amytal), pentobarbital (Nembutal), phenobarbital (Luminal), secobarbital (Seconal)
- *Benzodiazepines:* alprazolam (Xanax), chlordiazepoxide (Librium), clonazepam (Klonopin), diazepam (Valium), flunitrazepam (Rohypnol), lorazepam (Ativan), oxazepam (Serax), triazolam (Halcion)
- *Nonbenzodiazepine sedatives:* eszopiclone (Lunesta), zaleplon (Sonata), zolpidem (Ambien)
- *Opiates:* morphine, codeine, hydrocodone (Vicodin), oxycodone (OxyContin), methadone, fentanyl, meperidine (Demerol), and many, many mixtures containing these medications under various trade names

Psychiatry has not been alone in this dangerous and regrettable malpractice, as virtually every other discipline of medicine has prescribed and continues to prescribe *nonindicated* addictive medications to people with histories of alcohol and other substance use disorders. I emphasize "nonindicated" because there are clinical circumstances in which addictive drugs are, indeed, essential in the care of people with alcohol and other substance use disorders.

For the minuscule minority of circumstances in which addictive drugs are, in fact, indicated in the care of our patients with alcohol and other substance use disorders, the following guidelines should be, but rarely are, followed. In addition, in order to prevent physicians from initiating dangerous dependencies in people who have no previous histories of dependencies, the following guidelines are also mandatory. In the latter circumstances, the so-called "treatment" is all too often far more lethal and dangerous than the illness of the person who is being treated with the addictive medication.

1. The physician must allocate to and spend with the patient the significant time that is *always* required to review the *medical indications* for that particular addictive medication.
2. The physician must devote the considerable amount of the time that is *always* required to explain fully the *safe use* of that addictive

medication. This explanation must always include a full explication of medication doses, timelines for initiation and discontinuation, side effects of the medication, and the early manifestations of dependence on and abuse of that medication.

3. The physician must secure the *informed consent* of the patient, which includes a full communication of the reasons for its prescription to the patient, to the patient's family members, and to other physicians treating this patient.

4. The physician must continuously *monitor* the patient and the prescription practices of the patient throughout the course of treatment. This includes asking the patient directly in each meeting about the use of the addictive medication prescribed, inquiring whether or not *other* prescriptions have been written by other physicians, and confirming regularly the patient's medication use with his or her other physicians.

5. The physician must continuously monitor the patient to adjudicate whether or not the addictive medication remains effective and needed and *remind* the patient of the designated date of discontinuation.

6. The physician must *never "routinely" refill* any prescriptions—particularly for a medication that is addictive.

7. The physician must *discontinue* the medication as soon as it is no longer effective or required or can be replaced by a nonaddictive medication.

As the result of time constraints in the practice of medicine and/or because of medical negligence, the practice standard that I have outlined above is infrequently followed, and the physician, thereby, is complicit in initiating an addiction or aggravating a preexisting substance use disorder. Even though the ill-advised prescribing of addictive medications for anxiety, mood disorders, insomnia, pain, and other symptoms, syndromes, and various other purposes (e.g., dental work, routine postsurgical orders) is primarily perpetrated by nonpsychiatric physicians, members of AA have every reason to have serious reservations about psychiatry—to a point.

Many members of AA also accuse psychiatry of promoting antireligious, atheistic, nonspiritual biases in its treatment of people with alcohol use disorder. They also may believe that psychiatrists all too often blame or hold others responsible for alcoholism—particularly parents and other family members—and that we thereby shift the responsibility of maintaining sobriety away from the alcoholic person to others. They maintain that psychiatry focuses too much on "dredging up the past" while ignoring the present and future problems and issues concerning a person with alcoholism.

In the following section, the concerns and objections of some psychiatrists to AA are reviewed.

"Ancient" History, Part II: Psychiatry Perspective— "AA is a Cult!"

Almost every psychiatrist who treats patients who have current or historical problems with alcohol abuse has heard the following objections to AA from patients, families, colleagues, and students familiar with the organization.

From a patient, I was told,

> People in my AA meetings keep telling me to stop taking the antidepressant you have been prescribing me. They say that it is addictive—another *crutch*, no different whatsoever from alcohol. They say that the only thing that I need to do to stay sober is to keep coming to the AA meetings and that I am wasting my time and money on psychiatry. I am in a bind because I believe that the medication and your treatment have been really helping me, but so is AA.

A hospital-based psychiatrist who treats patients with psychotic disorders such as schizophrenia and severe bipolar disorder recounted,

> I am getting sick of AA members practicing medicine without a license. They insisted that a former patient of mine with chronic schizophrenia and alcoholism stop taking his antipsychotic medications because they said that they oppose "all mind-altering drugs." Well, he listened to them, stopped his olanzapine, and committed suicide by jumping in front of a subway train. I will *never again* refer another one of my patients to AA.

The wife of an outpatient with panic disorder and alcohol use disorder whom I referred to AA shouted the following at me over the telephone:

> Why on Earth did you send Paul to AA, Dr. Y.? Do you have any idea whatsoever what goes on in that cult? They badgered Paul into

stopping the Lexapro because they said he was going to get hooked on it. All they do is bombard him with their shallow, mindless, meaningless slogans. Now we are back to square one. He won't leave the house, won't go to work, and won't attend his cognitive-behavioral therapy. He had two panic attacks already this morning and is pleading with me to call 911 because he's convinced he's having a heart attack. He's about to fall apart, and you and I both know that's how he started up with alcohol in the first place. What the hell were you thinking when you sent him to AA? I'm just furious with you!

More than a few female patients whom I have referred to AA have complained,

> Every time I go to an AA meeting, someone hits on me—usually before or after the formal meeting takes place. I have tried to change meeting groups on several different occasions, but the problem always recurs. I know that AA frowns on sexual contact among members, but I can tell you it happens all the time to women, especially those of us who are new to the group. It's unbelievably annoying and interferes with the good things I get from AA.

From my medical students and psychiatry residents, I have repeatedly been asked the following:

> Why do you send so many of your patients with alcohol use disorders to AA? You are always saying that psychiatrists must practice evidence-based medicine. What's the evidence that AA works? How do we know it doesn't harm our patients? I did a Google search last night to review outcome studies about effectiveness of AA, and it isn't at all convincing. First of all, AA doesn't permit research on its members. Secondly, what little "outside" research has been permitted shows that as many as 95% of people drop out of AA after the first year! Have you read the review article by the Cochrane Collaboration? AA's own data say that about 75% drop out in the first year! We couldn't prescribe a medication with results that poor, so how in good faith can we refer patients to AA?

Similar to the criticisms of psychiatry by AA members, there is veracity and abundant justification to the concerns about AA that were expressed above. Without question, each example has occurred many times and continues to take place in sanctioned AA meetings by AA members. No different from physicians prescribing life-threatening addictive drugs to people with alcohol and other substance use disorders, AA members have told and continue to tell fellow members that they are no longer "clean and sober" because of their use of a psychoactive drug. In effect, these individuals in AA were and are dispensing medical advice without training or license.

Modern History, Part I: Comparing Psychiatry and AA

Membership/Eligibility

AA welcomes anyone who views himself or herself as having a problem with alcohol and wants to do something about that problem.

Psychiatry is a specialty of medicine, so all psychiatrists must be physicians with degrees in medicine from certified medical schools (M.D.) or colleges of osteopathy (D.O.). To become licensed, physicians must take three rigorous written tests, Step 1 and Step 2 during medical school and Step 3 during their internship following graduation from medical school.

In addition, on completion of their medical degree, which characteristically requires 4 years after graduation from college, psychiatrists must complete 4 years of training in an approved residency training program associated with a medical school and teaching hospital. Moreover, psychiatrists can also elect to subspecialize in addiction disorders, which requires 2 more years of focused training and research beyond residency. Thus, the latter group has a minimum of 10 years of medical and psychiatric training beyond college.

Certification and Licensure

AA is an international mutual aid fellowship. Comprising what has been called "a kinship of common suffering," it has no trained leaders or formal hierarchy. Thus, no certification or licensure of any sort is required throughout the organization.

American psychiatrists must be licensed in medicine and have been graduated from an approved and monitored residency program in psychiatry that is overseen by the Association of American Medical Colleges. In addition, most hospitals require that their medical staff receive specialty certification in their respective specialties, which in the case of psychiatry is from the American Board of Psychiatry and Neurology (ABPN), which also certifies neurologists.

To receive board certification in psychiatry, psychiatrists must be licensed physicians, have completed an approved 4-year residency training program, and take a rigorous two-part specialty examination in psychiatry. Part 1 of that certification examination is a 6-hour written test, which has approximately a 50% pass rate. After passing Part 1, the candidate for certification must take Part 2, an oral clinical examination, which is monitored by selected unpaid peers who examine the candidates on live patients or videotaped interviews of patients with psychiatric illnesses. Intensive study is required to pass both parts of the certification examination.

Finally, psychiatrists are required to participate in ongoing, yearly continuing education programs to maintain the medical licensure and recertification by the ABPN every 10 years.

Licensed and certified clinical psychologists and clinical social workers who practice psychotherapy also have extensive and demanding educational and training backgrounds, as well as licensure, certification testing, and recertification requirements. I regard the all-too-commonly dismissive, demeaning mischaracterization of psychiatrists, psychologists, social workers, and other trained mental health professionals as "air-brained, psycho-babbling, ineffective fools" as the prejudiced extension of the stigmatization of the mentally ill to those of us who devote our lives to caring for people with these conditions.

Structure and Delivery of Services

AA is free to all members. It does not formally raise money or solicit funds from members or others. Meetings are held in nearly ubiquitous locations and venues that are decided on by and are convenient for members. Anyone may attend an *open meeting* of AA, but only those with a problem with alcohol may attend a *closed meeting* of AA. Generally, meetings consist of members voluntarily telling their life stories—particularly how these relate to problems with alcohol—and discussions of what has been presented or one of the Twelve Steps of spiritual and character development that lead to recovering from problems with alcohol, which, along with the Twelve Traditions of AA, form the central philosophy of the organization. AA is not regulated by independent professional, state, or federal organizations.

Outpatient psychiatry is frequently fee-for-service delivered in a private office setting, but there are innumerable exceptions accounting for a significant percentage of treatment in not-for-profit systems such as state and county hospitals or community mental health centers, in medical school and religiously affiliated systems, and in prisons. From individual care to family therapy to group treatment to structured/manualized therapy to biologically based treatments including medicines, electroconvulsive therapy, regional transcranial magnetic stimulation, and deep brain stimulation with neurosurgically implanted electrodes, there is a vast range and variety of approved psychiatric care. All forms of treatment are monitored and highly regulated by professional associations, hospitals, and state and federal governmental organizations.

What Is and What Is Not Provided by Psychiatry and AA

- AA provides spiritually based group meetings for people who want help with alcohol. Through AA, individual "sponsors," who are members of AA with long histories of sobriety, are also available to counsel and support the recovery from alcohol dependence of other members on a 24 hours per day, 7 days per week basis.
- As previously listed, psychiatry provides a vast array of services for people with a broad range of psychiatric disorders, ranging from childhood conduct disorders to schizophrenia to personality disorders to alcohol use disorder to Alzheimer's disease to multiple combinations of so-called physical and mental illnesses.
- AA declares that it does *not* diagnose or treat its members; does *not* educate its members about alcohol; does *not* engage in or support research on alcoholism; does *not* keep records or official documents; does *not* support or provide social services; does not provide letters of reference to employers, parole boards, courts, attorneys, or social agencies; does *not* provide or support religious services or retreats; and is *not* protected by regulations enforcing confidentiality among members.
- Psychiatry is actively engaged in research and education about mental disorders including alcohol and other substance use disorders. Psychiatry participates in the prevention, diagnosis, and treatment of mental and physical disorders and keeps formal medical records and documents on all patients served. Psychiatrists are held to strict legal and professional standards and can lose their licenses and be prosecuted legally for infractions

thereof including negligence of diagnosis and treatment, boundary violations with patients, financial exploitation of patients, and breeches of confidentiality. As a component of medicine, psychiatry is *evidence based* and relies on rationality and scientific methodologies to guide its assessments and treatments. Psychiatry is a medical profession that is *not* based on religious beliefs or spiritual philosophies—beyond respect for patients, advocacy of patients, empathy-guided approaches and goals, rationality, and the desire to reduce the suffering of our patients while helping to prolong their lives and enhancing their quality of life.

Modern History, Part II: AA and Psychiatry Working Together

Because of—not despite of—the profound differences between AA and psychiatry, the two organizations make ideal partners in helping people who abuse alcohol. Although our organizational structures and therapeutic approaches are vastly different, our services are complementary, as each does different things in different ways to help our patients and members achieve similar goals. Given the fundamental complexity of alcohol abuse and dependence—which encompasses the full range of biological, psychological, social, and spiritual dimensions—it stands to reason that *there is no single approach or solution to conceptualizing, combating, and overcoming alcohol use disorder.* This reality has led to much of the confusion and controversy surrounding the comparative approaches and effectiveness of psychiatry and AA.

For a broad variety of reasons ranging from poor motivation on the part of the person with alcohol use disorder to malpractice and misfeasance on the parts of the psychiatrist or AA member, many people with alcohol use disorder do not get better and/or are actually harmed by their care. Not infrequently, both psychiatry and AA are judged by worst practices as opposed to best outcomes. How often it is when I am standing at an event with a group of physicians that someone walks up and says to the orthopedist in the group the equivalent of, "Thank you, Dr. Jones, for taking such good care of my father after he fell and broke his hip!" How rare it is in the same social settings for that same person to say, "And thank you, Dr. Y., for helping him overcome his chronic alcoholism, which led to him falling and breaking his hip in the first place." Again, this "oversight" can be understood as an extension of almost every society's profound stigmatization of people with alcohol use disorder and all other brain-based behavioral/emotional conditions—and of those among us who care for them. *The hidden truth is that many people with alcohol use disorder are helped significantly by both psychiatry and AA, especially when the two organizations work together.*

Another "hidden truth" is that, although many psychiatrists and members of AA do not support their corollary "sister organization," the two organizations have been officially working together for many decades. In fact, AA has worked closely with organized psychiatry and psychiatrists since it was founded. The following direct excerpts from official AA General Service Conference–approved literature titled "Three Talks to Medical Societies" by Bill Wilson, cofounder of Alcoholics Anonymous, corroborate the indelible historical connection between AA and psychiatry (Wilson 1958, pp. 5–22):

- "Our primary purpose is to stay sober and help other alcoholics to achieve sobriety."
- "I'm glad to say that psychiatrists in great numbers are referring alcoholics to A.A.—even psychiatrists who more or less specialize on alcoholics. Their understanding of alcoholics is now great. Their patience and tolerance of us, and of A.A., have been monumental."
- "In 1949, for example, the American Psychiatric Association allowed me to read a paper on A.A. before a section of its Annual Meeting. As these doctors specialize in emotional disorders—and alcoholism is certainly one of them—this act of theirs has always seemed to me a wonderful example of fine humility and generosity."
- "Thoughtful A.A. members everywhere realize that psychiatrists and physicians helped bring our Society into being in the first place and have held up our hands ever since."
- "We also realize that the discoveries of the psychiatrist and the biochemist have vast implications for us alcoholics. Indeed, these discoveries are today far more than implications."
- "We know that psychiatrists have sent us innumerable alcoholics who never would have otherwise approached A.A., and many clinics have done likewise."

- "We clearly see that by pooling our resources we can do together what could never be accomplished in separation, or in short-sighted criticism and in competition."
- "We frequently work with the psychiatrist and often find that he can do and say things to a patient which we cannot. He in turn avails himself of the fact that as ex-alcoholics we can sometimes walk in where he fears to tread."

Correspondingly, for more than 50 years, organized medicine and psychiatry, in their local and national continuing medical education and scientific programs, have acknowledged the value of AA and of psychiatrists' and primary care physicians' collaborating with AA and 12-step programs to care for people with alcohol use disorders.

Standard psychiatric textbooks used in medical schools, psychiatry residencies, and subspecialty fellowships in addiction medicine include sections describing AA and its benefits. These textbooks uniformly recommend the program as an invaluable therapeutic asset for many of our patients with alcohol and other substance use disorders. Many people who abuse alcohol—and their families—first turn to psychiatrists and family physicians for help, and the vast majority of psychiatrists and primary care physicians have, for decades, referred these patients to AA for care that is complementary to their medical treatment. And, perhaps most important, many psychiatrists and other physicians of all specialties—and their family members—who suffer from alcohol use disorder are active and enthusiastic members of AA, in the same fashion that AA members consult psychiatrists when they have not maintained sobriety when using "the Program" alone. And that was the circumstance when Mr. Clifford Bentsen consulted me about Mrs. Lydia Jensen, who had stopped going to AA meetings, was not performing optimally in her job, was damaging her family relationships, was spoiling her quality of life, and was harming her health with recurrent alcohol abuse.

In Addition to AA, What Is Required for Lynda to Become and Stay Sober? (Dr. Y.'s Perspective)

I postulated that the reason that AA alone had been unsuccessful in helping Lynda to maintain sobriety related precisely to what she indicated when she said,

But as my imagined future unfolded in real life, I found my past was cast with a sticky substance from which there was no easy escape and to which I was pulled again and again, like a swimmer unable to outswim a strong current no matter how furiously she paddles and kicks. Although I was now well settled into my formerly imagined future, I am not able to fully understand or let go of the patterns from the past that continue to hold sway over my present-day life.

In the early phases of Lynda's treatment, as we reviewed her childhood history, I conveyed the following to her:

Dr. Y.: Lynda, I don't believe that your alcohol dependency and disappointing relationships are the *direct* result of the profoundly stressful events of your early childhood. Paradoxically, there were benefits as a result of your challenges as a child, such as your motivation to succeed by making the most of the many gifts with which you are blessed. However, the *indirect* consequences of your childhood trauma, which comprise your unconscious distortions of the *meanings* of those events, have led to your alcohol abuse and to many of the other nettlesome problems that you face today.

Mrs. Lynda Jensen: Such as?

Dr. Y.: Such as when, after the death of your father, you had to move to a new school and a less affluent neighborhood. You were embarrassed to acknowledge to your peers that you were not like them. Your father had died, your mother was overwhelmed, your brother was failing, and your home was in disrepair. You incorrectly began to regard yourself as "damaged goods" that you would repair by working hard and being the best in just about everything. But you unconsciously resent having to work so hard and to be perfect just to feel worthwhile and worthy—particularly at the times when you have setbacks and when others let you down. That's when you retaliate—but always against yourself. And alcohol is your weapon of choice.

Lynda: Good heavens, Dr. Y. That's a lot to think about.

Dr. Y.: And to change.

Lynda: Change what? Should I work less hard?

Dr. Y.: Not at all. I was thinking that you will have to work harder than ever, but in different realms from job performance. First, you will have to work to change conclusions that you reached about yourself as a result of your childhood traumas. And second, you will have to examine your important relationships—and your *choices of important relationships*—to discover how these have been adversely affected by how you regarded yourself as damaged goods. I surmise that that analysis will lead to

> many insights and the need to make many important adjust-
> ments in your relationships. And none will be easy to make.
> **Lynda:** It seems like we have a lot to do, Dr. Y. And that's not all
> bad for a worker bee like me.
> **Dr. Y.:** Just what I was thinking, Lynda. Let's get on with it.

Alcoholics Anonymous' cofounder Bill Wilson wrote about AA, "We know, too, that psychiatry can often release the big neurotic overhang from which many of us suffer after A.A. has sobered us" (Wilson 1958, p. 21). I interpret this to mean that people with alcohol use disorder—like Lynda—often drink to help them deal with deep-seated, unconscious psychological conflicts, but when they stop drinking, those conflicts and their consequences persist. In fact, because the now-sober person's brain is no longer depressed by alcohol, the "neurotic overhangs," which I infer from Mr. Wilson's assertion to be the equivalents of "psychological hangovers," lead to the person feeling worse. The catch-22 is that people with alcohol use disorder like Lynda must stop drinking in order to be able to deal with the issues that had led them to drink in the first place.

You can't learn much new about yourself or make important changes in your life with a brain that is anesthetized with alcohol. One way out of this impasse is to attend AA to get help and peer support to become and remain sober while, *at the same time*, working in psychotherapy to understand the psychological underpinnings of your addiction and to change the dysfunctional manifestations of these conflicts in your everyday life and relationships.

Decision to Give Up Alcohol

How Mrs. Lynda Jensen Is Stuck in Pause

Utilizing the organizational structure of Table 3–2 (p. 29), let us now review the underlying reasons that Lynda is stuck in pause with alcohol.

Confusion: Lynda Was Not Clear or Precise About Where She Was Stuck

When Lynda began treatment with me, she believed that her principal, if not sole, problem was that she was unable to remain sober:

"I am an alcoholic." Partially correct, she alleged that her guilt, embarrassment, low self-esteem, and symptoms of anxiety and depression either were the toxic effects of alcohol on her brain or were related to the life chaos brought about by alcoholism. In the past, however, when she was able to stop drinking for varying periods of time, her self-esteem and symptoms did not appreciably improve—despite her regular and devoted attendance at AA. The reason for her recidivism has long been her deficient conceptualization of *where* and *how* she is stuck.

I liken Lynda's confusion about *where* she is stuck to that of the person with gambling disorder who believes, "If only I can hit the jackpot on my next big bet, all of my problems will be over." On the rare occasions when the gambler does, indeed, hit the jackpot, his multifarious life problems do not go away. His family continues to be disaffected; his personality disorders remain unidentified and unaddressed; he has no motivation to work a "regular job" with standard working hours and productivity demands; and he is devoid of an orienting life purpose, which leaves his days empty, unstructured, and dispirited. Lacking goals, meaning, and structure, he becomes terrified and confused. It is only a matter of time until he talks himself into placing another bet. And yet another, until he loses his winnings and, once more, goes into debt. And once more the gambler embraces his sustaining delusion: "If only I can hit on my next big bet, everything will turn out OK." Thus, gambling use disorder is the "fool's gold" for people whose lives lack meaning, purpose, spirituality, mature human involvement, and structure. As with Lynda, lacking insight about the true nature of their problems, they are "mining for gold in all the wrong places. And like the pathological gambler, Lynda (and the countless others who stop drinking without addressing other fundamental realms in which they are stuck) inevitably and invariably returns to drinking.

Ignorance: Lynda Did Not Understand Why and How She Became Stuck

Lynda did not appreciate the determining role of her traumatic childhood experiences on her emotions, behavior, important life choices, and relationships. Nor did she recognize the high toll that her day-to-day responses took on those choices and relationships.

Specifically, she did not understand how her traumatic childhood damaged her self-worth and engendered her fear of abandonment or how these factors combined to handcuff her ability to demand a fair deal in relationships. For example, she worked to exhaustion as the sole provider for the comfortable lifestyle that she and her spouse enjoy but seethed in silent rage as her retired husband did little, if anything, to help out around the house.

Superficiality: Lynda Had Not Discovered, Gained Insight About, or Addressed the Underlying Conflicts That Kept Her Stuck

The sudden, unexplained loss of her father left 4-year-old Lynda to her own devices to explain and deal with the repercussions of this loss, which led her to believe that she was somehow responsible for his death. She sought repair through perfection, control, and hard work, at the expense of resentment for having to work so hard just to feel deserving of acceptance and love.

Without understanding her conflict of *wanting to express her anger over having to work hard to be admired and accepted (by virtue of accomplishments)* while simultaneously *avoiding expression of her anger out of fear of rejection* (an approach-avoidance conflict), Lynda's internalized rage transformed into depression and self-destructive behaviors. Alcohol was the blunt instrument with which she numbed her rage and took revenge on others by attacking herself and destroying the confidence of others in her.

Indecision: Lynda Had Not Decided That She Wanted to Get Unstuck

Lynda knew that she liked the effects of alcohol but was not clear about what "alcohol does for me." She did not understand that beyond its euphoric and disinhibiting effects, alcohol artificially enhanced her self-worth and temporarily diluted her rage at having to work so hard to be perfect in order to feel worthy and accepted. Therefore, although she could decide to stop drinking, she did not know that she *also* had to decide to gain insight into the roots of her conflicts and to change many other derivative behaviors in order to *remain* sober.

Disorientation: Lynda Did Not Have a Clear Direction or Pathway to Get Unstuck

For two primary reasons, psychiatry is a particularly demanding profession, and psychotherapy is a particularly challenging modality of treatment. First, most people often come to treatment without a precise understanding of the full extent of their problems. Initially, Lynda believed that her primary, if not exclusive, problem was drinking. In treatment, Lynda discovered that alcohol is both a problem and a symptom of another primary problem. An individual cannot devise a plan to fix problems that he or she does not know exist. Second, the very organ that is impaired—the brain—must *acknowledge* the presence and relevance of these problems and *agree* that they merit repair. Thus, a "broken brain" must make the decision to change itself. It is not easy for a broken brain to understand and fix itself. I share the belief of many that it is impossible for a broken brain to repair itself when it is under the influence of alcohol and/or other mind- and mood-altering drugs.

After many failed attempts to stop drinking, Lynda discovered and accepted that there were fundamental unconscious conflicts that led to her drinking in the first place. As a general rule, when one must exercise the Power of No, there are usually at least two fundamental conflicts with which to deal: 1) the manifest behavior (or substance) that must be avoided (e.g., alcohol) and 2) the unconscious and unrecognized psychological conflict that led to the untoward dependency or behavior. Once these conflicts are identified, a strategy can be crafted to resolve both. Through discovering and accepting the validity of her pivotal unresolved conflicts, Lynda was finally able to *decide* to get unstuck from her alcohol use disorder by engaging the Power of No and the Power of Go.

Key Features of Lynda Jensen's Being Stuck in Pause

1. *How Lynda is Stuck:* Dependent on alcohol
2. *Goal for change:* Become and stay sober
3. *Central, unresolved conflicts:* 1) Likes alcohol and its disinhibiting effects; likes being responsible and in control (approach-approach); 2) wants to be admired and accepted by virtue of accomplish-

ments; resents (is angry at) having to work diligently to be admired (approach-avoidance); and 3) wants to express anger at pleasing others to be accepted; fearful that if she expresses resentment/anger, she will be rejected (approach-avoidance)

4. *Hallmarks of Lynda's being stuck*: Demoralization, shame, embarrassment, anger, resentment, self-deprecation, sadness, low self-esteem, dysthymia, and anxiety

5. *Binary problems/solutions*: Addiction/sobriety, anger/acceptance

6. *Critical decision points*: Don't drink; self-exploration, self-understanding, and change (cognitive and behavioral) through engaging in intensive psychotherapy

7. *Corollary factors required to achieve resolution:* Attend AA and intensive, insight-oriented psychotherapy to stop drinking, gain insights into conflicts, and make changes in the cognitions and behaviors that lead to and sustain drinking

8. *Resolution*: Stop drinking by utilizing the Power of No and understand and change reasons for drinking by utilizing the Power of Go

Discipline: Getting Unstuck Through the Power of No and the Power of Go

For the key principles of getting unstuck through the Power of No, see Table 3–6 (p. 43). Let's review these five principles as they apply to Lynda.

1. You must *stop* something that you like in order to *gain* something that you like more.

2. You are saying "Yes!" to something that you fundamentally want by saying "No!" to something else that you want less.

Not everyone is inclined to use alcohol to avoid addressing his or her central unresolved conflicts. As in most of medicine, the fertile loam of genetic/biological predisposition and distressing life experience is required to germinate the seed of alcohol use disorder. In addition to her father, who died of an alcohol-related medical disorder, her brother and many other members of Lynda's family suffered from severe alcohol use disorder. She was born with and carried with her a genetic vulnerability for alcohol abuse. Because medicine does not yet have a valid and sensitive laboratory test to pinpoint this genetic vulnerability, we rely on taking detailed and careful family and personal psychiatric histories of the patients whom we evaluate for this condition. One question that I *always* ask patients whom I believe may have vulnerabilities to alcohol abuse is the following:

> **Dr. Y.:** Do you remember how you felt when you took your *very first drink?*
>
> **Mrs. Lynda Jensen:** I was not a kid who got in trouble, nor did I push the limits. I stayed within a pretty safe zone of behavior. I had a few boyfriends and dates to dances but nothing really serious. I didn't drink until toward the end of my senior year, when my friend Bindy and I decided we should really give it a try so that we'd be "ready for college." That was our rationale. So, one night we planned to raid her parents' liquor cabinet. First we had a babysitting gig where all the adults left after having hosted a cocktail party. After the kids were asleep we started cleaning up and helping ourselves to the unfinished drinks. When we went back to Bindy's, we proceeded to the liquor cabinet as planned and continued our drink fest.
>
> After the first few gulps of alcohol my brain told me to keep going, to let it rip. I was looking for that altered state. I got sick, very sick, but a little voice inside me was already telling me that I definitely wanted to do this again. The next morning I had to get up and drag myself to my Saturday job at the local camera store. It was my first time of having to show up somewhere I needed to be with a hangover.

Aversive conditioning is a powerful force. Many people have told me that they became so sick after drinking too much the first time they sampled alcohol as a young person that thereafter, they had an aversion to alcohol. That was not Lynda's response. Despite becoming so ill from getting inebriated, "a little voice inside me was already telling me that I definitely wanted to do this again."

Similar to the response of Lynda, when I have asked other patients who have strong genetic loading for alcohol dependence about their first experience with alcohol, I have had the following responses:

- "For the first time in my life I felt what it must be like to be *normal*, just like everyone else."
- "I immediately began to plan how I was going to get my next

drink. I was 11 years old at the time, and I haven't stopped looking for that next drink over the last 23 years."

- "I felt like I could finally turn off my brain and stop worrying every second of the day."

- "I felt like 'myself'—whatever that is—for the very first time. I even considered changing my birthday to the day I drank my first drink."

- "My life changed at that very instant. I began to hang out with a different crowd in middle school who were mainly interested in getting high. Planning how and where to get high and getting high were essentially was all we did through high school and college—until we failed out. And we all failed out."

As I have tried to emphasize throughout this chapter and Chapter 8, alcohol is a powerful force with which to contend. It is always a mistake to take this adversary lightly, because if we do so, we will always lose our battle with the bottle. And my first step in the treatment of my patients with alcohol use disorder is to help them to acknowledge and accept that they "really like alcohol."

Once Lynda was able to appreciate how much she liked alcohol—and why—she was able to choose what she liked *more:* alcohol or her children, alcohol or her husband, alcohol or her job, alcohol or her health, alcohol or her self-esteem, and alcohol or her life. These were classic approach-approach conflicts, and she said "yes" to her life, which meant saying "no" to alcohol. Once she had made her decision about what she wanted more, she could proceed to implementing her choice of the Power of No through discipline— paradoxically one of Lynda's strengths—with the help of ample servings of the Power of Go.

3. A *none or all* binary choice is required to achieve success. Moderation does not work in this case.

As indicated throughout this chapter and Chapter 8, for complex biological, psychological, social, and spiritual reasons, one can *never* underestimate the Power of Alcohol. No one with Lynda's family and personal history of alcohol use disorder can "drink in moderation." That is a myth or just another self-deception of someone who is stuck in pause. The word *moderation*, as it applies to alcohol use, is halfway between "No" and "Go," the classic, dangerous middle ground of someone who is stuck in pause. For whatever reasons or excuses, any person with a strong history of alcohol use disorder who believes that he or she can drink in moderation has not decided to stop destroying his or her life. Typically, people with histories of alcohol use disorder who try to drink in moderation have all the hallmarks of being stuck in pause, including persistent ruminations about *when, where,* and *how much* to drink, and, thereafter, guilt, shame, and embarrassment when they inevitably drink too much or behave poorly while drinking. Both AA and psychiatry agree that for people with histories of alcohol use disorder, alcohol is an all or none choice. A binary decision. A compromise approach rarely, if ever, works.

4. The Power of Go is *always* required to achieve the Power of No.

The list of corollary activities that Lynda must initiate and maintain to sustain her sobriety is long and continues to be enlarged. Initially, these obligations (to herself) included attending almost daily meetings of AA and engaging in intensive psychotherapy. Working hard *in* psychotherapy to gain insight is important, but effort *outside* the clinical office to apply this insight in order to *change* patterns of thought and behavior is even more important. Just like when a car is stuck in a muddy ditch, figuring out how it got stuck and where it is stuck is required to get it out of the ditch. But unless one uses these discoveries to take action with a tow truck or winch, the car will remain stuck in the ditch. Insight alone does not bring about meaningful change. Taking focused action based on insight is required to get unstuck. This applies to attending AA as well. Sitting in the AA meetings is not sufficient: Lynda must "work the Program." She must take to heart what she has learned from fellow members and apply this knowledge in her own life. Thus, both psychotherapy and AA require the Power of Go on an ongoing basis.

For example, in treatment Lynda discovered that her low self-esteem and fear of abandonment led her to overwork to please her spouse. Although her husband superficially suggested that she work less and take more vacations, he did not go to work himself; overspent on his clothes, hobbies, and trips; and hardly lifted a finger to help out around the home or with family finances. He was living on easy street in the most expensive neighborhood in town, and Lynda was paying for, paving, and sweeping that road. The Power of Go was required for Lynda to communicate clearly her concerns and angry feelings to her spouse and to insist that his exploitative, self-centered behaviors cease. Given her fears of rejection and abandonment, this aspect of the Power of Go has been far more difficult for her to accomplish than the discovery and insight component of psychotherapy. At the present time, Lynda's husband, Bernard, is joining her periodically for couples counseling with me. For the first time ever, she is openly communicating with Bernard about her anger and dissatisfactions as they involve him and their relationship. In the most recent session, she discussed how upset she has been that he has placed all the financial burdens of family support on her, even though he is a highly qualified professional and would have no trouble securing employment. Bernard has been a willing participant and has been making effort to change his self-centered behavioral patterns. As would be expected, Bernard has ample issues for Lynda to address, including behaviors related to her perfectionism and lofty, unreasonable expectations of him and other people.

5. A reprioritization of time and a restructuring of daily schedules are usually required to become unstuck.

Lynda is the prototypical, overly responsible, high-performing high-level executive in an international megabusiness. Her calendar is forever overflowing. Although she is consummately efficient and hardworking, there are never sufficient hours in a day for her to accomplish her self-imposed duties. And none of her efforts is ever wasted because each project is "essential." In addition, her work requires frequent traveling. Each of these factors makes attending daily AA meetings and flying to Houston to attend regular psychotherapy sessions with me impractical—or, as she initially stated, "practically impossible." However, unless Lynda exercises the Power of Go to restructure her priorities, which would require that she spend more time on recovery and less time working on her job and pleasing others, she will not remain sober for long.

At first, Lynda thought reprioritizing her time and efforts seemed to be untenable and "self-centered." However, in treatment, she determined the following:

- "My family, my health, my job, and my self-esteem are most important to me."
- "Although it is now obvious that I also love alcohol, my returning to drinking will destroy all of my highest priorities."
- "I have finally chosen what I love most: my family, my health, my job, and my self-esteem."

Thus, the decision to restructure her time and priorities to attend AA and regular psychotherapy made some sense. It has been more than 50 years since Lynda "had figured out how to improve my lot in life and be accepted. I would use my superior intelligence and outwork everyone. I would become the very best at everything I did." Understanding the origins and costs of that ancient decision is enabling Lynda to redraft and reengineer her priorities.

Trudging Along (Lynda Jensen's Perspective)

I am writing this at 24 months+ of sobriety and have never felt better in my entire adult life. What happened this time around that has led to a more solid and joyous recovery? I can't explain exactly why I didn't make it in the past because I don't fully understand all of the reasons myself. I really wanted to quit and sincerely attempted to countless times. I now believe that sobriety and recovery are part of an ongoing process, and sometimes it takes a number of tries before fully "getting it." Recovery is progressive, as is the disease itself. By "getting it," I mean coming to a complete understanding and deeply held acceptance of what it truly means to be alcoholic and what you need to do on a continuing basis to stay well. There are layers of denial and old ideas that one must wade through and replace, and sometimes we can go only so far at a particular time. Just like a cancer patient who may need several rounds of chemotherapy to arrest the cancer, some of us need more than one stint in treatment. And some people with cancer need new medications and new approaches to treat their illnesses, as Dr. Y. and his approach have provided for me.

The book of *Alcoholics Anonymous* ("The Big Book") refers to members of the fellowship meeting one another in sobriety as we "trudge the Road of Happy Destiny" (Alcoholics Anonymous 2001, p. 164). I had quite a negative reaction when I first read this passage—is this what my new life would become, one of trudging? It did not sound very enticing. Now, more than 2 years sober, I am gaining a deeper appreciation and acceptance of what it means to trudge. As I plod along each day, staying true to a routine that ensures my sobriety and keeps me rooted and balanced no matter what chaos is going on around me, I am reassured. I just keep trudging along, happy to have something I am trudging for and toward, looking to help fellow travelers where I can. As I continue down this path the problems in my life seem more manageable, even simpler, and gradually things are getting better. I no longer look for the fast track or quick fix in recovery. I accept the process. There is something uplifting, even spiritual, in this trudging. I continue on because I made an absolute commitment to sobriety and I finally accept that this is what it takes, daily trudging. It is simple, but not easy.

For me to finally make this absolute commitment, I needed to undergo a deep, transformational change on a spiritual level. Something had to reach into my innermost core and shake it all up so that I could see and feel with a fresh perspective.

The "need" to feel better is an essential theme of my addictive voice. For me to live comfortably as a sober person, I am learning how to live comfortably in my own skin and not run away from fear, anxiety, or other negative emotions. As they say in AA, "there is a lot more to quitting drinking than quitting drinking," which I hadn't fully appreciated in the past. Some of my character traits or leanings of mind that I am beginning to understand and work on with the help and guidance of Dr. Y. and through working the AA program include the following:

Oversensitivity

I magnify external and internal signals and tend to take things personally. It is as if the volume is always turned up to high. I have an exaggerated sense of the things I must do and the relative importance of getting it all done. I often feel pressured by the passage of time, such as feeling I don't have enough time to perform successfully and wishing I could freeze time or at least make it slow down until I am fully ready to show up. Alcohol seemed to work beautifully earlier on in turning down the volume and muffling the sound of the continuous ticking of the clock in my head. Ultimately, as my drinking progressed, I crossed the line from slowing down or muffling time to killing it.

Thirst for Creative Connections

I have a strong yearning to experience expansiveness and creativity and a sense of connection to something bigger than myself. I want to shed the burden of self. Alcohol in earlier times seemed to release within me that sense of expansiveness and connection, bringing to the fore buried emotions and creative insights. Although that perception of alcohol's effects may have been at least partially true in my earlier phases of drinking, in later phases the tables turned and alcohol brought with it only darkness, contraction, loneliness, and isolation.

Perfectionism

I've had trouble knowing when good is good enough. This fits in with my sense of needing to slow down time because there is never enough time to do things perfectly. I am gradually learning to show up as I am with the best I can do on the basis of the time and resources available. I come up for air more often without needing to use alcohol.

Victim Mentality

I have acted from a belief that bad things can and probably will happen to me without warning. I am übervigilant and have a tendency to alternate between wanting someone to protect me from being in harm's way and then being bitterly disappointed and hurt if he doesn't. Being a victim always provided a ready excuse to drink, as I'd tell myself alcohol was the only thing I could rely on to bring relief.

Avoidance

I don't like head-on confrontations in personal relationships; they feel too risky. So I lie to myself and pretend that things are OK when they really aren't. I call this false acceptance. I see this now as a form of self-deception, of trying to turn blue into green by declaring it so. Through avoidance I have reinforced my victim role by not confronting situations that were sometimes intolerable. Alcohol fueled the flames of avoidance. I am learning now to take the risk of being more honest with myself and others, of trying to see things the way they really are, not just the way I want them to be, and to authentically communicate my feelings and opinions.

Transition Difficulties

I've always had difficulty transitioning from one situation or encounter to another—from home to work and vice versa, from one city to another, from being with people to being alone, from Sunday to Monday morning and the ensuing work week, and so forth. I get stuck wherever I set my focus, and moving on feels like having to undergo a major process of uprooting and replanting. These transition challenges are closely related to my perfectionism and difficulties with time. Using alcohol helped me let go.

At the core, all of this trudging supports a spiritual makeover. The Big Book declares we are given "a daily reprieve contingent on the maintenance of our spiritual condition" (Alcoholics Anonymous 2001, p. 85). That idea scares away a lot of people because they associate spirituality with the religion they were fed growing up and may have long ago rejected. The brand of spirituality referenced is not religious in a traditional sense, however. For me, it is about finding something greater than myself, more transcendent than my mind that harbors my addictive voice.

Over time, I am learning to be appropriately confident in my sobriety but not step over the line into overconfidence or complacency. I no longer live in fear that my alcoholism will leap out and capture me like a scary monster in the forest, but at the same time I realize I need to pay proper homage to the power of the disease and continue to submit myself to the daily work and routine of recovery. I try to find the proper space within the tension between confidence and humility, strength and caution, and effort and letting go, all with gratitude and grace.

Finding this zone is what I imagine it is like to catch the perfect wave—very tricky but unspeakably wonderful when experienced. I start most days asking the collective spirit (my higher power) for help in staying sober and for the strength, persistence, and willingness to trudge the road. I also give thanks for another day to practice and grow in this new way of life. At the end of my day, I thank my higher power for another day of sobriety. I review the day for things I can improve on in the areas of honesty, fear, resentment, selfishness, and judgmental thought.

I was recently in Paris, a city I have often visited and which I deeply associate with food and wine. So close was my association that I had wondered whether I would even enjoy Paris without being able to drink the wine. This was a test, not only of my sobriety, but of my ability to fully enjoy life without my old stand-by. My second evening there, safely tucked away within my cozy room after a long and busy day with my family, I was infused with an exquisite sense of freedom. I was not drinking in Paris, I was staying true to my commitment, and I was so utterly happy. I felt lifted up into an expanse of light and joy as I realized I could go anywhere, do anything. I was no longer held back by the chains that had for so long kept me captive.

And all I really have to do is keep on trudging. Simple, not easy, but definitely doable.

References

Alcoholics Anonymous: The Story of How Many Thousands of Men and Women Have Recovered From Alcoholism, 4th Edition. New York, Alcoholics Anonymous World Services, 2001

American Foundation for Suicide Prevention: Facts and figures. New York, American Foundation for Suicide Prevention, 2014. Available at: http://www.afsp.org/understanding-suicide/facts-and-figures. Accessed February 1, 2014.

American Psychiatric Association: Diagnostic and Statistical Manual of Mental Disorders, 5th Edition. Washington, DC, American Psychiatric Association, 2013

Centers for Disease Control and Prevention: Alcohol-Related Disease Impact (ARDI). Atlanta, GA, Centers for Disease Control and Prevention, 2014. Available at: http://apps.nccd.cdc.gov/DACH_ARDI/Default/Default.aspx. Accessed May 15, 2014.

Jørgensen CH, Pedersen B, Tonnesen H: The efficacy of disulfiram for the treatment of alcohol use disorder. Alcohol Clin Exp Res 35:1749–1758, 2011

Kendler KS, Prescott CA, Neale MC, et al: Temperance board registration for alcohol abuse in a national sample of Swedish male twins, born 1902 to 1949. Arch Gen Psychiatry 54:178–184, 1997

Knapp CM, Ciraulo DA, Kranler HR: Neurobiology of alcohol, in The American Psychiatric Publishing Textbook of Substance Abuse Treatment, 4th Edition. Edited by Galanter M, Kleber HD. Washington, DC, American Psychiatric Publishing, 2008, pp 111–127

Maisel NC, Blodgett JC, Wilbourne PL, et al: Meta-analysis of naltrexone and acamprosate for treating alcohol use disorders: when are these medications most helpful? Addiction 108:275–293, 2013

Mokdad AH, Marks JS, Stroup, et al: Actual causes of death in the United States, 2000. JAMA 291:1238–1245, 2004

National Highway Traffic Safety Administration: Traffic safety facts 2012 data: alcohol-impaired driving. Washington, DC, U.S. Department of Transportation, December 2013. Available at: http://www-nrd.nhtsa.dot.gov/Pubs/811870.pdf. Accessed February 1, 2014.

Sinclair JD: Evidence about the use of naltrexone and for different ways of using it in the treatment of alcoholism. Alcohol Alcohol 36:2–10, 2001

Wilson, B: Three Talks to Medical Societies. New York, Alcoholics Anonymous World Services, 1958, pp. 5–22

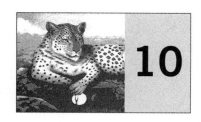

10

Stuck in Pleasing Others, Part I (Discover): The Case of Eleanor Lai

When Anorexia Nervosa Is Complicated by Child Physical and Psychological Abuse

A revolution is not a dinner party, or writing an essay, or painting a picture or doing embroidery; it cannot be so refined, so leisurely, and gentle, so temperate, kind, courteous, restrained and magnanimous.
—*Mao Zedong*

Flowers from hell—real blood has watered them,
Blood mixed with animal sweat, with parting tears.
—*Huynh Sanh Thong*, Flowers From Hell, *1984*

"I began to examine every inch of my body to check how fat it is. I still do it all the time. I started to obsess about every morsel that goes into my mouth, and I still do. I began to hate my body and hate myself, and I still do."

The Case of Eleanor Lai: D1 (Discover) Assessment Component

Presentation for Treatment

The call came on New Year's Day from Dr. Pamela Klinger, Chief of Nephrology at one of the large, private not-for-profit teaching hospitals where I am on the clinical faculty.

> **Dr. Pamela Klinger:** Good morning, Stuart. I am referring you a tough one this time. Her name is Eleanor Lai, and she is a 20-year-old college sophomore. Her parents are both physicians. Her mother, Dr. Ruth Lai, is a well-known businesswoman who owns a large chain of dialysis clinics throughout the region, and her father, Dr. Leonard Lai, is a nephrologist. For years he has attended almost all of our department's updates and continuing medical education courses, but I don't think I have ever heard him say a word to anybody. He has an excellent academic background, but he just sits in one of the back rows and takes notes.
>
> Leonard Lai called me to tell me that Eleanor has been admitted to the neurology service for a workup of weakness and weight loss. Both parents are very unhappy with their daughter's care by neurology—particularly because they couldn't find anything wrong with her physically beyond the symptoms I just mentioned. Dr. Lai said that Eleanor's doctors now think she should be evaluated by a psychiatrist right away. He asked my opinion about whether he should do so. I told him that it's a good idea and gave him your name. Can you take her on?
>
> **Dr. Y.:** I am happy to. Thank you for the referral. Do you know anything more about her?
>
> **Dr. Klinger:** All I know is that she's been here for about 10 days, is 5 feet 10 inches tall, and weighs 97 pounds.
>
> **Dr. Y.:** I'll see her this afternoon.

"Who's There, Please?"

I later learned from her electronic medical record that Eleanor Lai had received multiple laboratory tests and consultations to evaluate her weight loss, muscle wasting, and weakness of undetermined cause. There were no abnormal findings beyond her weakness and low weight. Although anorexia nervosa was a primary diagnostic consideration of the neurology team at the time of her admission, a psychiatry consultation was not ordered. Routinely, a psychiatrist would have been called the first day for a patient with Eleanor's clinical presentation. I postulated that the fact that standard hospital protocols were not followed would become a valuable clue to solving the mystery of how Eleanor became ill and how to help her recover. Stopping by the nurses' station before proceeding to the patient's room, I encountered Mrs. Sandra Hall, the head nurse on the Neurology Unit.

Dr. Y.: Well hello, Sandra. It's been a while since we have worked together.

Mrs. Sandra Hall: Oh, we are working together now, are we Stuart? Funny, no one asked me. I know that you are here to see Eleanor. Please don't drag me into that morass.

Dr. Y.: Since the family is not happy with their daughter's care thus far, it is probably best that we not discuss her case until after I meet with the patient. Otherwise they might believe that I am biased: a company man conspiring against their better judgment about how their daughter should be treated. However, I do think it would be a good idea if you would join me for my first meeting with the patient, if you can spare the time. I would very much appreciate your perspective of our interaction.

Mrs. Hall: You just want a witness, don't you, Stuart?

Dr. Y.: This is not your first rodeo either, is it, Sandra?

Hanging from the handle of the door to Eleanor Lai's hospital room was a sign that read, "Please Knock." Obligingly, I knocked at the door, and, after a moment's delay, a woman's voice responded loudly through the closed door:

Voice from hospital room: Who's there, please?

Dr. Y.: Dr. Yudofsky from Psychiatry.

Voice from hospital room: The patient is not available.

Dr. Y.: With whom am I speaking?

Voice from hospital room: Dr. Ruth Lai, the patient's mother.

Dr. Y.: Good afternoon, Dr. Lai. When would be a good time for your daughter to visit with me?

Dr. Ruth Lai: I do not know.

Dr. Y.: I will leave my professional card at the nursing station. The number of my administrative assistant is on the card, and she will be able to help arrange a time that is convenient for your daughter. I very much look forward to meeting you both.

"Game on!" was the thought that came to my mind as I returned to the nurses' station with Mrs. Hall.

Mrs. Sandra Hall: As I guess you are aware, there is no reason on Earth that Eleanor couldn't meet with you right now. Nothing else is on her schedule today. All she has been doing for the last week is lying in her bed and reading fashion magazines. Her mother had a portable bed moved into the room and has been staying with Eleanor day and night. She almost never leaves Eleanor by herself—certainly not when nurses and doctors are seeing Eleanor. Nothing can happen with Eleanor without going through Dr. Lai first. What should we do now?

Dr. Y.: Please make a brief descriptive note in the chart about what just happened. I will do the same. Please have another nurse give my professional card with my contact information—including my cell phone number—to Eleanor. Not to Dr. Lai. And then we'll wait.

Mrs. Hall: Wait for what?

Dr. Y.: To climb on the bucking bronco.

We did not have to wait very long. At 11:00 P.M. that evening, I received an emergency page from Dr. Craig Aaronoff, the hospital's Chairman of Neurology, on whose service Eleanor was a patient.

Dr. Craig Aaronoff: I am sorry to bother you this late, Stuart, but we have a big problem. The mother of one of your patients on our service has filed a complaint against you and our department.

Dr. Y.: What did the mother say that "we" did wrong?

Dr. Aaronoff: She said *you* acted unprofessionally. That you insulted her daughter and were impolite to her.

Dr. Y.: Did she specify?

Dr. Aaronoff: Yes. She alleges that you scared her daughter by calling her daughter "crazy." She said that you were disrespectful to her as a professional by telling her to work through a secretary in your office and not permitting her to deal directly with you. She also said you screamed profanities at her when her daughter was indisposed and not able to meet with you.

Dr. Y.: Anything else, Craig?

Dr. Aaronoff: I did learn from nursing that you had asked Mrs. Hall to accompany you and that she was present for the entire interaction through the closed door. As you might imagine, she has an entirely different story from Dr. Lai's. The mother doesn't know that yet. Ultimately, I don't think anything will come of their complaint. It's one of those "she said," "we said" deals.

Dr. Y.: The key is in the "we," Craig.

Dr. Aaronoff: You lost me, Stuart.

Dr. Y.: Dr. Ruth Lai was not the only person inside that closed door. At some point Eleanor will have her say.

The following afternoon, I was asked to meet with Mrs. Yolanda Mitchell, the Director of Patient Services at the hospital. She had already met with Dr. Ruth Lai and Mrs. Hall. I recounted to her my version of the episode.

Mrs. Yolanda Mitchell: Have you spoken with Mrs. Hall since this complaint was filed?

Dr. Y.: No, I have not, nor did I access the medical record to look at her note.

Mrs. Mitchell: Your account is absolutely consistent with that of Mrs. Hall. However, Dr. Lai's version is totally different.

Dr. Y.: Where does this go from here?

Mrs. Mitchell: I would like for this to be settled without Dr. Lai filing a formal complaint to the Texas State Medical Board against you and against the hospital. Do you have any ideas?

Dr. Y.: Did Dr. Lai file a *written* complaint about me and this episode with the hospital?

Mrs. Mitchell: Yes.

Dr. Y.: Very good. Please let her know what you have found out thus far regarding your investigation of this episode, including Mrs. Hall's testimony. Also, please communicate that I regret this misunderstanding and that the family is upset. Finally, please tell her that I would like to meet with her, her husband, and Eleanor to resolve the issue to the satisfaction of everyone and to proceed with the care of her daughter. My sole, nonnegotiable, requirement is that Eleanor joins us for this meeting.

Believe it or not, Mrs. Mitchell, Eleanor does actually exist beyond the presence and influence of her mother; she is the identified patient, she is an adult, and she has not given me permission to speak with any family member about her care. If Dr. Lai agrees to the meeting, which I believe is unlikely, I would also like you to join us for that meeting. In any case, Mrs. Mitchell, I believe that this complaint will be resolved soon.

The Elephant in the Room

Even without the benefit of being able to meet with the designated patient, the vital elements of this case were becoming increasingly clear. Anorexia nervosa is a lethal illness, with the highest mortality rate for young women among all psychiatric disorders. Notwithstanding Eleanor's dangerously low weight and the seriousness of her other medical signs and symptoms, Dr. Ruth Lai was disregarding medical advice and diverting attention of the medical team from her daughter to herself.

One of the great privileges of my medical and psychiatric education was being taught about anorexia nervosa by Dr. Hilda Bruch, the leading pioneer of her era in the conceptualization and treatment of this condition. After I became a psychiatrist, I collaborated with Dr. Bruch on the treatment of many young women with this disorder. Dr. Bruch embraced the omnipresent interplay of biological, psychological, and social influences in every person with anorexia nervosa and emphasized that the issue of "control" was central to every case, as well.

In this instance, Dr. Ruth Lai had seized control over the medical care of her daughter. Eleanor's participation in her own treatment, for all practical purposes, had disappeared—just as she was doing in the physical sense. I postulated that her mother's hijacking of Eleanor's self-agency was most likely the central dynamic in the etiology of Eleanor's illness, and changing that power dynamic would be essential to her treatment and recovery. By setting up a power struggle between me and her, Dr. Lai was preventing me from establishing a relationship with Eleanor.

Without having the opportunity to meet with the patient or her family, I could only *speculate* about the sources of Dr. Ruth Lai's motivations. The following are the three possibilities that I considered to be most likely:

1. *Dr. Lai is an anxious and frightened mother.* She is fearful that without her controlling Eleanor's medical care, something dire will happen to her daughter.
2. *There is a cultural dimension to Dr. Lai's concerns.* Dr. Lai spoke English with a pronounced accent that appeared to me to be of Asian origin. In many—although certainly not in all—Asian cultures, people with mental illnesses can be highly stigmatized. Additionally, psychiatry is not a well-regarded discipline, and psychiatrists are vastly underrepresented among medical specialists in most Asian countries. For example, there are only 20,000 psychiatrists in China, or 1.5 psychiatrists per 100,000 people. That is approximately 10% of the ratio of psychiatrists per capita in the United States (Cyranoski 2010).
3. *Dr. Lai has a serious mental illness,* ranging from a personality disorder to a psychotic disorder. For reasons that were uncertain to me, she clearly distorted what had occurred during our brief encounter. Was the problem related to poor reality testing (psychosis), or did she deliberately lie (personality disorder)?

How Dr. Lai reacted to my request to meet with Eleanor and both parents would help refine my understanding of which, if any, among these hypotheses applied.

1. If the third possibility were true, it was possible but still not likely that Dr. Ruth Lai would persist with her intention to report me and the hospital to the Texas Board. Unless she were psychotic, a medical professional would understand the futility of this approach and its high potential to backfire.
2. If the second possibility were operant, Dr. Ruth Lai would see to it that neither I, nor any other psychiatrist who was independent of her control, would be in a position to care for her daughter.
3. If the first possibility prevailed, there would be a small chance that Dr. Ruth Lai would accept the meeting that I had proposed, which would provide an opportunity for her to be reassured, for us to make amends, and for me to move forward with the evaluation and treatment of her seriously ill daughter.
4. If there were a combination of these options, the most avoidant behavior between or among the possibilities would prevail. Importantly, if ever Eleanor and I were permitted to meet, each option that pertained would need to be addressed at some point in her care.

About 2 hours after my meeting with Mrs. Mitchell, she called me.

Mrs. Yolanda Mitchell: I just finished speaking with Dr. Ruth Lai in her daughter's room. I told her what we had learned from Mrs. Hall and your offer to meet with her, Eleanor, and Eleanor's father at their convenience.

Dr. Y.: And what did she say?

Mrs. Mitchell: She said that Eleanor had told her that she wanted to leave the hospital this morning. Dr. Lai also said she decided not to pursue her complaint further—although she is still upset over your behavior. I indicated to her that most likely Eleanor would need to be discharged "against medical advice," and she was OK with that.

Eleanor Lai was discharged that morning against medical advice. The Neurology Service volunteered to arrange outpatient follow-up with Psychiatry and Dietary Services, but Dr. Ruth Lai declined to accept either referral.

A Call in the Night

At approximately 1:30 A.M. 17 days later, I was awakened by my pager.

> **Page operator:** You have an emergency call from a Dr. Leonard Lai. He says you know who he is. He also said that the call could not wait until the morning.
>
> **Dr. Y.:** I have not spoken with him up to this point, but I will take the call.
>
> **Page operator:** I will put him through right now.
>
> **Dr. Leonard Lai:** I am so sorry to disturb you, Doctor, but I worry that my daughter is going to die. Eleanor does not eat food for 2 weeks. She only drinks water.
>
> **Dr. Y.:** She probably should be readmitted to the hospital. Will she sign in voluntarily?
>
> **Dr. Leonard Lai:** She says she will go to your office. She will not go back to hospital.
>
> **Dr. Y.:** Will her mother permit her to see me?
>
> **Dr. Leonard Lai:** I do not care about my wife. My daughter will die soon. Please, Doctor. I will bring her to your office now.

I gave Dr. Lai the directions to my office in the Texas Medical Center and told him to come there immediately.

The Elephant Speaks

It was a chilly, blustery January morning in Houston when I met Dr. Leonard Lai and Eleanor in the lobby of the Baylor College of Medicine office building. Dr. Lai was wearing a faded blue windbreaker jacket that I thought might be a bit too thin to protect him from the cold wind. To my surprise, Eleanor appeared elegant in a green woolen trench coat that was draped fashionably about her tall frame. She was strikingly beautiful. Prior to our meeting, I had braced myself to encounter an emaciated young woman—a living skeleton painfully reminiscent of pictures of the liberated survivors in Nazi concentration camps. As she was wrapped, Eleanor more closely resembled a fashion model.

Her eyes darting furiously, Eleanor conducted an intense, thorough visual examination of me and our surroundings. Our disparate trio remained silent in the elevator and stepped out onto the fourth floor and down the antiseptically modern and angular corridors leading to my office. The office is sparsely decorated in early twentieth century arts and crafts furnishings. I sensed, somehow, that the recognition of the stark contrasts among the three of us, between the old and new, among incongruent pasts and uncertain futures, was lost only on Dr. Lai, who seemed resigned to his role as a taciturn, nonparticipating prop. He did, however, speak up almost inaudibly.

> **Dr. Leonard Lai:** Distinguished Professor, my daughter says she wants to see you by herself.
>
> **Dr. Y.:** That's fine with me, Dr. Lai. I believe it is best that Eleanor is in control of her treatment. So if you will excuse us.

After she was in the office and the door was closed, Eleanor briefly diverted her systematic laser gaze from me to the furnishings and then spoke.

> **Eleanor Lai:** I am so, so sorry for how you have been treated by me and my family. I know my mother misrepresented totally what you said to her in the hospital. I heard every word. And now my father dragged you out of bed so early in the morning just to see me. I'm so embarrassed, and grateful that you would still agree to see me.
>
> **Dr. Y.:** It is my great privilege and pleasure to meet with you, Eleanor. And I understand that your parents would be very worried about you. Do you share their concern?
>
> **Eleanor:** No, I do not. They're obsessed with my weight and with what I do and don't eat. They actually believe I'm about to die. Nothing could be further from the truth.
>
> **Dr. Y.:** Do *you* think you need to see a psychiatrist, Eleanor?
>
> **Eleanor:** Actually, I'm not sure. I really don't know what psychiatrists do. But I do know that I don't need to see you about my weight or about what I'm eating.
>
> **Dr. Y.:** Most people don't know what psychiatrists do. I will do my best to explain, at all times, what I am thinking and trying to accomplish. And why. If you aren't sure what I'm getting at, please ask me.
>
> I agree fully that you don't need to see me because of your weight or what you are eating. I am certain that I will find what you eat and how much you eat to be the least interesting, least captivating aspect of you. It's only when your weight becomes so low that it threatens your health that I am compelled, as a physician, to help you deal with it directly. Do you think you are at that point right now?
>
> **Eleanor:** No, I don't. In fact, I feel as big and fat as an elephant. Or a whale.

Caring for People With Eating Disorders

Although Eleanor and I had been conversing for only several minutes, her comment about feeling so overweight marked a critical juncture in our work together. Because she had not removed her overcoat, I could judge her weight only by her facial appearance, a visual measure that can be highly misleading. From what I could tell, she clearly was very thin, but I did not know if she were in immediate medical danger. It would be my professional and legal responsibility to come to that determination before she left my office that morning, an objective conclusion that might require a physical examination and certainly would necessitate my weighing her.

As stated in previous chapters, I believe that it is best to initiate therapeutic relationships with a patient by learning as much as possible about the *person*, beyond his or her problems. This principle establishes that our relationship is based not on a patient's deficiencies but, rather, on his or her uniqueness, which includes strengths, interests, proclivities, and potentials—as well as his or her psychiatric problems. If I were to go for the bait that Eleanor cast toward me— "I feel as big and fat as an elephant"—by asking her how much she weighed or even by commenting that she did not appear to me to be fat, I would have likely embarked with her on a familiar, tried-and-trodden path of power struggles with authority figures such as her parents, her teachers, and her primary care physicians. This is territory that she knew quite well and a battle that she knew that she would win. All that she had to do was not swallow what I was dishing out, and she would prevail.

> **Dr. Y.:** I am guessing that you already spend too much of your mental energy thinking about how much you weigh or about what you should or should not eat. What a waste of your fine brain. Let's talk about you and not about what goes in and out of your body.
>
> **Eleanor Lai:** You guessed right, Dr. Yudofsky. That's about all that I think about these days. Can you tell me why?
>
> **Dr. Y.:** I don't know you very well and believe it to be premature for us to get into that topic, Eleanor. But since you asked, let's discuss it for only a minute or so.
>
> I will venture another guess. You are preoccupied with food and your weight for at least two reasons. First, your preoccupation is a distraction—a counterirritant, if you will. So you won't

have to experience and deal with powerful feelings with which you are uncomfortable. Second, you have ceded the authority over your life to others because you don't have the courage to stand up for yourself. You try to please them at the expense of doing what you want. The one area of your life that you have retained control over is what goes into your mouth. So your obsession with eating and your weight is all about power and control.

Eleanor: I'm not quite sure what you're talking about. But it sounds interesting and worth thinking about, which I can assure you that I will do. Thank you. I didn't expect you to even try to answer my question. Could you answer just one more question right now about my eating?

Dr. Y.: Yes, I can try.

Eleanor: Do you think you can make me stop obsessing about food and getting too fat? Even though I think I'm OK, I'm pretty miserable these days. I feel like a lost cause.

Dr. Y.: No, I *can't* make you stop obsessing. More than that, I won't even *try* to make you stop.

TREATMENT PRINCIPLE 9

Mental health professionals should avoid getting into power struggles over weight and diet with their patients with eating disorders. Such interactions, which are about the patient's need for control, reflect therapeutic attention away from the underlying conflicts that have led to the eating disorders and will interfere with the therapeutic alliance between patient and clinician.

Dependency and Transference

Closely aligned with "control" is "dependency." The many young patients with anorexia nervosa whom I have treated have waged a battle with themselves that is camouflaged as a struggle with a controlling caregiver, usually their mother or father. Their lifelong experience of being informed by someone else what they like, being told what they should do, being advised what is best for them, etc., has created an addictive dependency on authority figures who believe they have all those answers. These children have not been afforded the opportunity to learn by trial and error how to make up their own minds about what they like and don't like, what they want to do and don't want to do, etc., so they depend on their parents and others to make those decisions for them. Ambivalent about their dependencies, they also rebel against their parents by setting up power struggles over what they do and don't eat and how much they weigh. In this way they achieve a pseudo independence. Although their parents may be helpless in forcing them to maintain a healthful diet, weight, and lifestyle, the patients are still basing their actions and decisions on their parents' reactions.

After these patients are in treatment, this conflict will invariably be transferred to the psychiatrist—usually by the patients persuading their clinicians to promote and accept their dependency on them. If the therapist is so persuaded, the "treatment" is comparable to that psychiatrist prescribing morphine to a patient who is addicted to heroin. Same problem, different powder—now in a white-coated capsule. They try to turn their doctors into omniscient authorities on what is and what is not best for them who will make important decisions for them and, thereby, replicate the conflict and dysfunctional relationship they have with their parents. If a therapist is so engaged, nothing will change. Treatment will become all about weight regulation.

I endeavor to counter this transference in every interaction. When asked my opinion about what they should like, do, or decide, I will say, "How would I know? You are the world's authority on what you do and don't like. I don't know what's best for you. You are the world's authority on you." When asked if I can make them better, I bluntly say, "No."

> **Eleanor Lai:** Are you saying that I can't get better?
> **Dr. Y.:** Not at all. What I am saying is that I don't have the power or the ability to *make* you better. However, I can help you decide whether or not you want to change. And, if you decide to change, I can help you do the hard work to bring about those changes. But you have all the power to change and must do all the heavy lifting.
> At long last, Eleanor, please tell me about yourself—beyond your weight.

TREATMENT PRINCIPLE 10

Because eating disorders often reflect patients' conflicts between dependence and autonomy, mental health professionals should avoid assuming the roles of *omniscient advisor* or *decision maker* for their patients.

From China, With Time and Toil

Escaping starvation in their small rural hamlets, all four of Eleanor's grandparents went as penniless teenagers in search of work to Chengdu, a city in western China that was just beginning its boom into modernity. And work they did in endless hours of tedious hand labor for pitiful wages. Hoping that their children would lead less miserable lives than they, Eleanor's grandparents sacrificed mightily to support and advance the lots of their children. Like so many before and after them, her grandparents believed that the sole route to the emancipation of their children was through formal education, a luxury that had always been beyond their own reach.

Spurred by their own wretchedness, Eleanor's grandparents more than encouraged, they *insisted* that her parents stay the course of China's brutally competitive education system that would lead to a promised land of clean-fingernailed employment. Education would open to their children the front doors of those brand new Chengdu skyscrapers that, clinging to flimsy bamboo scaffolding, they had built and, crawling on naked knees, whose floors and toilets they continued to clean with their ungloved hands. When you are illiterate and impoverished parents in Chengdu, so desperate is your life and so intense is the competition for admission to universities for your children that the pursuit and pathway to education become indistinguishable from who your children are and why you exist.

Both Ruth and Leonard met as first-year students at Sichuan University, one of China's oldest and most prestigious institutions of higher education. Even at age 18, they both were veterans of many academic wars. They had survived the vicious classroom competition, had endured the grueling years of preparation for admission tests, and had overcome the overwhelming odds against their acceptance to Sichuan University. Although they had attained their goal in vastly different ways, the reward for this competition was the same: even harder work and stiffer competition at the university.

Both were enrolled in the 7-year medical track at Sichuan University when Ruth spotted Leonard during their first year. Almost immediately she forged an alliance with Leonard that was based on their differing personal strengths. Thin, shy, and bookish, Leonard glided effortlessly through the demanding classes, crowded science labs, and taxing tests to the top of their class. He was passionately interested in the subject matter, and this interest and passion drove his hard work. Concepts entered his mind easily, and they did not escape. Thus, he never was harried about completing assignments, nor was he anxious about tests, nor did he study late into the nights before the dreaded term examinations.

A taut tangle of ambition, anger, and enterprise, Ruth was driven by her desire for security, dominance, and recognition. She also wished to please her father, who believed that it was his responsibility as a parent to ensure that his daughter was graduated from a prestigious Chinese university. His motivational methods were extreme discipline and deprivation of the "distractions" of fun, play, and enjoyment. Corporal punishment was *de rigueur* when expectations were not met. For Ruth, the subject matter was incidental to her goal and the underlying concepts were challenging to master and retain. Her grades in her first year at the university were barely passing, but in her second year, she corralled Leonard to help her with her daily assignments and to prepare for tests. Throughout their remaining years at the university, Leonard was indentured as Ruth's full-time personal tutor. In their fourth year, Ruth determined that it was time for them to marry, and Eleanor was born 1 year thereafter. The three lived with Leonard's parents, two brothers, and grandmother in a two-room flat in a soot-coated cinderblock apartment building that was nearly invisible in a forest of other identical, graying, decaying, and despairing edifices.

A vestige of Mao Zedong's Cultural Revolution, the lot of physicians in China, despite their education, intelligence, hard work, and sacrifice, is little better than that of struggling hand laborers like the Lais' parents. Ruth yearned for far more. She wanted Leonard and herself to be rich doctors in America. Ruth badgered their parents into scraping together nearly every cent that they had managed to save during their lifetimes of toil in order to procure passage for the three of them to the United States. Leonard, who graduated first in his class, was invited to remain at the university as a junior faculty member, and he desperately wanted to do so.

> **Dr. Leonard Lai:** Ruth, I do not want to leave China and be away from our families. They have done so much for us, and we can help them have better lives in their old age. Also, I will not be good as a practicing physician. It is better that I stay with the university to do research and teaching.
>
> **Dr. Ruth Lai:** I married a fool and a Maoist. The pay in China for a university teacher is nothing, and I will make nothing working like a dog in some government hospital. In America doctors are rich. They work for themselves and not the government. We can buy Eleanor a big home with a yard and will send money back home to our families.

Dr. Ruth Lai Makes Her Move

Ruth prevailed and arranged jobs for both of them as nighttime laboratory technicians in a small hospital in rural Iowa. Although they were not eligible to practice as physicians, these jobs authorized them to live and work in the United States as permanent residents with green card status. They would not be eligible to take residencies in medical specialties in the United States without passing the formidable Federal Licensing Examination (FLEX) tests required for the licensure of all physicians in America. During weekdays, with baby Eleanor in tow, they traveled 60 miles by bus to and from Iowa City. There, they took English language classes and preparatory courses for the FLEX tests.

Furious with Leonard when she did not pass the written FLEX examination on her first attempt, Ruth assailed,

> **Dr. Ruth Lai:** Since I have to take care of everything else, you could at least make sure this *one* thing goes well for us. Making sure I pass this test is the only thing I have ever asked you to do. And you failed. You are worthless.

Leonard received the equivalent grade of 250 (a passing grade is 140; the top grade is 260) on the written component of the current version of the FLEX, the United States Medical Licensing Examination (USMLE). This is a remarkably high score for the top students at the best American medical schools and a result that is nearly unheard of for an international physician who is just learning English. Ruth failed the test with an equivalent grade of 90 and took the written FLEX examination three more times without improving her failing score.

> **Dr. Ruth Lai:** This government is as corrupt as ours in China. They don't want me to practice medicine. They won't let me pass the test, and your help is worthless. So there is no use trying again. But they won't stop me. I have read where doctors can make fortune by running clinics in Texas for patients with kidney disease. You love chemistry, so you must specialize in nephrology. You will treat the patients, and I will run the clinic. Now you must apply to take your residency in Texas.

Nephrology is a subspecialty of internal medicine. The process of becoming certified in this subspecialty is to take 4 years of residency training and pass board certification tests in general internal medicine to be followed by completing 2 years of subspecialty training in nephrology. Although admission to premier residencies in internal medicine is generally difficult for graduates of medical schools outside of the United States, the training director of the program at the University of Texas Southwestern Medical School in Dallas took note of Leonard's academic achievements. He was accepted to their program in internal medicine and, later, into their fellowship in nephrology. He excelled throughout his training.

Ruth did not squander the 6 years expended during Leonard's residency and fellowship training. She found work in the billing and collections department of a large Dallas-based dialysis company, and this proved to be an ideal position for her to learn the financial fundamentals of this business. In due time, Ruth gained expertise in Medicaid and Medicare reimbursements for dialysis and determined ways that the company could substantially increase its billings to and collections from the government. Incrementally, she was promoted to positions of increasing responsibility and authority and eventually became the business manager of the organization. In that position, through ruthless attention to maximizing billing and minimizing expenses, she dramatically increased profits of all the clinics. In the pursuit of profit, she became equally despised by the clinic doctors, who believed she was increasing their so-called "efficiency" at the expense of good patient care, and by federal regulators, who contended, but could not prove, that she was devising elaborate schemes to overcharge the government for patient services. The proprietors of the clinic, however, could not be more pleased with Ruth's performance, and, at her continuous prodding, they rewarded her with a high salary and annual performance bonuses.

Dr. Ruth Lai's American Dream

Leonard also found success in Dallas. Diligent, scholarly, compassionate, and self-effacing, Leonard was beloved by his patients, fellow residents, and physician supervisors. He was selected for the research track during his nephrology fellowship and demonstrated both scientific acumen and creativity in his independent research work. He wrote several papers that were published in excellent medical journals. At the conclusion of his training, he was offered a research position on the faculty, which he passionately wished to accept.

> **Dr. Ruth Lai:** You are still the same idiot that you were in China. You are still a Maoist and haven't learned anything in America. I have already made other plans. We are moving to Houston this summer.

Ruth had made a bold business proposal to the owners of the Dallas chain of dialysis clinics. She believed that there was an unusual opportunity to open a similar chain of clinics in the suburbs surrounding Houston, which were among the most rapidly growing regions in the country. She would manage the clinics, while Leonard would serve as their medical director. The proposal was bold in that, in addition to their receiving generous salaries and performance bonuses, the Drs. Lai would have 51% ownership of the Houston chain. Additionally, she put forward that the Dallas group would entirely fund the start-up and infrastructure costs—including billing, medical informatics, and marketing. She also proposed that the new enterprise would begin with three clinics and increase by a clinic a year over the succeeding 5 years. During her intense negotiations with the Dallas company's owners, attorneys, and bankers, Ruth would not budge on her terms.

> **Dr. Ruth Lai:** If you don't take my offer, I will do it anyway. I am sure I can get funding for the Houston project from many other sources, and I will also go into competition with you in

Dallas. As you know, I understand the business very well, and Leonard will have no trouble recruiting the best young nephrologists from the university. He is well respected there.

Ultimately, the company conceded, and Ruth, Leonard, and 8-year-old Eleanor moved to Houston.

True to her word and consistent with the timetable of the business plan, Ruth opened, developed, and operated the new dialysis clinics in the suburbs of Houston. The company made local and national news as being among the most innovative and successful new businesses in the medical field. Within 6 years she had accumulated sufficient wealth and credit to buy out the minority Dallas owners, with their only nonnegotiable term being that neither Dr. Ruth Lai nor her husband would be able to own or operate a dialysis clinic within a 50-mile radius of Dallas. So virulently had she harassed them with demands, contract renegotiations, and disputes during the 5 years of their partnership that the Dallas group was relieved to have Dr. Ruth Lai gone—despite their having made a great deal of money from their association with her.

Ruth took full advantage of a fragmented, poorly developed medical marketplace in and around Houston. With her increased capital, she rapidly expanded her capitalistic empire. In time she developed and managed the largest chain of outpatient dialysis services in the nation. In addition to running her enterprise with ruthless efficiency, she forged new models of service delivery by forming joint ventures with hospitals in secondary markets throughout Texas, Louisiana, and Florida. These dealings, in turn, led her to branch into other related medical businesses, including providing laboratory, imaging, and pathology services for small, independent hospitals. As Medical Director and Director of Quality Assurance, Dr. Leonard Lai also delivered a vital service to the company. He truly cared about the patients whom the clinics served and was highly knowledgeable about the most advanced and effective technologies of laboratory diagnosis and patient care. The net result was that the services that their company, Gulf States Medical Systems, provided were superior to most of the others in smaller marketplaces and rivaled those offered by the large not-for-profit systems in metropolitan areas.

Eleanor's Childhood

Huiquing

Eleanor's earliest memories were as a young child living in Dallas, where her family had moved when she was 3 years old. Chinese was her native language, as it was spoken exclusively by her parents at home and often by Huiquing, who cared for Eleanor when her parents were away at work. The 25-year-old sister of a graduate student at the University of Texas Southwestern Medical School, Huiquing was gentle, affectionate, and permissive and was terrified of Dr. Ruth Lai. Like the magnetized tips of a compass, the consciousness and attention of both Eleanor and Huiquing were drawn irrepressibly to the iron will and steel presence of Dr. Ruth Lai, whether or not she were physically present in the small garden apartment that was their world.

As far back as Eleanor could recall, she and Huiquing were loving allies and co-conspirators in trying to fulfill the unquenchable daily demands of her mother. Huiquing's responsibilities were numerous: cleaning the apartment, doing the laundry, shopping for food and household supplies, preparing all their meals, tutoring Eleanor in English and arithmetic, and seeing to it that Eleanor was dressed meticulously and acted perfectly. Eleanor had a single task: to be the perfect child. But neither Huiquing nor Eleanor could ever get it right. There was always a speck of dirt on a cabinet, a misaligned crease on a garment, or a bruise on a piece of fruit, with its cost to be deducted from Huiquing's wages. Eleanor's manners and appearance were never quite right: a sprig of wayward hair trespassing her eyebrow, her voice too shrill, her shoulders slouching, chewing her food "like a cow." Even worse, Eleanor was always falling short when on display to her mother's group of wealthy Chinese American friends or important business associates.

Although there was a television in the Lai home, both Eleanor and Huiquing were forbidden to turn it on.

> **Dr. Ruth Lai:** I don't work all day like a dog to pay for you to sit around and watch TV, Huiquing. You do not have time for that foolishness. I want Eleanor to know how to read and do arithmetic before she starts school.

Had it not been for her love of Eleanor and had she been able to bear the guilt of abandoning her to "the Dragon," as they both called Ruth in secret, Huiquing would have rather gone hungry than undergo the daily terror and tyranny of the Dragon. A master tactician, Ruth understood that her child was the fragile living chain that bound both her husband and Huiquing to their unbearable servitude and to her. Just before Eleanor was to start kindergarten, Ruth moved the family to a much larger apartment in a fashionable building in the Highland Park area of Dallas. On showing Eleanor her new bedroom for the first time, her mother said,

> **Dr. Ruth Lai:** I am working so hard and spending all of my money so you can go to a fine school in a rich neighborhood. Everything I do in my life is for you and not for me. All I ask is that you not waste your time, and I expect you to be the best student in your new school.

Not having been permitted to play with the local children or having attended preschool classes, Eleanor was shy and intimidated when she began kindergarten.

> **Eleanor Lai:** It was as if I were dropped onto an alien planet. I didn't know how to interact with the other children, who were singing songs and playing games that were totally unfamiliar to me. All I wanted to do was sit by myself until it was time to go home to Huiquing.

After the first week of classes, Mrs. Wren, Eleanor's kindergarten teacher, summoned her parents to a conference.

> **Mrs. Louise Wren:** I don't believe that Eleanor is adjusting well to school. She hardly says a word and does not interact at all with the other children. Would you permit her to be evaluated by the school psychologist?
>
> **Dr. Ruth Lai:** Absolutely not. She is just like her father; he doesn't speak a word either. I don't care how she plays. The most important is that she works hard and gets the best grades.

Although Eleanor remained shy and cautious, within 6 months she had adjusted to her new school and felt safer and more comfortable relating to her classmates. Ruth also became more socially active as well. She joined the Dallas chapter of the National Association of

Professional Women, where she befriended Mrs. Alicia Monroe, who owned several retail medical equipment and supply stores. In addition to learning from Mrs. Monroe about business opportunities through government funding and regulations, such as electrically powered wheelchairs and scooters (Medicare) or electronic lifts to access public pools (Americans with Disabilities Act), their conversation focused on their children.

> **Mrs. Alicia Monroe:** We finally broke into the Ivy Leagues with our third child, Alan, who attends Princeton. We were so naïve with our two oldest.
>
> **Dr. Ruth Lai:** Please explain, Alicia.
>
> **Alicia Monroe:** Did you ever hear about "The Rule of Three"?
>
> **Dr. Ruth Lai:** No.
>
> **Alicia Monroe:** The Rule of Three is about getting accepted to the best colleges, like Princeton, Yale, Harvard, or Stanford. It says that your child has to be outstanding in at least *three* areas—grades, college boards, and a special talent. Just having straight A's and 800s on your SATs won't cut it at this level. They can fill their classes 10 times with kids like that. And Ruth, don't believe what anyone tells you about "community service." For the Ivies and Stanford, community service doesn't mean much of anything without being the best in the other three categories.
>
> **Dr. Ruth Lai:** What kind of "special talent"?
>
> **Alicia Monroe:** We're not talking about making your own pie crust here. We're talking *real* talent. The best thing is to be an incredible musician, artist, or dancer, and you can't get them started soon enough. How old is Eleanor?
>
> **Dr. Ruth Lai:** Almost six.
>
> **Alicia Monroe:** I hope the horse isn't already out of the barn. Alan started playing piano when he was four.

That evening, Ruth returned home in a panic-driven fury. She found Eleanor in her bedroom. With Huiqing sitting by her side and crayons in her hands, Eleanor was at her desk, quietly absorbed in drawing a picture of a camel.

> **Dr. Ruth Lai:** You both are lazy idiots! All I do is work, and all you do is sit around my house and play. That will change right now. Huiqing, I don't want you to sit down any more when you are at work. Why should I pay you a salary when you are resting or playing? Eleanor, I am going to throw away all your

stupid toys and silly books tonight. Pictures of dumb animals won't get you into Princeton.

The next day Eleanor was enrolled in a music school, which, thereafter, she attended every day after school and throughout the summer. For at least 2 hours a day, she was also expected to practice on the rented Yamaha piano that occupied much of the space in the living room of their apartment.

In recalling her responses to this episode in a treatment session, Eleanor brought my attention to two traumata:

> **Eleanor Lai:** Can you imagine how Huiqing and I felt all the time, Dr. Y.? So many times when we were quietly enjoying ourselves doing something completely innocent, mother would burst in on us in a rage. It was like a terrorist bomb going off in a café where people are laughing, talking, and drinking coffee. I could never feel relaxed or safe in my own home. Or I should say, my mother's own home. I was always looking over my shoulder to check to see where she was and what her mood was at the moment. The only time that Mother was consistently kind to me was when we were around other people—especially people who she thought were important. Like at a dress-up social event. Then, she was a completely different person. But if I made a mistake in front of her friends, she would really make me pay for it later when we got home.
>
> One more thing, Dr. Y., Mother never once asked me if I *liked* playing piano. The only thing she cared about was if I were good at it. No, that's not true. She didn't really care how well I played, only if I were better at it than all the other children. But there were always kids with more talent than I had. I think that I might have liked playing piano if it weren't only about competition. As it is, I hated everything about playing piano. Even these days I get anxious if I see one.

Off to Houston

Ruth had kept the move to Houston secret from Huiqing until the day before they were leaving:

> **Dr. Ruth Lai:** We are going to move to a new city tomorrow, and your services will no longer be needed. I will pay you through the end of the week, even though you don't have to come to work on Thursday and Friday.
>
> **Huiqing:** What about Eleanor? Can I call her and come visit her?

> **Dr. Ruth Lai:** She is 9 years old and doesn't need you anymore. She will be very busy in her new school, and so happy in her beautiful new house.

Eleanor was not told that they were to leave Dallas until the moving truck and packers had arrived the next morning.

> **Eleanor Lai:** One day a giant moving truck pulled up to our apartment. It was only then that my mother said, "I bought you a big, beautiful house in Houston. It has a big backyard, and your bedroom is bigger than our whole apartment here." My first question to her was if Huiquing had a big bedroom too. My mother said that Huiquing decided not to come with us because she wanted to stay in Dallas with her brother.
> Mother forbade me from calling or writing her, so I never got to say goodbye to my beloved Huiquing. I was devastated and cried myself to sleep for months and months. I still miss her terribly and am terrified when I see moving trucks. Sometimes, when I am in a mall or on a busy street, I see someone who looks like Huiquing. My heart starts racing, until it breaks when I figure out that it is not her. I think about her all the time.

Transition, Transformation, and Labels

Ruth, Leonard, and Eleanor did not walk to Houston from Dallas, as did their peasant parents in straw sandals from the scrubby Sichuan Province countryside to Chengdu. Nor did they squeeze onto a single scuffed Naugahyde seat in a Greyhound bus, as when the three new immigrants to America had traveled, penniless, from the Port of San Francisco to Muscatine, Iowa. And they did not fly to Houston on a discount flight on Southwest Airlines, as they had done from Iowa to Dallas, Texas.

Clad in a Chanel suit freshly purchased from Neiman Marcus, Ruth regally maneuvered her family in her new Mercedes-Benz S-350 toward their beautiful new home in Kingwood, Texas. Looking almost petite under the towering ceiling, a new Steinway grand piano had replaced the rented Yamaha upright that had suffocated in the minuscule living room of their former Dallas apartment. Tall, lean, and resplendent in a John Galliano silk dress that was framed by her Philip Lim contrast-trim coat, Eleanor was placed in the front seat on the passenger side of their new carriage from Stuttgart.

Her father was relegated to the backseat, where he read the most recent issues of *The Journal of Nephrology* in his thin, faded-blue Kirkland windbreaker jacket from Costco. On the 4-hour drive to Houston, Leonard didn't look up once from his journals to peer out the window of the new car to catch a glimpse of his new city. That was not where he "lived."

Founded in 1970 as a joint venture between the Exxon Corporation and the venerable King Ranch, Kingwood is a 14,000-acre master-planned community on the outskirts of Houston. About 200,000 people live within its 10-mile radius. Proximate to what is called the Energy Corridor of Houston, Kingwood has a large, affluent white-collar population of engineers, scientists, and technicians. The strip malls around this suburb proved ideal locations and growth areas for Drs. Ruth and Leonard Lai to open up their first three dialysis clinics. Ruth also carefully researched Kingwood's public schools, which are known for their academic excellence. Although Eleanor was not yet in middle school, each year her mother kept close track of the number of graduating seniors from Kingwood High School who went to Ivy League colleges, especially to Harvard. She annually posted their names and pictures on the bulletin board that she had placed prominently in front of the desk where Eleanor did her schoolwork.

The cultural transitions are not easy for immigrants and refugees who come to America from countries that have strong traditions in feudalism and/or totalitarianism. It is especially difficult for newcomers to our society to determine *value* in a free-market system so dominated and distorted by marketing. As new arrivals to our country gain wealth, they try to avoid being cheated by *buying by the label*. They pay high prices to *get the best*, and they wear their labels on the outside to confirm the wisdom of their decisions to themselves and to display their newly attained power to others.

Along with the many changes associated with her move to Houston and becoming the CEO of a highly profitable company, Ruth assumed a new persona. So immediate was the anguish of poverty, class immobility, and the gritty toil of the Old World that, as have innumerable immigrants to America of all races and national origins, Ruth feverishly pursued the New World's labels, products, and institutions of wealth and power. She realized full well that her own bitter sacrifices and those of her parents and peasant ancestors were about to pay off. She and Eleanor were on the threshold of becoming members of the ruling class in the most powerful country on Earth. No longer a rag puppet with her strings being yanked by the rough and punishing hands of China's new lords and emperors, the Communist Party leaders, Ruth was finally in the position to control her own fate and those of many others. At long last, she would become an empress, and Princess Eleanor was destined to be the most sparkling jewel in her crown.

Houston prides itself on its openness, opportunity, and diversity, and Ruth quickly understood that she could become one of the city's icons in all three of its most cherished realms. She became an active participant in and generous benefactor of many of Houston's worthy cultural organizations, including the Houston Fine Arts Museum, the Houston Symphony, and the Texas Asia Society. Frequently, she was formally recognized for her success by business organizations and professional women's societies and was featured in many articles in local and national news and business publications. As the sun insists that the obedient moon orbit glowingly about him in reflected homage to his resplendence, Ruth positioned her shy, exquisite daughter by her side at almost all of the many social occasions that she attended.

Performance

With classes, extracurricular activities (including piano lessons, practice, and recitals), and homework, Eleanor, like so many of her classmates in Kingwood, was a busy child. Unlike her peers, however, Eleanor was not permitted to go to parties or to have friends over to her house "to hang out." Nor was she permitted "to live better through electricity" by spending hours talking on her cell phone or friending on Facebook or listening to popular music on an iPod or playing video games or watching TV. Her mother considered such activities frivolous and distracting from Eleanor's primary mission of being accepted to an Ivy League college, preferably Harvard. Although her grades and standardized test scores were outstanding, Eleanor was having trouble with the third component of "The Rule of Three." She did not win the top prizes at piano recitals, nor did she receive the class award in music at Kingwood Middle School. Frantically upset, Ruth met with Mr. Keith Simms, Eleanor's piano instructor.

Dr. Ruth Lai: I pay you more than $400 a week for Eleanor's piano lessons, and she has not won a single prize. What is her problem? What's *your* problem?

Mr. Keith Simms: Eleanor is a wonderful student, and I think that she is doing very, very well. She seems to enjoy playing piano, and everybody in the music school just adores her.

Dr. Ruth Lai: I don't pay $400 a week for Eleanor to have fun or be popular. She needs to play piano so well that Harvard accepts her.

Mr. Simms: Pardon me, Dr. Lai, but I don't understand what you are telling me.

Dr. Ruth Lai: Just what I said. She has the best grades and tests in her class, but she needs to be the best in piano to get into Harvard.

Mr. Simms: Eleanor has wonderful rhythm, practices diligently, and has a great attitude. She plays piano very, very well. However, the pianists that Harvard accepts are at what we call "the conservatory level." That will not be possible for Eleanor.

Dr. Ruth Lai: What are you saying? Why am I wasting all of my money on piano?

Mr. Simms: I don't believe that you are wasting your money, Dr. Lai. For the rest of her life, Eleanor will always have the knowledge and pleasure of music. What I am saying is that she does not have the talent to play piano at the most elite level.

Dr. Ruth Lai: Why did you wait so long to tell me she's no good? To steal even more money from me?

Mr. Simms: Eleanor is a very good young pianist—just not the prodigies that are accepted to Harvard and Yale for their musicality. I do have one suggestion, however. Every now and then before our class begins, I have watched Eleanor dancing for fun with her friends in the school. She is an absolutely superb dancer—a natural. She is graceful, flexible, and coordinated. She also is beautiful and has the perfect body type for ballet. I believe that Eleanor has real talent and potential as a dancer, Dr. Lai.

Without saying goodbye or thanking Mr. Simms, Ruth stormed out of the music school and immediately called her friend, Mrs. Alicia Monroe, and told her what had just transpired.

Dr. Ruth Lai: I feel that I have been cheated. I have wasted all my time and money for nothing.

Mrs. Alicia Monroe: This is a serious problem, Ruth. I'm not certain what to do at this point. This is a real long shot, but is Eleanor good at any sports?

Dr. Ruth Lai: Who has time to play games? Besides, she is a frightened little rabbit, just like her father. Her piano teacher said he thinks she has talent for dancing.

Alicia Monroe: That's probably worth checking out. Let me do some research about where to go in Houston, and I'll get right back to you.

About a week later Alicia Monroe phoned Ruth with information about the acclaimed Houston Ballet Academy (the Academy) and with contact information of someone at the Academy who would meet with Eleanor. An appointment was scheduled for the next week. Although the Academy begins to accept students at age 4, and although 12-year-old Eleanor had not had any formal dance experience, the interviewer asked Eleanor to do some freestyle dancing to popular music. On the basis of what the instructor saw, Eleanor was accepted on the spot to the preballet course that met 2 days per week. After several months, Eleanor began taking private lessons in ballet the other days as well.

Eleanor Lai: Next to Huiqing, being able to stop piano and do dance is the best thing that ever happened to me. I just love every minute of it.

By age 14, Eleanor was accepted to Houston Ballet's 6-week Summer Intensive Program, where she was instructed 8 hours per day, 6 days per week by the Academy's senior teachers and company dancers. At age 16, she had surpassed the best of her peers at the Houston Ballet Academy, was being taught by the company's ballet masters and leading dancers, and was making regular appearances in the company's performances. She was finally ahead of the curve on the "special talent" component of The Rule of Three for gaining admission to an Ivy League college. However, the time required for dance instruction and practice and traveling back and forth to Houston from Kingwood was beginning to impinge on Eleanor's academic performance. That dilemma was solved when Eleanor auditioned for and was accepted into the ninth-grade class of the Houston High School for the Performing and Visual Arts (HSPVA).

Although HSPVA is a magnet school of the Houston Independent School District, Eleanor was one of the few students who was admitted from outside the Houston School District on the basis of her high grades and talent. Her mother made it quite clear to Eleanor, who loved dancing and performance, that she would be permitted to remain at HSPVA only if her grades and scores on standardized tests remained at the top.

> **Dr. Ruth Lai:** I'm not sending you to this school to play and waste time like the other kids. You are not at this school to become a dancer but to get accepted to Harvard. On weekends there will be no dance, only study and going to the tutor for your SATs.

Battement

During her sophomore year of high school, Eleanor and several other student dancers from her high school and the Houston Ballet Academy auditioned for the Summer Intensive Program of the preeminent American Ballet Theatre (ABT) in New York City. Eleanor was the only dancer her age from the southwestern region who was selected, and this afforded her the opportunity to spend a month under the tutelage of ABT's master teachers and company dancers. She would live in supervised housing with a selected group of other young dance students from around the world. Initially, her mother was adamantly opposed to Eleanor "being on her own" in New York. She discussed the issue with her friend and advisor from Dallas, Alicia Monroe.

> **Dr. Ruth Lai:** I won't let Eleanor live with other children and run wild in New York City without my supervision.
>
> **Mrs. Alicia Monroe:** The American Ballet Theatre is a big deal. It is one of the foremost international ballet companies. You can't set the terms for them, Ruth, like you would for a small hospital in Laredo, Texas. Attending that program and getting a recommendation from their artistic director could be Eleanor's ticket to Princeton or Harvard. Let me check into this before you say no.

True to her word, Alicia Monroe contacted the director of the Program in Dance at the Lewis Center of Princeton University, where her son had attended college. They had a long and pointed conversation, which she later recounted to Ruth.

> **Mrs. Alicia Monroe:** I have important news for you, Ruth. We are on the right track with Eleanor. I just spoke to the head person in dance at Princeton, and she asked a lot of questions about

Eleanor—her background in dance, her grades, what she looks like, how tall she is, and a bunch of other stuff. By the time we were finished, I got the feeling that she was trying to get me to help her recruit Eleanor to Princeton. She was actually *selling* me, if you can imagine such a thing!

Anyway, she told me what I had thought—going to the Summer Intensive Program in Dance of the American Ballet Theatre in New York is a *big, big* deal! They only take the best of the best—and most of those don't even apply to colleges. They either go to conservatories or go on to dance professionally with some elite dance company. You have to let her go. Think of it as an investment—like opening up another dialysis center.

Reluctantly, Ruth permitted Eleanor to go to the New York City program. In her treatment, Eleanor described her conflicted feelings about being alone for the first time as follows:

Eleanor Lai: When my mother walked out of my dormitory room to go back to Houston, I became panicked. I didn't know whether I should jump up and down with joy or run after her to go home. That was the first night in my life that I spent apart from my mother.

Eleanor's experience in the Summer Intensive Program of the ABT in New York was just that: intense. Despite being among a group of America's finest ballet dancers in her age group, she more than held her own in the classroom and in the studio. Inheriting her father's temperament, selflessness, intelligence, work ethic, and focus, Eleanor was a teacher's dream. She listened carefully to and followed precisely their instructions. Unlike so many other gifted young athletes and performers, she was neither temperamental nor "pouty" when she made mistakes. It was evident to both her instructors and classmates that Eleanor's talent for dance was at the very top of the group. Tall, lean, and lithe, Eleanor was also the most beautiful among the young women dancers.

Eleanor was oblivious to and in no way prepared for the competitive retribution of her dancemates, each of whom had been accustomed to regarding herself as the prima ballerina assoluta. Her superiority being Eleanor's sin, they consolidated their otherwise shaky group cohesion by excluding her. She became the classic scapegoat. Unworldly and eager to please, Eleanor was easy prey for the pack of spurned prima donnas. Calling Eleanor "Goody Two-

Slippers," the young ballerinas made her the brunt of their jokes, jibes, and pranks. They would not invite her to join them on their "adventure walks" around New York City, to sneak out with them at midnight to jazz bars that served liquor, or to go to the movies that their parents would not let them see at home.

> **Eleanor Lai:** It was terrible, Dr. Y. I would walk into the common area of our dormitory, and they would suddenly stop talking. During class they would look at me, whisper to each other, and laugh. The more I tried to fit in and get them to like me, the worse it seemed to get. I was miserable and couldn't understand what I was doing wrong.
>
> **Dr. Y.:** It was not what you were doing *wrong*, Eleanor, it was how you are *right*. They saw admirable qualities in you that they could not find in themselves. Wrongly, they thought that they could fix themselves by destroying you. The danger to you would be if you would oblige in order to fit in and please them.
>
> **Eleanor:** What do you mean by "oblige," Dr. Y.?
>
> **Dr. Y.:** By doing their work for them. By tearing yourself down.
>
> **Eleanor:** I didn't know *what* to do. Even though I just loved the dance program, I hated all the rest of it. To my surprise, I couldn't wait for the program to end and to get back home.

Buying by the Label

In the last month of Eleanor's junior year at HSPVA, Mrs. Cornella Arnsbarger, a college counselor, scheduled a meeting with Eleanor and her parents to review the college application process. Atypically, Mrs. Arnsbarger also invited two other participants.

> **Mrs. Cornella Arnsbarger:** Thank you all for joining us today. We are primarily here to discuss Eleanor's undergraduate educational options and to answer your questions. Given Eleanor's unique talents in dance, I have also taken the liberty to invite Ms. Constance Martin, the director of our school's dance program, and Mr. Arnaud Durand, the Associate Director of the Houston Ballet Academy.
>
> We have only good news today. As you know, Eleanor has always been a straight-A student, and her College Board scores are nearly perfect on both the aptitude and achievement sections of the tests. In addition to her splendid accomplishments in dance, she is also bilingual in English and Chinese, which is quite attractive to colleges these days. To make a long story short, I am confident that Eleanor can be accepted to the in-

stitution of her first choice. What we need to discuss and decide today is not just the colleges to which Eleanor will apply, but also the *type* of undergraduate education that she will choose.

Dr. Ruth Lai: What do you mean by the "type" of college she will choose?

Mrs. Arnsbarger: If she wishes to continue to pursue dance seriously, it might be better for her to consider a conservatory, such as Juilliard in New York or the Boston Conservatory. Let's have Mr. Durand's input at this point.

Mr. Arnaud Durand: Ms. Martin and I concur that Eleanor is at the very top of America's high school dancers. We also know that her potential to grow in dance is virtually limitless. To meet that potential, we believe that it is imperative that she attend a dance conservatory—either in America or abroad.

Dr. Ruth Lai: I don't want Eleanor to be a dancer. Dancing is to have fun. It is a hobby. She has no future in dancing. She will be a doctor or a businesswoman—or do both like I do.

Mr. Durand: She cannot continue to dance at her current level, much less improve, unless she concentrates entirely on her dancing. If she goes to a standard college, she will lose too much ground. And there will be no turning back. On the other hand, if Eleanor attends a conservatory for several years and decides that a career in dance is not for her, she will be able to attend college at that point without a problem.

Mrs. Arnsbarger: Maybe we should ask Eleanor what she would like to do.

Dr. Ruth Lai: Eleanor is a child. She doesn't know what she wants. She has no money to pay for college or dance school. I will pay and I will decide where she will go. My only question is can she get accepted to a best school like Harvard, Yale, Princeton, or Stanford?

Mrs. Arnsbarger: I have total confidence that Eleanor will get into any school she wants to attend. The questions to be answered are what does she want in a particular school and what is the best school to meet those expectations?

Dr. Ruth Lai: Good. Finally we are getting somewhere. I have the answer to both those questions: Harvard.

Crimson Breaks

Eleanor was accepted to Harvard University through its early decision application process. As dictated by her mother, she would take courses to fulfill the premedical science requirements and to qualify for a minor in either business or economics. Even before Eleanor's first day of college, her mother was laying plans for her postgraduate education.

> **Dr. Ruth Lai:** I found out that Harvard accepts a few of the very best college graduates for a joint degree from Harvard Medical School and the Harvard Business School. You get to go to both schools at the same time. Perfect training for you to join me in my business. My company is getting very, very big. And you know that your father is no help to me. He is worthless.
>
> **Eleanor Lai:** What about my dancing?
>
> **Dr. Ruth Lai:** Very good question, Eleanor. You are finally learning something. I checked out that question very carefully. Harvard Medical School and Harvard Business School don't care about The Rule of Three. If you make straight A's and get perfect scores on your medical school and business school entrance tests, you will get accepted. Special talent doesn't mean much, especially when you graduate top in your class from Harvard University. They are so smart to know that dancing is a waste of time.

Unscheduled Time

Apart from her intellectual gifts and excellent academic background, Eleanor was totally unprepared for what she was about to experience in college. There were so many "firsts." Primary among the remarkable changes in her life was that, for the first time, she had unscheduled time. Prior to college, every moment of her time was scheduled by her mother and devoted to "accomplishing something" or "getting somewhere." Heretofore, traveling to school, attending classes, going to dance practice, coming back home, doing homework, and studying for tests constituted her life. "Free time" and "fun" were alien concepts. Eleanor was shocked that at Harvard, there was sufficient unscheduled time that having fun seemed to be the primary objective of many of her classmates.

In consultation with a career counselor from Houston, Ruth chose the courses that Eleanor would take during the first and second semesters of her freshman year at Harvard. She was to take 16 credits of the courses that were standard for most premedical students with science majors. The counselor suggested that Eleanor fulfill her foreign language requirement with Chinese: "This will be an easy A for her. Best of all she will prop up her grade point average while giving her extra time to spend on her more difficult science classes."

Intellectually and temperamentally favoring her father, Eleanor demonstrated the same superior organizational and scientific flair that he had shown a generation ago at Sichuan University. Both predisposed to and experienced in time management, she did not feel the same pressure that many other high achievers endure in Harvard's competitive academic environment. Arriving early to all classes, systematically completing her written and reading assignments, and efficiently preparing for both classwork and examinations far ahead of deadlines enabled Eleanor to have both excellent grades and, for the first time in her life, an abundance of free time. An unachievable dream for most of her classmates, free time became more of a burden and challenge to Eleanor than her classwork.

Dance

Harvard offers several credit-granting courses in dance that Eleanor pointed out to her mother and to the career counselor when they were reviewing the course catalog.

> **Dr. Ruth Lai:** No more dance, Eleanor. We got what we needed from your dancing. It has always taken up too much of your time, and you will not have time at Harvard to waste on things that won't get you into medical school and business school.

Although Ruth was not going to be able to be on site in Cambridge to monitor her daughter's every move, she had Eleanor's access code to her personal e-mail account and demanded copies of her official college records. Therefore, Eleanor would not be able to enroll in credited dance courses or do much else without her mother finding out. What Ruth did not know was that most of the students at Harvard communicated through their new Harvard e-mail addresses, to which she would not have Eleanor's password. Eleanor soon learned about the abundant noncredit dance offerings in which she could participate. After ruminating about how her mother would react if she found out, Eleanor finally decided to enroll in Ballet III and several other noncredit modern dance and physical conditioning courses and classes. She also joined the Harvard Asian American Dance Troupe, a student-run organization that embraced the full spectrum of traditional and modern Asian dance.

Eleanor's technical superiority, effortless grace, and artistic beauty in all of these dance forms did not escape notice by Harvard's performing arts faculty, student dancers, and audiences. How each of these dance constituents responded to Eleanor's gifts comprised a projective test of their personalities, self-esteem, and character. Their reactions spanned a continuum from awe to envy, from appreciation to enmity, and from pleasure to lust. And all created problems for Eleanor, who wanted to please everyone.

Male Classmates

Word quickly spread among her male classmates that Eleanor was among the "hottest freshmen." Given Eleanor's height, toned body, and carriage, the Harvard athletes took special notice. They speculated that she was on either the basketball or volleyball team and did not hesitate to approach her. Asked so frequently "Do you play a sport?" and unpracticed in small talk, Eleanor developed a standard, cryptic reply: "No, I'm a dancer." In no way deterred, her multitude of admirers promptly asked her out, and, not wanting to disappoint, she indiscriminately accepted. Never having dated and uncertain about what *she* wanted in most important domains, Eleanor was entering what for her was dangerous and uncharted territory.

> **Eleanor Lai:** I had no idea what I was doing, Dr. Y. These guys would ask me out and tell me to meet them at their fraternity house at hours that I was usually asleep. I didn't have a clue about what was going to go on there, how I was supposed to dress or act. I got whatever information I could from my roommates and just went there, hoping for the best.
>
> **Dr. Y.:** Did you get what you hoped for, Eleanor?
>
> **Eleanor:** No, just the opposite. It was horrible. It was loud and crowded. Nearly everyone was drinking beer, and some were even smoking cigarettes or marijuana. Most people seemed to know each other, but I didn't know anyone. I could barely hear what my dates were saying, and they usually were drunk. The only part I liked about it was the dancing.
>
> **Dr. Y.:** Did you drink as well?
>
> **Eleanor:** No, but they kept encouraging me to drink and asking me why I didn't. When I told them I couldn't because I was underage—the drinking age in Massachusetts and Texas is 21—they couldn't believe their ears. They thought that I was joking; I was always so embarrassed. The worst part was when I wanted to go home. My dates who hadn't passed out always tried to keep me from leaving. Physically. A few even tried to kiss and fondle me out in the open or drag me into their rooms. I think they were quite surprised about how strong I am.

Dr. Y.: How so?

Eleanor: For some reason almost all of the guys who asked me out at first were members of the football, lacrosse, or ice hockey teams. They are very strong and didn't expect me to be as strong as I am. I had to kick away one guy who wouldn't let go of me, and his friends thought I broke his leg. After that episode, which was in the third week of school, I decided not to go out at all. Even though I was asked out so many more times, I didn't accept one more date until my sophomore year. There are lots of nice men at Harvard, Dr. Y. Do you know why I only seemed to be asked out by these aggressive athletes?

Dr. Y.: I believe I do, Eleanor. When you first arrived at college, you were especially shy and retiring. Most of your Harvard classmates could sense and would respect that. In other words, you did not give off the verbal or nonverbal cues that you were interested in going out. Therefore, the ones who asked you out were a "select" group who either didn't pick up your signals or, if they did, they didn't care. They were more interested in what *they* saw and what *they* wanted. What they saw was a beautiful, poised young woman. And what they wanted was sex. Many athletes, although certainly not most, can be highly self-assured, self-centered, and assertive. I assume that those were the ones who were the first to ask you out.

Eleanor: That makes sense. After my third week at Harvard, my solution to the dilemma was to say no to *everybody* who asked me out. I told them that I needed to study.

Dr. Y.: Sometimes "all-or-none" solutions are the best way to go. In this case, I do not believe it to be so.

Eleanor: But I couldn't tell who I could trust, Dr. Y.

Dr. Y.: I don't believe that to be true, Eleanor. I have every reason to believe that you are super at reading people. It isn't that you were unable to tell whom you could trust but that you could read them *too well*. And you didn't want to *displease* them. Therefore, you couldn't say "no" to anyone. That is, until you were physically assaulted. It shouldn't have gotten to that point in the first place. By stopping dating altogether, you missed out on getting to know more respectful and suitable young men. You also didn't gain experience with dating. You pay a huge price for having to please everyone.

Female Classmates

Unlike most other freshmen, Eleanor did not know any Harvard undergraduates before she arrived there. Consequently, her first friends were the four other coeds with whom she shared her dormitory suite. Reasoning that Eleanor could get help from other pre-med Harvard students (as she had done with Leonard at Sichuan University), Ruth made a special request that Eleanor have premedical students or science majors as roommates. As the year progressed, Eleanor's roommates grew to resent her efficient and tenacious work habits, her high grades, and, especially, her attractiveness to men. Three of the young women were substantially overweight and the fourth was almost a foot shorter than Eleanor. When Eleanor innocently confided to her roommates how much she disliked going to the library because she was always "being hit on by the guys," they secretly hated her. They were never asked out. Much more subtle, creative, and vindictive than the high school dancers who taunted Eleanor during her summer program at the American Ballet Theatre, her Harvard roommates adopted the timeless strategy of "killing her with kindness."

Perennially monitoring others for their approval, Eleanor correctly picked up that her roommates didn't like her, but her modesty prevented her from understanding why. She tried to do everything possible to please them and to fit in.

Eleanor Lai: Nothing I did could make them like me. All they would comment on was how I skinny I looked or how little I was eating. I didn't know how to answer them. Eventually, I dreaded coming back to my room.

Dr. Y.: What exactly would they say?

Eleanor: I'll give you some examples, Dr. Y. But first you have to understand that, as a dancer, I know how much I should weigh and how I should look physically. My dance teachers made that very clear to all of us. Until this year, my weight had been stable since I was 15 years old. These are things that they would say routinely, even before I had lost any weight:

"Aren't you going to eat *anything* tonight? We won't let you go to bed until you finish every bite of the pizza we got for you."

"We just bought two quarts of Ben and Jerry's Chunky Monkey Ice Cream. We won't enjoy it unless you eat it with us."

"You look like you lost so much weight; are you sure you are OK?"

"I thought you exercised already this morning. Are you going again?"

"You have so little on your plate. Is that all you're eating for an entire day?"

The worst part about it was that they were always monitoring my every move and judging me. I like to be invisible, but I was always on display. I had no choice but to stuff myself. By the end of the first semester I had gained over 25 pounds. The funny thing is, Dr. Y., the boys kept asking me out anyway. It didn't seem to make any difference to them that I had gained so much weight. But it did to my mother when my parents came to visit me in Cambridge for Thanksgiving.

Harvard for the Holiday

Most students at Harvard University go home to be with their families for the Thanksgiving weekend. The main exceptions are the international students, many of whom are invited to the homes of their American friends and classmates for the holiday. There are also a few American students who cannot afford to travel home. It is not an ideal time to visit the campus, which is pretty much shut down and deserted. After immigrating to the United States, Ruth and Leonard did not celebrate holidays—either their native Chinese or American ones. When, as a little girl, Eleanor asked her mother why they didn't eat turkey on Thanksgiving or put up a Christmas tree, her mother would reply,

> **Dr. Ruth Lai:** We don't believe in holidays. When everybody else is having fun and wasting time, we catch up and get ahead. Holidays are for lazy and stupid people. The only thing they do in China is celebrate holidays.

Growing up, Eleanor had felt particularly lonely during holidays because she missed being with her friends and going to school. She was also aware that her classmates were home having fun with their families and friends while she was home alone completing assignments, studying for tests, and practicing piano or dance. Therefore, she was prepared to be alone on campus during her first holiday at Harvard. About 1 week before Thanksgiving, Eleanor received a call on her cell phone from her mother.

> **Dr. Ruth Lai:** I will come to visit you on Thursday. Our clinics are shut down for 4 days except for emergencies. Your father insists on coming too. He wants to look at the Medical School libraries and laboratories.

Having learned from years of experience the futility of arguing with or opposing her mother, Eleanor said nothing. She realized that most of the "things" that other parents came to do and see on campus—meet with their children's friends; attend student performances or athletic events; and visit art galleries, buildings, libraries, and classrooms—would all be shut down. She also understood that although her mother was coming to check out if Eleanor were following all of her rules, her father was coming to Harvard to be with her. Although Leonard did not speak much and never openly expressed acts of affection, Eleanor knew that he loved her dearly—beyond anything or anyone else in his protracted universe. Eleanor also knew that he missed her beyond words or physical expressions, as she did him.

As was her practice, Ruth did not provide Eleanor with specific details about when she would arrive. Around noon on Thanksgiving Day, Eleanor received a call on her cell phone.

> **Dr. Ruth Lai:** I am downstairs with your father. The door is locked, and no one is here to let me in. I pay too much money in rent for your room, so I should have my own key. Come down here right now and unlock this door.

Fortunately for Eleanor, she was in the study area of her dormitory, where she had been preparing for the next week's inorganic chemistry laboratory. Immediately on opening the door, her mother shouted,

> **Dr. Ruth Lai:** What did you do to yourself? You are as fat as a pig. I thought that you came to Harvard to become a doctor like your mother, not to waste all your time stuffing your mouth.

Because they had not made reservations in a local hotel, Eleanor's parents spent nearly all of their time during the next 3 days in Eleanor's dormitory suite. They slept in her roommates' beds and purchased food in a local grocery store. But Ruth did not "waste time." She systematically went through all of Eleanor's graded coursework and tests and reviewed all of her e-mail messages in her Harvard account, which did not take her long to discover. The grades on the coursework and tests were all high A's, but she did not comment on that to Eleanor.

> **Eleanor Lai:** I was totally devastated, Dr. Y. Mother learned from my Harvard e-mails that I was dancing again and was furious

that I was doing *anything* behind her back. Most of the weekend she threatened to withdraw me from Harvard and to take me back home with her to Texas and put me to work in their clinics. Believe it or not, the worst part of it all was how she kept criticizing me about my weight. She went over every part of my body and emphasized how disgusting each part of me looked. How disgusting I looked being so fat. I kept thinking that I was so fat that I was making everybody who saw me sick to their stomachs. I became even more self-conscious than I usually am.

I have always been forbidden to cry in front of Mother. She thinks it's weak and self-indulgent. But from the moment she left my dormitory room until now, I have not stopped crying when I am alone. Since I came home for the Christmas holiday, she has not left me by myself.

Dr. Y.: May I assume that this is when you started to worry about your weight and what you look like?

Eleanor: I began to examine every inch of my body to check how fat it is. Especially my thighs and stomach. I still do it all the time. I started to obsess about every morsel that goes into my mouth, and I still do. I began to hate my body and hate myself, and I still do.

Reference

Cyranoski D: China tackles surge in mental illness. Nature 468:145, 2010

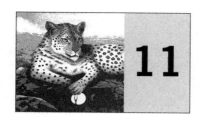

11

Stuck in Pleasing Others, Part II (Decide and Discipline): The Case of Eleanor Lai

An Introduction to Supermentalizing

Those who deny freedom to others,
deserve it not for themselves;
and, under a just God, can not long retain it.
—*Abraham Lincoln, Letter to Henry Piers, 1859*

My very chains and I grew friends,
So much a long communion tends
To make us what we are: even I
Regain'd my freedom with a sigh.
—*George Gordon, Lord Byron, "The Prisoner of Chillon"*

"When I dance, I'm at peace. I lose myself in the music and the movement. I have always believed that dancing is my natural state of being."

The Case of Eleanor Lai: D2 (Decision) Treatment Component[1]

The Maoist That Roared

The history of Eleanor Lai that was detailed in Chapter 10, "Stuck in Pleasing Others, Part I (Discover)," was secured during our initial 3-hour meeting and the treatment sessions thereafter. As I had indicated to Eleanor at the beginning of the first session, my professional responsibilities required that I weigh her and do an abbreviated physical examination to determine if her life were in danger because of weight loss.

> **Eleanor Lai:** You can't imagine how uncomfortable I feel by having you weigh me, Dr. Y.
>
> **Dr. Y.:** I can try to imagine, Eleanor. You probably feel violated, like when your mother violates your boundaries.
>
> **Eleanor:** Totally.
>
> **Dr. Y.:** I will try to understand your feelings, Eleanor, but I must meet my responsibilities as your physician. I look forward to the time when your weight is sufficiently safe that neither of us has to go through this. But *that* time is in the future and will depend on *your* decisions and actions. Now let's go to the examination room.

When Eleanor removed her voluminous overcoat, the physical effects of her self-imposed starvation became obvious. She was clearly emaciated, as confirmed by her weight of 96 pounds. Beyond her weakness and muscle wasting, my physical examination did not detect any immediate life-threatening somatic signs, but she was clearly on the cusp of danger.

> **Dr. Y.:** Eleanor, your weight is such that I will need to see you daily until you are at a safe weight. If you agree, I'd like to invite your father to join us in my office so that we can discuss and begin to come to terms with short-term and long-term treatment plans.
>
> **Eleanor Lai:** I agree.

---

[1]As indicated throughout this book and exemplified in my care of Eleanor Lai, when mental health professionals take a psychiatric history, patients experience this process as therapeutic. Conversely, our knowledge of patients' psychiatric histories continues to expand throughout their treatment.

With that, I walked into my waiting room and asked that Dr. Leonard Lai meet with Eleanor and me.

> **Dr. Leonard Lai:** Is my daughter going to die, Dr. Yudofsky?
> **Dr. Y.:** If we all don't agree on a workable treatment plan, Eleanor's health and safety are, indeed, in imminent jeopardy.

I outlined a short-term treatment plan that required the following of Eleanor:

- To meet with me on a daily basis—including weekends—for 1 hour per visit
- To have a physical examination with an internist on a weekly basis until she weighed 114 pounds
- To be weighed by me every day until she weighed 114 pounds and, thereafter, on a monthly basis until her weight has been stable for 6 months
- To be hospitalized immediately if, after 1 week, she were to weigh less than 96 pounds
- To be hospitalized immediately if, after 1 month of treatment, she were to weigh less than 100 pounds

Although she was apprehensive, Eleanor agreed to the short-term treatment plan, which I later transcribed and had both her and her father sign. Eleanor and I would continue to discuss and formulate a long-range treatment plan over the next week.

> **Dr. Y.:** Thank you for buying into this plan. What do you suggest we do regarding Dr. Ruth Lai?

Following a long silence, Eleanor spoke.

> **Eleanor Lai:** Mother does not even know that we are here. She will go berserk when she finds out. One thing for sure, when she finds out that I came to see you without her, she will torture me and Daddy every minute. Mother won't go along with anything that she does not control completely. She won't pay for my treatment, and she won't let me travel to your office from Kingwood. I will be lucky if she ever lets me leave the house again.

> **Dr. Leonard Lai:** I will not let you die, Eleanor. Your mother calls me "stupid Maoist." But I am not stupid, and I am not a communist. Capitalists get things done, not make false promises. I can fix the problem.
>
> **Dr. Y.:** What do you suggest, Dr. Lai?
>
> **Dr. Leonard Lai:** Ruth does not care about her husband. She does not really care about her daughter. She does not care about sick people. She only cares about money. She tries to make everyone a slave to get her more money. But she is the servant to money. It is time now for Eleanor and me to become free from her. We will leave her home and rent an apartment in Houston. Eleanor will come see you from that place and not go home again.

Leonard went on to disclose that he and Ruth were each 50% owners of their company, Gulf States Medical Systems, a holding company with more than several dozen dialysis units, nine private community hospitals, and several professional associations for the physicians who work in these facilities. She agreed to that arrangement on the advice of her tax attorneys, who explained that otherwise, the tax implications would be enormous if either of them were to die suddenly in an accident. Their attorney, Mr. John Connors, also explained that Texas state law does not permit hospitals or their officers to employ physicians, but licensed physicians can hire other physicians in professional practice organizations (PPOs). Ruth did not have a Texas license. Additionally, she did not want the doctors who worked at Gulf States Medical Systems to have any independence. Most importantly, she wanted to maximize her profits from their work. Therefore, she arranged that Leonard would own the PPO and collect on Part B, or the physicians' fee component of Medicare and Medicaid, which pays for much of dialysis.

> **Dr. Leonard Lai:** Most of our money is in the company. I invest assets, not Ruth. Ruth is a bully, not a scholar. I study financial markets all the time and make much money from investments. I don't care much for money, but I am good at analysis.
>
> **Dr. Y.:** Does either of you believe that it is at all possible that Dr. Ruth Lai can participate constructively in Eleanor's treatment?

Like suppressed people living under totalitarian regimes responding when asked political questions by journalists from the free world, Eleanor and her father stared back at me in agonized deliberation. They knew the answer but, fearful of repercussions, were reluctant to respond openly and honestly. Finally, Leonard said,

> **Dr. Leonard Lai:** Ruth loves money more than she loves Eleanor. She is also arrogant. She is not smart enough to know that she will lose much money if she fights me when I save my Eleanor.
>
> **Dr. Y.:** Please explain to us exactly what you mean, Dr. Lai.
>
> **Dr. Leonard Lai:** She will not give up control of Eleanor. Ruth will threaten and bully, but she cannot win. I control the PPO and can close down the business right away by removing all the nephrologists. No nephrologist would ever work for her.
>
> **Dr. Y.:** I have two questions, Eleanor. How do you feel about opposing the will of your mother, and what do you prefer to do at this point?
>
> **Eleanor:** I am terrified by my mother. She has tortured me, literally, every time I have tried to go against her wishes. But I can't go on like this anymore.
>
> **Dr. Y.:** What *exactly* do you mean, Eleanor, by the word "literally?"
>
> **Eleanor:** You don't know this, Daddy. Mother would kill me if I ever told you. She hits me all the time. Very hard. Since I was a very little girl. She probably hit me when I was a baby, but I can't remember back that far. Whenever I was not perfect as a little girl, she would beat me with a belt. Often over how I looked or over a grade on paper that wasn't perfect. She never beats me when you are around. When I became a teenager, she just slapped me in the face—hard—when she was mad at me. She hit me 2 months ago in my dorm room at Harvard when she found out that I was dancing behind her back. She hit me many times in the face. You were outside getting groceries.

Stunned by what he had just heard, Leonard dropped his head into his faded blue windbreaker. He then stood up from his chair, walked over to Eleanor, and embraced her. He and his daughter held each other tightly and sobbed. And sobbed. Finally, he looked up, brought his daughter's face to his and said,

> **Dr. Leonard Lai:** I failed you, Eleanor. Your mother is right about one thing. I have been a very weak and stupid man. I will fix that right now.

No Accidents

Leonard was not the valedictorian of his large, bright, and competitive class at Sichuan Medical College without reason. Nor were his gifts of intelligence, logic, and reasoning limited exclusively to science. Nor did he become chief resident in one of America's premier internal medicine residency training programs without demonstrating initiative, independent thinking, and the capacity to work with others. There are no accidents. Leonard's waters run deep.

As I requested, Leonard detailed his plan to "fix" things for his daughter. He indicated that on leaving my office, he and Eleanor would drive directly to his bank, where there were several large business accounts in his name that he used to operate the PPO. These accounts were set up primarily to pay salaries for the physicians in the PPOs associated with Gulf States Medical Systems. He would remove a substantial sum from the accounts and, that day, open a personal account in another bank that he would keep secret from Ruth.

Next, he would consult the company's outside lawyer, Mr. John Connor, whom he liked and trusted. Mr. Connor specializes in business law and medical corporations. He also planned to call a nephrologist whose wife is an attorney specializing in family law (i.e., a divorce lawyer). Finally, that day he would rent an apartment near my office in which he and Eleanor could reside for the near future.

> **Dr. Y.:** What do you feel and think about this plan, Eleanor?
> **Eleanor Lai:** I am terrified and totally in favor of it. I don't care if I ever see my mother again.
> **Dr. Y.:** So you don't want to try to work with her in any way?
> **Eleanor:** There is no point, Dr. Y. Including her in my treatment would ruin the treatment. It might even be dangerous. She will try to stop me in any way she can—and that includes physically. I want to escape from her for once and for all.
> **Dr. Y.:** You are over 18 years old and have the legal authority to make your own decisions. I will do my best to support you in what you choose to do.
> **Eleanor:** Then I choose to live with my father and to have nothing more to do with my mother. I want to get well.

True to his nature, Leonard proceeded diligently with what he had proposed. That afternoon he met with John Connor. On hearing the background and reviewing the corporate legal documents that Leonard had brought with him, Mr. Connor responded as follows:

> **Mr. John Connor:** I have several other recommendations to make, Leonard. You need two more lawyers in addition to me. I will

work with you and Eleanor on the business side. You also must have a personal attorney who is smart and tough. I predict you will need a restraining order to keep Ruth away from you and Eleanor—and probably even from Eleanor's shrink. I know the best person for that job.

Most importantly, don't hire your friend's wife as your divorce lawyer. Hiring a friend for a job like this rarely works out. She will try to "make nice" and will get rolled over by Ruth and her lawyers. I will get you Jerry Westerman. He's the meanest son of a bitch in the state of Texas. I can assure you that he takes no prisoners in a divorce case. He'll be a good match for Ruth.

Sorry about all the lawyers, but there is a ton of money involved, and the dissolution of your company and your divorce will be all-out wars. You will need the best advocates when you deal with Ruth. No polite country club lawyers. They can't be afraid of a street fight. As you know, I have dealt with Ruth for years, and she is cheap as hell and as mean as a snake. And she won't fight fair. I never told you, Leonard, but my firm always had to fight with her over our legal bills. She didn't think she had to pay us anything. She'll fight you for every last dime, but Jerry will fight her for every penny.

The good news, Leonard, is that you are in a very strong position, both legally and financially. You are about to become independently wealthy, meaning you will be both wealthy and independent.

Dr. Leonard Lai: I will do just what you say, John. I am not afraid of Ruth.

Diagnosis and Treatment

Decision

Eleanor agreed to meet daily with me for the next 2 weeks to establish her definitive psychiatric diagnosis and to fine tune our treatment plan. Eleanor fully met the official DSM-5 diagnostic criteria for anorexia nervosa (307.1 [F50.01]) (American Psychiatric Association 2013) as evidenced by the following:

1. Deliberate and severe restriction of food despite her significantly low weight
2. Intense fear of gaining weight and becoming fat
3. Distorted body image: although skeletally thin, she saw herself as obese

In addition, Eleanor exhibited the following:

1. Lack of insight about and denial of the fact that she was so thin
2. Self-esteem being intimately linked to her weight as opposed to her many positive qualities and accomplishments
3. Fear of *losing control* as manifested by any gain in weight
4. Intense, excessive exercise regimen
5. Extreme social anxiety and self-consciousness in public
6. Secretive, idiosyncratic eating patterns

Regarding her distorted body image, Eleanor was especially preoccupied with the fear that her buttocks and thighs were "disgustingly fat" and would examine them in the mirror repeatedly. Directly after eating anything, she would palpate her body parts obsessively to determine if they had "grown bigger." Objectively, her thighs and buttocks were emaciated by all reasonable and realistic standards.

Although she certainly met the official standards for the disorder, Eleanor did not demonstrate all of the classic "associated features" of anorexia nervosa. Importantly, she was in overall good physical health. She did not induce vomiting or take laxatives or diuretics, nor was there evidence of a loss of bone mineral density. Additionally, she did not have major depression, which is so commonly associated with this condition.

Eleanor exhibited symptoms associated with two anxiety disorders: obsessive-compulsive disorder—with symptoms principally related to her concerns about food, weight, body size and shape, and exercise—and social anxiety disorder. I therefore initiated a selective serotonin reuptake inhibitor type of antidepressant for the treatment of these conditions.

As alluded to previously, my primary "technical challenge" in the initial stage of treatment was to establish a constructive therapeutic alliance with Eleanor in the face of her life-threatening weight loss. The principal threat to a successful outcome would be that our treatment would devolve into a power struggle between the two of us over her weight. This struggle would be a toxic reflection of her historic battle to individuate from her mother. My principal tools in the face of this challenge were clear communication with Eleanor of our treatment goals and process accompanied by psychodynamic interpretations of the inevitable clashes that would emerge between us.

Avoiding wars requires much more subtle and imaginative tactics than fighting wars, and this is particularly true when a person is in mortal combat with herself. In our second meeting, I asked Eleanor the following question:

> **Dr. Y.:** When is your mind at peace?
>
> **Eleanor Lai:** I'm not sure I understand your question, Dr. Y.
>
> **Dr. Y.:** You have told me how unsettled your mind is. You ruminate about food and your weight; you have told me how self-conscious you are when you are around people and about how much you worry about what they think of you later on; you have told me that you never feel safe in your home, especially when your mother is around. But I don't know anything about the circumstances when your mind is at peace. When do you feel safe and happy?
>
> **Eleanor:** When I dance, I'm at peace, Dr. Y. I lose myself in the music and the movement. Even when I am learning a difficult new piece, I feel pleasure and not pressure. I have always believed that dancing is my natural state of being.
>
> **Dr. Y.:** Then you must dance to be alive, Eleanor, and we must work together to make that happen.

At the time of this discussion, Eleanor weighed 96 pounds. Her body mass index was 14.5, which, according to the Centers for Disease Control and Prevention and the World Health Organization categories for thinness in adults, is in the "extreme" range. She would need to weigh 109 pounds to move into the "moderate" category. "Severe," meaning "severely thin," is between the "moderate" and "extreme" categories. With this as background, our discussion of anything involving Eleanor's need to gain weight would be within the context of what *she* wants most—to dance—thereby reducing our power struggles.

> **Dr. Y.:** Do you have much opportunity to dance these days?
>
> **Eleanor Lai:** Not in a formal way. I was no longer permitted to dance with the two Harvard dance companies I had joined. Truth be told, although fun, neither of these venues was very challenging to me. I certainly wasn't learning much new or growing as a dancer.
>
> **Dr. Y.:** Why weren't you permitted to dance?
>
> **Eleanor:** In December I was called aside by Professor Evans, the faculty supervisor of the Harvard Asian American Dance Troupe. Professor Evans told me that several of the other dancers in my group had asked to meet with her privately. They told her that they were worried that I was getting too thin and that I might be sick. I was absolutely mortified when Professor Evans told me these things.

Dr. Y.: Please elaborate, Eleanor.

Eleanor: Dancing is something I do to "lose myself." To be happy. It mortifies me to think that people are watching me and judging me when I am lost in dancing. But I was so oblivious to it. It makes me feel that I have to be on guard all of the time.

Dr. Y.: Just like when you were a defenseless little child at home with your mother.

Eleanor: Exactly! I'd be having fun doing something harmless— like coloring pictures—when she would sneak up behind me and scream at me. Or, if she was in a really bad mood, she would hit me hard on the back of my head.

Dr. Y.: You were powerless then, but not now. That is, unless you sneak up and attack yourself like you are doing now with self-imposed starvation.

Identification With the Aggressor

Eleanor's self-directed tyranny can be traced back to millennia of feudalism that her peasant ancestors endured. From being the chattel of feudal landlords to being ravaged by ruthless foreign invaders to the more recent so-called Cultural Revolution of Chairman Mao, her ancestors had long suffered despotic oppression. For countless centuries, their eyes were fixed on the masters, whose needs, ire, and whims carried life and death implications for them. And the eyes of Eleanor's "survivor" ancestors were not closed when tens of millions of their less fortunate fellow Chinese peasants were slaughtered or died of starvation under Mao Zedong. Her grandparents understood full well that their fates would be no different should they be disobedient to Mao's Communist Party successors.

Although the concept of *identification with the aggressor* has been reinterpreted in many ways to mean many different things, I believe that Hungarian psychoanalyst Sándor Ferenczi's original 1932 description of the term has the most merit in understanding Eleanor's psychological problems. Ferenczi described the unconscious processes by which victims adapt to chronic trauma and abuse—at a considerable cost. He posited that the maltreated individual submits to the will of the perpetrator by forsaking his or her autonomy—in feelings, thoughts, and behavior. The victims come to believe that they are responsible for and deserve the abuse they suffer, and thus they punish themselves when they do not meet the expectations of others. Their form of "identification" is to turn the tyranny of the abuser on themselves through constant self-monitoring and self-reproach. Additionally, having lost all awareness of their own wants, needs, and priorities, they feel especially vulnerable to all criticism and abandonment—even by the abusing party. Thus, they become obsessed with pleasing others and are overly compliant and easy to exploit.

Beginning with Anna Freud, more modern interpretations of identification with the aggressor have more application to Eleanor's mother and her abusive grandfather than to Eleanor. In this case, identification with the perpetrator is an unconscious defense mechanism by which the victim mitigates fear and the perception of danger by *becoming like the abuser.* Notorious examples of this form of identification include the so-called Stockholm Syndrome, which involved bank employees who were held hostage for 6 days in a bank vault during a failed robbery attempt in Stockholm, Sweden. These hostages developed positive emotional attachments to the robbers, whom they grew to admire and defend. This parallels the case of heiress Patty Hearst, who assumed the radical beliefs of and began to rob banks with her kidnappers. This form of identification with the aggressor can be understood as *traumatic bonding,* or a way that an individual can cope with abuse by rationalizing it to be justified and even constructive. Both physically and psychologically mistreated by her father, Ruth adopted his attitudes and approaches that, in turn, she applied with a vengeance to her husband and daughter.

Why would Eleanor have such a radically different reaction to abuse from that of Ruth's to the abuse of her father? My answer is that Eleanor inherited the biological temperament and the cognitive and behavioral predispositions of her modest, compassionate, and brilliant father. Thus, on the basis of their genetic/biological predispositions, the same experiential stimulus would yield diametrically different responses from Ruth and Eleanor. This can help explain why different siblings in the same family exhibit widely different reactions to the same stresses (Yudofsky 2005, pp. 352–366).

With this understanding, I continued the discussion with Eleanor of how we should deal with her life-threatening weight loss.

Dancing for Pounds

Dr. Y.: What is your current standing with Harvard?

Eleanor Lai: Professor Evans had me evaluated by the Health Service after the girls in my dance company complained to her about me. I have completed my first semester of my sophomore year, but I can't reenroll without a letter from a doctor that it is safe for me to return.

Dr. Y.: What do you want to do?

Eleanor: I don't really know for sure. I was pretty miserable most of the time that I was there, and I really missed dancing at an advanced level. On the other hand, I did enjoy the courses that I took. The subjects were very interesting, and the professors are fantastic.

Dr. Y.: As I see it you would like to do both—to go to Harvard and to dance with a professional company.

Eleanor: How is that possible?

Dr. Y.: When I was on the faculty at Columbia, I became aware that there were joint programs for Columbia and Barnard undergraduates with Juilliard. Of course, these programs were for selected students with special talents in musical performance. I suspect that something similar is also possible at Harvard. We would have to look into it when you get better.

Eleanor (*with a mischievous gleam in her eye*): You mean that I can eat my cake and stay thin too?

Dr. Y.: You have a wonderful sense of humor, Eleanor. We should have a great time solving your puzzle together.

Eleanor: Although I hate to think about it, how much weight do you think I will need to gain to dance in a conservatory and to be let back into Harvard?

Dr. Y.: I calculated that you will have to weigh a minimum of 114 pounds.

Eleanor: That is terrifying to me, Dr. Y. Not only will I look like an elephant, but I don't believe that I can stop gaining weight once I start. When I gained all that weight at Harvard, I started eating compulsively. Especially when I was anxious or upset.

Dr. Y.: Then we must work to understand these feelings and how to deal with them.

Together, we calculated and discussed how many calories she would have to ingest per day to gain 18 pounds in a reasonable period of time. We also acknowledged that she would need to consume at least that many calories to sustain a safe weight once she returned to the physical rigors of an advanced dance regimen. We estimated that if she maintained a diet of about 3,500 calories per day, she would probably gain from 1 to 2 pounds per week. At that rate, it would take about 3 months before she would dance again. Fortunately, as a dancer, Eleanor was familiar with the topic of diet. Additionally, gifted in science and mathematics, Eleanor knew and understood the principles of nutrition. As are so many people with anorexia nervosa, she was both interested in and knowledgeable about food—which carried both positive and negative repercussions. The upside was that she knew how to gain weight in a healthful fashion, and the downside was the risk of her becoming even more preoccupied with food, eating, dieting, and her weight.

> **Dr. Y.:** Would you permit me to engage a dietitian to work with you on your weight-gaining regimen? You and I can set your goals and rely on the dietitian to help you get there. Even though you and I know a good bit about diet, it is more productive for us to work on other things.
>
> **Eleanor Lai:** Such as what?
>
> **Dr. Y.:** What causes you to be so fearful of losing control and how you can go about gaining control of things that are important to you—which will include how you look and feel about yourself. I also believe that we need to do a lot of work on your propensity to try to please everyone.

Eleanor agreed to meet regularly with a dietitian, who would report to me weekly about her weight status. Eleanor petitioned Harvard for a year's leave of absence, which was approved. She also met with Mr. Arnaud Durand of the Houston Dance Academy, who agreed that she could practice daily with the company dancers when I determined that it was safe for her to do so. So that she did not spend too much time alone, she volunteered to work as a translator and tutor in the Harris County Independent School System (the Houston public schools) for students who had recently emigrated from China and Taiwan. In the meantime, she would meet with me in daily psychotherapy, with her father joining us on selected occasions for joint sessions.

Opening Doors

With the advantage of her superior intellect and motivation to return to dancing, Eleanor made great progress during her first 2 months of treatment. The following discussion took place during one of the joint sessions with her father:

> **Dr. Leonard Lai:** Eleanor and I are having much fun together. We go to symphony, to watch ballet, to museums, and write letters to her grandparents in China. My parents are too old to use computers or cell phones, but they are no longer too poor. Ruth never let me send them any money, but now I send much

money to my family and to Ruth's family. They can live in bigger apartments now and eat good food. One day soon Eleanor and I will go back to China to visit them.

Ruth is not much problem anymore. My attorney does audit, and he finds that Ruth was cheating on bills to government for Medicare and Medicaid. We report it to government right away. She is in big, big trouble. Will pay big fines and may go to jail. Not much time for Ruth to bother me and Eleanor. I am now "whistle blower," so have immunity. We are safe.

Dr. Y.: What are your plans, Dr. Lai?

Dr. Leonard Lai: Will take about a year for lawyers to fix business and to divorce Ruth. Then I will sell business to large company. Then I will go work in your medical school. Take care of patients, teach, and do research. What I always want to do. Spoke to chairman of medicine and dean of medical school, and it is all set up. Will work in county hospital.

How is Eleanor doing, Professor Y.?

Dr. Y.: How are you, Eleanor?

Eleanor Lai: Dr. Y. won't tell me how I'm doing, Daddy. It drives me crazy. He thinks I am the best judge of that. I think I am OK. I have gained 12 pounds, and it scares me to death. I still hate the way my body looks. I worry that I won't be able to stop gaining weight when I reach my target. Most of all, as you know, I love teaching the kids. They are the highlight of my life, and I can't wait to go back to the dance company next month.

Dr. Leonard Lai: Does Ruth try to bother you, Dr. Y.?

Dr. Y.: I don't have Eleanor's permission to speak with her mother. Were I to do so without Eleanor's expressed approval, I would be in violation of federal HIPAA [Health Insurance Portability and Accountability Act] regulations. I wasn't even around when Dr. Ruth Lai showed up at my office and demanded to speak with me. She raised a big ruckus, so security was called to remove her from the medical office building premises. A restraining order was executed by the general counsel of the medical school, and security will notify me if Dr. Ruth Lai enters any school or hospital properties. As far as I know, she hasn't tried anything further.

Ironic how she and I have changed places behind the closed door, isn't it?

Stuck in Pleasing

If you think that it is possible that you may be "stuck in pleasing," which I also term in this chapter being an "overpleaser," the following self-report scale—The Stuck in Pleasing Scale (see Table 11–1)—will help you determine whether or not it is likely that you are.

Eleanor's Need to Please

The following dialogue took place during a session several months into Eleanor's treatment:

> **Eleanor Lai:** I hate to have to ask you this, Dr. Y. My students are going on an overnight trip to Austin next Tuesday, and the principal of the school has asked me to come along as their adult chaperone. The kids have been begging me to go with them. I stayed awake most of the night worrying whether I should ask you if I can miss our appointment on that day.
>
> **Dr. Y.:** What exactly are you worrying about?
>
> **Eleanor:** Just about everything. If you would be mad at me. If you would think I didn't appreciate your help. Or if you would feel that I was being disrespectful to you.
>
> **Dr. Y.:** What would *you* like to do, Eleanor?
>
> **Eleanor:** I don't even know, Dr. Y. I don't want to disappoint the principal, and I don't want you to be mad at me. Situations like this just drive me crazy.
>
> **Dr. Y.:** How could you know what I would "think" until you asked me? Let's talk some more about how you try to please everyone, Eleanor.

Over the course of her entire treatment, Eleanor and I reviewed the origin and far-reaching ramifications of her overpowering need to please others. These are summarized below.

Childhood origins of Eleanor's need to please others:

- Since she was a small child, Eleanor was physically and emotionally brutalized by her mother.
- Eleanor did not feel safe or protected in her own home.
- Eleanor was hypervigilant in monitoring her environment and her mother's moods for impending abuse.
- Eleanor's mother was inconsistent in inflicting her punishments.
- Eleanor could not rely on her father to protect her from her mother's abuse.
- Eleanor believed that she could avoid maternal abuse by being perfect and through perfect performance.

TABLE 11-1. The Stuck in Pleasing Scale

The following scale is in the form of a self-report questionnaire that will help you determine whether or not you may be "stuck in pleasing" or an "overpleaser."

I. Please check the *best* answer to the following questions	Almost never	Sometimes	Nearly always
1. I dress for myself, not others.			
2. I rapidly get over being criticized.			
3. I stand up for myself when I'm right.			
4. I like "ruffling people's feathers."			
5. I say "yes" when I want to say "no."			
6. I consider my own needs first.			
7. I express my anger when I feel angry.			
8. I say what's on my mind.			
9. I don't "second-guess" my decisions.			
10. I decline when people ask me to do them favors.			
11. I ask for help when I need help.			
12. I overlook my minor mistakes.			
13. I return my food in a restaurant when I don't like the way it's prepared.			
14. I express my opinions even when they aren't welcome.			
15. I return items to the department store when dissatisfied.			
16. I undertip waiters and cab drivers when service is poor.			
17. I am my strongest advocate.			
18. I try to be the person in charge.			
19. I defend myself when attacked.			
20. I value what I think of myself more than what others think of me.			
II. Total			

TABLE 11-1. The Stuck in Pleasing Scale *(continued)*

III. Scoring the Stuck in Pleasing Scale

Add up the numbers that you checked: 1 point for "almost never," 2 points for "sometimes," and 3 points for "nearly always."

If your total is 30 or below, it is *probable* that you are stuck in pleasing (an overpleaser).

If your total is between 30 and 45, it is *possible* that you are stuck in pleasing (an overpleaser).

If your total is 45 or more, it is *unlikely* that you are stuck in pleasing (an overpleaser).

Source. Copyright © Stuart C. Yudofsky, M.D., 2015.

Adult ramifications of Eleanor's need to please others:

- Eleanor believes that it is her responsibility to make everyone around her happy.
- Eleanor will do almost anything to avoid disappointing others.
- Eleanor endlessly scans others for validation that she is pleasing them.
- Eleanor experiences unbearable anxiety and insecurity if she believes that she has displeased someone.
- Eleanor tries to control the thoughts and feelings of others by overdoing things.
- Eleanor tries to control the thoughts and feelings of others by overwhelming them with kindness.
- Eleanor prioritizes the needs of others over her own.
- Eleanor is unable to "say no" or refuse requests made of her by others.
- Eleanor is uncomfortable with leadership or directing others.
- Eleanor is vulnerable to manipulation by others.
- Eleanor is overworked and often exhausted.
- Eleanor is constantly self-effacing, apologizing, and self-critical.
- Eleanor feels insecure, unworthy, and unsafe—even when praised.
- Eleanor cannot relax or be generous to herself.
- Eleanor has difficulty knowing what she wants.
- Eleanor will not advocate on her own behalf.
- Eleanor cannot make important decisions involving her future.

- Eleanor has low self-esteem.
- Eleanor has poor self-definition.
- Eleanor is unhappy.

As summarized in Table 11–2, these features of pleasing others that are exhibited by Eleanor are also common in and representative of other people who are stuck in pleasing others.

TABLE 11–2. Twenty common features of people who are stuck in pleasing others

---

1. They believe that it is their responsibility to make everyone around them happy

2. They will do almost anything to avoid disappointing others

3. They endlessly scan others for validation that they are pleasing them

4. They experience unbearable anxiety and insecurity if they believe that they have displeased someone

5. They try to control the thoughts and feelings of others by overdoing things

6. They try to control the thoughts and feelings of others by overwhelming them with kindness

7. They prioritize the needs and wants of others over their own

8. They are unable to say "no" or refuse requests made of them by others

9. They cannot function as leaders or direct others

10. They are vulnerable to manipulation by others

11. They are overworked and often exhausted

12. They are constantly self-effacing, apologetic, and self-critical

13. They feel insecure, unworthy, and unsafe—even when praised

14. They cannot relax or be kind to themselves

15. They have difficulty knowing what they want

16. They will not advocate on their own behalf

17. They have difficulty making decisions

18. They have low self-esteem

19. They have poor self-definition

20. They are unhappy

Early on in her treatment, I asked Eleanor to fill out the Stuck in Pleasing Scale, and she scored 22, which is one of the lowest scores my patients have ever recorded on this scale. The only items to which she answered "sometimes" were "I say 'no' when I mean 'no'" and "I say what's on my mind." She checked "almost never" on the other 18 items of the scale. Therefore, it was highly probable that Eleanor was stuck in pleasing at the time that she completed the scale.

Key Features of Eleanor Lai's Being Stuck in Pause

1. *How Eleanor is stuck:* Overpleasing others
2. *Goal for change:* Determine and act on what she wants
3. *Central, unresolved conflicts:* 1) Wants to be in control; wants to please others (approach-approach) and 2) wants to be powerful; is fearful of rejection and abandonment (approach-avoidance)
4. *Hallmarks of Eleanor's being stuck*: Underachievement, anxiety, frustration, identity confusion, self-deprecation, low self-esteem, dysthymia, poor health, depleted interpersonal relationships
5. *Binary problems/solutions*: Self-starvation/healthful diet; prioritizing others/prioritizing self
6. *Critical decision points*: Adhere to 3,500 calorie diet; self-exploration, self-understanding, and change (cognitive and behavioral) through engaging in intensive psychotherapy
7. *Corollary factors required to achieve resolution:* Work with a dietitian on gaining and sustaining a healthful weight; intensive, insight-oriented psychotherapy to adhere to diet, gain insights into conflicts, and make changes that lead to autonomy and self-reliance; develop and apply mature social skills
8. *Resolution:* Return to and sustain the minimum weight of 114 pounds and develop self-agency utilizing the Power of No and the Power of Go

Getting Unstuck Through the Power of No and the Power of Go

Discipline

For a summary of the key principles of the Fatal Pauses 3-D Method of Getting Unstuck Through the Power of No and the Power of Go, see Table 3–6 (p. 43).

Let's review the first four principles individually as they apply to Eleanor.

1. **You must *stop* something that you like in order to *gain* something that you like more.**
2. **You are saying "Yes!" to something that you fundamentally want by saying "No!" to something that you want less.**

From our first session, Eleanor monitored me closely to determine what I wanted from her and whether or not I were pleased with her. She oriented her relationship with me as follows: 1) to determine what I expected from her, 2) to do everything possible to meet these presumed expectations, and 3) to have me make decisions that directly affected her that were determinations that she should have made for herself. These behaviors, of course, relate to her formative relationship with her mother.

As indicated in the following dialogue that occurred during her first visit, I was aware, early on, of Eleanor's need to please and began to address it right away.

> **Dr. Y.:** OK, Eleanor. We agreed that for the first 2 weeks you will come to see me every day. What is the best time for you to have your sessions?
>
> **Eleanor Lai:** I will come *any* time you are available. I know how busy you are, Dr. Y. I feel so guilty about taking up so much of your time when so many other people need your help.
>
> **Dr. Y.:** How do you know all of these things about me? We just met and you haven't asked any questions about me or my practice.
>
> **Eleanor:** I'm so sorry. I didn't mean to be presumptuous. Please forgive me. What I was trying to say is that, at this point, I have nothing else to do. I want to come any time that is convenient for you and fits with your schedule.
>
> **Dr. Y.:** Surely, Eleanor you must prefer getting up at a certain time. And don't you have other things that you would like to do during the day? When will be best for you?
>
> **Eleanor:** It really doesn't matter to me. I feel so privileged to be able to see you. I just hate your having to waste so much time on me. I know that your other patients are much more deserving than I am. I really, really want to come any time that is best for you.

Growing Pains

For most patients with anorexia nervosa, their angry feelings, acts of defiance, and desperation to control themselves and others are expressed most evidently and almost exclusively in their eating behaviors. They also try to control others by constantly trying to please them, which can become somewhat "wearing" for those close to them. By gaining weight in order to dance, Eleanor was giving up something that she thought that she *wanted*—to restrict her food intake and be very thin (and her misperception of being in control)—for something that she *wanted more*—to dance and feel alive. By relinquishing some of the defensive and distracting behaviors associated with food deprivation, she was certain to become more aware of her angry feelings. And, in turn, being angry would make her very anxious. Second, by trying to change her constant crusade to control people through pleasing, she also would feel anxious by "being at the mercy of their displeasure." Again, defenses are partially successful, unconscious thoughts and behavioral patterns that are in place as defenses from anxiety. No matter how gradually Eleanor proceeded, I would be suspicious and incredulous about whether she were truly changing if she did not become anxious. In this therapeutic circumstance, anxiety is a signal of vulnerability brought about by change and growth. And Eleanor became very, very anxious. The following is an interchange that we had about 4 months into her treatment.

> **Eleanor Lai:** Dr. Y., I think I am getting worse. I apologize to you because you are spending so much time trying to help me. But I just can't get better.
> **Dr. Y.:** What makes you think you are getting worse?
> **Eleanor:** Because I am anxious all of the time. I know that I have no right to complain, and I apologize for complaining all the time. But my anxiety is almost unbearable.
> **Dr. Y.:** What do you know about lobsters, Eleanor?
> **Eleanor:** About lobsters? I'm sorry, Dr. Y., did I hear your question right?
> **Dr. Y.:** You heard me correctly, Eleanor. Let's talk about lobsters. Do you know what they look like after they have been recently hatched?
> **Eleanor** (*disbelievingly*): I don't think I know, Dr. Y. I go to Harvard, so I should know the answer. I'm sorry.

Dr. Y.'s Lobster Metaphor for Change and Growth

Not long after hatching and being released from its mother to fare for itself in the cold, immense, and dangerous ocean, a "baby" lobster has assumed its exact adult form. At only ¼ inch in length, the morphology of the tiny infant is identical to that of a 100-year-old lobster that is more than 3 feet long and can weigh more than 50 pounds. Even though it has a hard, calcified shell for protection, a ¼ inch newborn lobster is vulnerable to being eaten by nearly every omnivore that is bigger than it is. And that is a long list.

The problem is that lobsters' shells are both protective and confining. Lobsters must shed their protective shells in order to grow. A lobster sheds its protective/confining shell through a process called *molting*, which occurs about 10 times in its first year of life. This molting process takes several days, during which time the lobster is soft, unprotected, and vulnerable to even more predators—no matter what size. Almost anything with a mouth can take a bite out of a molting lobster.

For safety, a lobster hides out during molting. It also eats ravenously during molting and grows rapidly until such time as it secretes a new calcium shell and can go back out in the open ocean a bit more safely. Over a long period of time of change and growth, a lobster becomes progressively safer from most predators other than humans. A lobster will shed its shells and grow new ones about 30 times before it weighs 1 pound.

> **Eleanor Lai:** Are you saying that I'm like a lobster, Dr. Y.?
> **Dr. Y.:** As you know from your science studies, Eleanor, we share many genes with all other living things. But what I am really saying is that you should expect to feel vulnerable and anxious as you change.

3. A *none or all* binary choice is required to achieve success in getting unstuck. In most cases, moderation does not work.

Eleanor's need to please pervaded almost all aspects of her interactions with other people. Consequently, her saying "no" to pleasing others was more integral and fundamental to her "being" and personality than most other types of maladaptive behaviors—such as smoking or gambling—are for other people. Additionally, as with all eating disorders, an all-or-none approach cannot apply. A person cannot stop eating altogether, nor can she exercise no restraint whatsoever with regard to eating.

Additionally, when applied *in moderation* to selected instances and situations, pleasing others can be positive and constructive—a true "win-win" behavior. After all, if one were to please only oneself, one would be narcissistic and devoid of altruism.

Therefore, Eleanor and I assumed a *moderate and gradual approach* to resolving her problem of trying to please all people all of the time. We began by highlighting and working on examples of her trying to please me in our therapeutic relationship. Once learned, the principles were then applied gradually to parallel situations in her current daily life, which primarily involved her job tutoring middle school students whose families were recent immigrants from China.

> **Eleanor Lai:** I need your help, Dr. Y. I've been driving myself crazy trying to buy a present for my supervisor at work. She is giving a party to celebrate Chinese New Year, and I know it is appropriate to bring a gift. I just can't decide what to get for her.
> **Dr. Y.:** How have you been going about deciding on the present?
> **Eleanor:** I spend hours upon hours looking for the present in stores and on the Internet, but I can't decide on the right gift. When I get close to deciding, I either find something wrong with it, or think I might find something better if I look longer. Mainly I worry that she won't like what I get for her. It would be much, much easier for me if I could buy everything in the store and have a truck bring it to the party. I drive myself completely crazy.

Through the lens of Eleanor's current dilemma, we engaged in a protracted discussion about 1) the origins of her need to please; 2) what she was trying to accomplish by pleasing; and 3) why pleasing was, as she indicated, "driving me crazy." We had gone over each of these factors previously, but, like all learning, psychotherapy requires repetition. And having a specific issue with which to deal enhances the learning process.

Eleanor was learning in psychotherapy that, as a child, she tried to feel safe by pleasing her mother at all times. We reviewed how, as do other children, she had tried to use her own behavior to influence the mood, feelings, and behavior of her mother. However, she experienced less success and more frustration than most others who are fortunate to have safe, supportive, and nurturing families. Additionally,

Eleanor was trying to find "the perfect gift" for her supervisor in order to control how the supervisor felt about her. Not only was that a difficult task for Eleanor, who did not know very much about her supervisor's interests and personal life, but Eleanor's frustrating experiences with her mother left her pessimistic to the point of being fatalistic about finding a gift that would really delight her. Therefore, Eleanor's self-imposed task was so formidable that she could not complete it. Ultimately, she was unable to decide on a gift. It is no wonder that Eleanor contemplated not going to the party at all, even though she liked her supervisor and thought that she might have a good time.

We all know that a certain degree of pleasing others can help us accomplish important personal goals. Eleanor knew this from experience as well. Eleanor was universally well liked and, by most objective standards, quite successful. Thus, to help Eleanor decide to abandon excessive pleasing behaviors that she believed "paid off in the long run," I continuously searched to find creative ways to cast her pattern of overpleasing in a distasteful light for her.

> **Dr. Y.:** Did your mother give gifts?
>
> **Eleanor Lai:** I never received any gifts that I wanted from her. She would buy me beautiful things to wear but not things that I would have chosen for myself. They were mainly things that she thought would impress her friends and clients. Mother always said that having food on my plate and a roof over my head were more gifts than I deserved.
>
> **Dr. Y.:** Did your mother give gifts to others?
>
> **Eleanor:** Only when she wanted something from somebody.
>
> **Dr. Y.:** What specific examples come to mind?
>
> **Eleanor:** When mother was in the process of purchasing a hospital, she would buy these very expensive gifts for the big shots who ran the hospital. I know this because, as a little girl, she would let me go with her to the fancy department stores where she bought these gifts, and I was jealous that she was buying these great presents for other people and not for me. Mother would also get hugely expensive gifts for people who could help me get some type of piano or dance award or into a good college. I was terribly embarrassed in my junior year of high school when she gave my college counselor a gift certificate to an expensive spa.
>
> **Dr. Y.:** You're talking more about *bribes* than about gifts. Perhaps you are trying to bribe your supervisor into liking you with that gift you can't decide on.

Eleanor: I never thought of it like that, Dr. Y. And I don't like thinking of myself doing something devious like that. As you know, I don't want to be anything at all like my mother.

Dr. Y.: Then we must find ways to help you stop trying to control how others think about you through overpleasing them. This will take time and effort and will also involve our finding ways for you to value and be more accepting of yourself. The more you value and accept yourself the less important it will be for you to overdo the pleasing of other people.

4. The Power of Go is *always* required to achieve the Power of No.

To avoid becoming seriously, perhaps fatally, ill, Eleanor had to stop her strict limitation of her daily caloric intake (i.e., utilize the Power of No). To achieve this goal, the Power of Go was required in multiple areas. First, she had to "show up" and work hard in our regular psychotherapy sessions, where her recovery activities would be advanced and coordinated. Too often in contemporary medicine, the patient becomes overwhelmed and lost amid constellations of specialists ordering and conducting profusions of tests from galaxies of office locations. Care becomes unfocused and goals are unmet. My responsibility was to make certain that this did not occur by co-ordinating her medical care, or Eleanor would not survive. Eleanor's job was to show up and work hard—both in her treatment *(discovery* and *decision)* and outside her treatment sessions *(discipline)*.

Second, Eleanor was obliged to work closely with a dietitian and to adhere exactingly to the nutrition and weight gain regimen that was prescribed. Given how mortified and ambivalent Eleanor was about gaining weight, she had to assert the Power of Go with every bite of every meal that she was required to ingest. No ruminating or fighting with herself about "What should I eat?" or "How much should I eat?" or "When should I eat?" That part of her being stuck would be overridden by the dietitian. Until she achieved and main-tained a safe weight for at least a year, Eleanor's executive function-ing regarding her diet would be removed and delegated to her dietitian, who, in turn, functioned under my oversight. Although El-eanor's being at a safe weight was my medical responsibility, to avoid power struggles and advance psychotherapy, I tried to remain at some distance from day-to-day issues regarding her eating and diet.

Eleanor's responsibility in this realm was to employ the Power of Go to follow the diet explicitly as directed. No questioning, no hesitation, no revision, no exception. This might seem overly severe and infantilizing, but Eleanor required a well-nourished, healthy brain—in addition to the rest of her body—to do the hard work—both in and outside of psychotherapy—that was required for her to save her own life and make so many fundamental changes. This approach, by the way, is the most compassionate because Eleanor was misguided and miserable using her own tactics, which primarily involved control of eating.

Third, Eleanor would work with me in her treatment to identify specific patterns of behavior that were associated with her overpleasing others. After we identified these patterns, we would devise a plan for her to remediate each specific overpleasing behavior. This was by far the most difficult aspect of her treatment, and Eleanor would have to utilize the Power of Go in her interpersonal relationships to execute each element of the plan. A prototypical example of this component of our treatment is as follows:

> **Eleanor Lai** (*clearly upset*): I had one of the worst days of my life today. The mother of one of my students complained about me to my supervisor. She said that I was upsetting her daughter. I don't think that I can ever go back to work there again.
> **Dr. Y.:** Try to calm down, Eleanor, and tell me what happened.
> **Eleanor:** My supervisor told me that the mother complained that I had been overstepping my bounds with her daughter. Believe it or not, Dr. Y., it had to do with what the girl was eating for lunch.
> **Dr. Y.:** Oh, I believe it, Eleanor.
> **Eleanor:** This isn't funny Dr. Y. I am *seriously* upset. You try to make a joke about everything!

TREATMENT PRINCIPLE 11

Humor, when not distracting, is an essential component of psychotherapy. It is a gentle way of providing perspective. *Humorless* treatment is *dead* treatment.

Eleanor was responding to this specific situation—and nearly every circumstance in which there is direct or implied criticism of her—as if it were a catastrophe. Manifestly, her over-the-top reactions relate directly to her mother's having only one response—unfettered attack—when she was upset with Eleanor—regardless of how minor or major the "transgression."

Additionally, I refused to permit Eleanor subtly to control my reactions and responses by her self-imposed set of rules of etiquette and politeness. I did not agree with her that this event had to be a crisis—even though that was how she experienced it. She would learn that our relationship could survive disagreements.

Finally, I was also delighted that Eleanor was feeling sufficiently self-confident and comfortable in our relationship to "give it back" to me, which I so richly deserve.

> **Eleanor Lai:** Now if you can be serious for just one minute, Dr. Y., that girl is only 13 years old and already is about 50 pounds overweight. She keeps bringing sweets in from home and not eating what's offered in the cafeteria lunch, which would be much more nutritious and far less caloric. For several weeks, I have been bringing in more healthy snacks for her to try. Mostly fresh fruits and some vegetables—like carrots and celery—for her to munch on. Yesterday, I caught her secretly throwing away the food I brought in, so I asked her not to do that anymore. I think that she has been throwing my food away all along. Anyway, she became very upset with me and started crying. She must have told her mother about it later on. The mother called the principal of the school today and complained about me. She is scheduled to meet with the principal tomorrow, and the principal wants me and my supervisor to attend the meeting.
>
> **Dr. Y.:** Did your supervisor know that you were bringing in food for the girl?
>
> **Eleanor:** Oh yes! Just about all of our students are very poor. All the teachers bring in books and supplies and other things for the kids. I asked my supervisor beforehand if I could bring in some healthy food for the child, and she had approved it.
>
> **Dr. Y.:** So what's the problem, Eleanor?
>
> **Eleanor:** You just don't understand. I just can't face that mother. I shouldn't have interfered in the first place. It's really none of my business what she gives her daughter to eat. Or what her daughter eats or doesn't eat. I'm such an idiot.
>
> **Dr. Y.:** What do you plan to do tomorrow, Eleanor?
>
> **Eleanor:** If I can get myself to go to work in the first place, I will apologize to the mother and promise never to bring in anything else for her child. Even worse, I can't bear to face my su-

pervisor for causing all of this trouble. I will offer to resign from my job, if that helps.

In our treatment session that day Eleanor and I painstakingly dissected each element of her crisis, with specific attention to whether or not *she* deeply believed that she had done something wrong. She ultimately concluded that she was doing her job responsibly as a caring educator and had followed all of the school's guidelines. She also understood that her extreme emotional response was directly related to childhood feelings about the many times she was blindsided by her mother's enraged disapproval and abuse when Eleanor had been trying to do the right thing all along. Her assignment for the meeting the next day was 1) not to remain silent during the meeting, 2) to communicate clearly to her student's mother her reasons for bringing in the snacks for the child, 3) to stand her ground in defense of what she believed she had done appropriately and in good faith, and 4) *not to apologize* for anything that she did not believe she had done wrong.

Eleanor Lai: I just don't think I am capable of doing that, Dr. Y. You know that I never stand up for myself.

Dr. Y.: If you don't believe that you have done something wrong, Eleanor, apologizing is a form of lying. You would be lying in order to try to control how the mother of your student feels about you. It is more valuable and ethical for you to try to explain to her why you are concerned about her daughter's diet and health.

The meeting the next day went well. Eleanor spoke up about her concerns over her student's unhealthful diet and what she was trying to accomplish. She was supported by her supervisor and the principal, who explained to the mother that health education was an important part of all students' education. In treatment, Eleanor and I identified her many other maladaptive behaviors that were directly linked with her need to please others. We developed specific actions utilizing the Power of No and the Power of Go that she would have to undertake to change these behavioral patterns. Enumerated as explicit rules to follow in Table 11–3, these actions and changes embody two general areas: overpleasing others and underpleasing herself. I believe that these remedies will also apply to many other people who have problems with overpleasing others.

TABLE 11–3. How to overcome overpleasing others and underpleasing yourself

1. Stop apologizing
2. Stop being self-effacing
3. Stop automatically agreeing with people
4. Stop monitoring people for their happiness
5. Stop taking responsibility for the happiness of other people
6. Stop looking to others for self-validation
7. Stop making excuses
8. Don't overreact to criticism
9. Limit monitoring others for their reactions to you
10. Limit overthanking others
11. Limit doing favors
12. Make decisions on the basis of what *you* want and feel is right
13. Accept the gratitude of others
14. Accept the compliments of others
15. Say "no" when you mean "no" and stand by it
16. Say what you are thinking and feeling
17. Express what you believe
18. Consider your own needs in addition to those of others
19. Consider your own preferences in addition to those of others
20. Protect your boundaries
21. Protect your time
22. Stand by your decisions

Table 11–4 summarizes in their most abbreviated forms eight principles and techniques that Eleanor had to learn, work on, and apply in order to take action on the 22 rules listed in Table 11–3.

In summary, Eleanor's work in and outside of treatment has been to identify opportunities in her daily interpersonal interactions that require that she exercise the rules, guidelines, and techniques summarized in Tables 11–3 and 11–4 and take action accordingly. In treatment we monitor and discuss both missed and met opportunities for change. Eleanor summarized this work as follows:

TABLE 11–4.	Guidelines and techniques to overcome overpleasing others and underpleasing yourself

1. Look for and become more aware of many of your automatic/reflexive responses aimed at pleasing others.

2. Before acquiescing to the requests of others, "buy some time" to consider whether or not you want to do what is being requested of you by others. No automatic compliance.

3. Acknowledge (to yourself) that you have the right to consider what you *want* to do in your responses to the wishes and requests of others.

4. Accept that you have a choice about whether or not to acquiesce to the expressed and implied wishes of others.

5. *Discover* what you actually want and do not want to do.

6. *Decide* what *you* want to do and not to do regarding the requests and wants of others and then do (or don't do) it.

7. Stand by your decisions and actions without apology.

8. Learn to accept and deal with any negative reactions or "push back" from those whom you may have disappointed.

> **Eleanor Lai:** I hope you realize, Dr. Y., that this is the hardest thing that I have ever tried to do.
>
> **Dr. Y.:** The price of freedom is always high, Eleanor. But so are the toll and toil of slavery.
>
> **Eleanor:** Stop being so preachy and dramatic, Dr. Y. You're making me sick to my stomach. I think I might even prefer your failed attempts at humor.
>
> **Dr. Y.:** I don't apologize for who I am—no matter how disgusting I may be.
>
> **Eleanor** (*with mischievous irony*): *May* be...? For every rule there is an exception, Dr. Y. And for the "don't apologize" rule, *you're* that exception. You *should* apologize.
>
> **Dr. Y.:** Are you the same nice, sweet Eleanor who didn't make a peep behind that closed hospital door?
>
> **Eleanor:** I hope not!

Introduction to Supermentalization

Problems

In her third month of treatment, Eleanor initiated the following dialogue as she was walking into her session:

> **Eleanor Lai:** What's wrong, Dr. Y.? Are you upset with me for some reason?
> **Dr. Y.:** I'm not upset with you, Eleanor. Why do you ask?
> **Eleanor:** You just look like you're upset today. I just assumed that I had done something wrong or disappointed you somehow. I'm sorry if I did.

I am not casual about my practice of psychiatry. Believing that it is essential that I do not distract my patients or call unnecessary attention to myself, I try to avoid such interference in many ways. For example, I make an effort to be consistent in my dress and appearance by wearing a white coat and similar styles of ties, shirts, glasses, etc., during every work day. By maintaining an upbeat, positive demeanor, I try not to permit the inevitable occasional stresses from my work or personal life to leak into sessions with patients. I regard this as being no different from other professions where leadership and discipline are required, such as piloting a commercial plane, acting on stage, adjudicating a case in federal court, teaching a prekindergarten class, or coaching a Major League baseball team.

Just prior to my meeting with Eleanor that morning, I had been called by the psychiatry department's director of residency training "to alert you that we are having a problem with one of our third-year residents." I was disappointed with the behavior of that resident and its effects on his care of patients. Given the scope of my administrative responsibilities, it was a relatively minor issue, but somehow Eleanor had picked up that I was disturbed.

> **Dr. Y.:** You have radar, Eleanor. I am somewhat upset by a problem that one of our trainees is having. I am sure that it will turn out OK. I didn't realize that my feelings were that apparent.
> **Eleanor Lai:** Oh, you'd be surprised about what I pick up on, Dr. Y. Most of the time I wish I didn't. But I can't help it.

This was not the first time that Eleanor had detected and was distracted by relatively minor changes in my mood and demeanor. I found the accuracy of Eleanor's "special sensitivity" to me unsettling and mildly annoying. However, in a circuitous route, it helped to explain clinical observations and answer a theoretical question that I had long pondered: Why do many people with severe problems related to overpleasing others have good self-esteem, generous, supportive families, and no significant histories of childhood abuse or trauma?

Although Eleanor certainly had very low self-esteem that was directly related to her history of being abused by her mother, she did not have a trace of several types of personality disorder that also are commonly tied to a history of childhood trauma and poor attachment to a parent. My link to answering this question came through an exploration of the concept of *mentalization*, which I will review briefly in the next section.

About Mentalization

Mentalization is a concept used in psychology and psychiatry that refers to a person's ability to understand the current mental state of oneself and others during interactions and relationships. A simple way of defining the term is *holding mind in mind* (Allen et al. 2008, p. 3). Mentalization enables a person to be aware of the mental state of others while simultaneously being conscious of his or her own psychological reactions to that person and his or her state of mind.

People with certain psychiatric disorders have difficulties mentalizing. These problems with mentalization are detailed in the following sections.

Hypomentalization

People who exhibit *hypomentalization* (also termed *undermentalizing*) attend primarily to what is going on in their own minds but have profound difficulties with attending to what is going on in the minds of others with whom they interact (Crespi and Badcock 2008). They often are not facile at interpreting social cues such as facial expressions, eye gaze, or body language. As a result, they tend to think and respond to others in concrete ways and have difficulties in seeing things from other people's points of view.

Because they are focused solely on their own immediate thoughts, wants, and needs to the exclusion of others, people with autistic spectrum disorders do not relate well to most others. For example, a 7-year-old child with autism might forcibly take away a toy from a classmate without considering, noticing, or caring how that action will upset or otherwise affect the other child. The profound problems that people who hypomentalize have in participating in group settings relate to their underinterpreting and, therefore, ignoring the mental states and behaviors of the others in their group.

Hypermentalization

Hypermentalization (also termed *overmentalizing*) is excessive, inaccurate mentalizing (Sharp et al. 2011). It occurs when a person becomes oversensitive to and overvigilant of what is going on in the minds of others. Hypermentalization is the result of distortions and misinterpretations of the mental states of others, which leads that individual to feel insecure or unsafe. Psychoanalysts and research scientists Peter Fonagy and Carla Sharp have been pioneers in our understanding of this state (Fonagy et al. 2000; Sharp et al. 2007, 2011). They posit and have scientifically demonstrated that some people with certain types of personality disorder, such as borderline personality disorder, have difficulties with mentalization that stem from personal histories of having experienced childhood trauma and abuse. As children, they have had difficulties making secure attachments with their caregivers, and as adults they suffer from the effects of having poor mentalization skills. For example, they might *misinterpret* what is going on in the minds of others and, consequently, become confused, fearful, or irritated. On the other hand, most people who have had the benefit of secure attachments usually demonstrate normal mentalization functions.

People with certain types of psychoses, especially schizophrenia, also have severe problems involving *hypermentalization*. These individuals have brain-based deficits that impair their perceptions (hallucinations) and their interpretations of reality (delusions), and consequently, they often feel vulnerable, unsafe, and fearful. Many structural and functional brain differences have been identified involving people with schizophrenia. Functional brain imaging research conducted by investigators in the Menninger Department of Psychiatry of Baylor College of Medicine has also demonstrated that people with borderline personality disorder have abnormalities in the anterior insular region of the brain. This impairment has been linked to the following dysfunction: "…norms used in perception of social gestures are pathologically perturbed or missing altogether among individuals with BPD [borderline personality disorder]" (King-Casas et al. 2008, p. 806). People with hypermentalization have problems participating in group settings that relate to their overinterpreting and, therefore, distort the mental states and behaviors of the others in their group.

Impaired Mentalization: Nature and Nurture

Extensive evidence from basic neuroscience research and from functional brain imaging in humans has confirmed that not only does brain biology profoundly affect human experience but also human experience affects brain biology and brain structure. Most people with severely impaired mental functions have *both* biological/genetic predispositions *and* experiential stresses. Nonetheless, there are exceptions to this general rule. Some people with autistic spectrum disorder or schizophrenia have severely impaired mentalization skills but do *not* have identifiable hereditary histories or neurobiological dysfunctions. Similarly, some individuals with borderline personality disorder do *not* have histories of childhood trauma or abuse. Interestingly, although Eleanor's childhood trauma was nearly identical to that of many people with borderline personality disorder, she did not meet diagnostic criteria for that condition nor for any other type of personality disorder. In fact, she demonstrated almost none of the traits that are characteristic of personality disorders.

Over the past 40 years I have cared for and known people who have significant problems with overpleasing others but who have grown up in loving, supportive, nurturing families. Accordingly, I am led to ask, "Can biology and/or life experience influence mentalization in other ways that lead to overpleasing others, along with all of its characteristic features and problems?" I believe that I have learned the answer to this question with a concept that I have termed *supermentalization.*

Supermentalizers

Supermentalizers: A Misnomer

I have long believed that the term *mentalization* and all of its related verbs, gerunds, participles, and other grammatical forms are misnomers. People with impairments of *mentalization* not only have incapacities in keeping the *minds* of themselves and of others in mind but also in taking into account their own *feelings* and those others.

Therefore, many people with impairments of so-called *mentalization* have major problems with compassion and empathy. Examples include people in the severe range of autistic spectrum disorder; selected, but not all, people with psychotic disorders; and certain others who have personality disorders, the most obvious being antisocial personality disorder and narcissistic personality disorder. Although several key researchers are quite aware that mentalization-based disorders involve *emotion blindness* as well as mind blindness, the focus of most research and clinical work is on the cognitive dysfunctions associated with mentalization. Nevertheless, I will bow to convention in order to enhance communication by labeling the condition we are now discussing *supermentalization.*

What Is Supermentalization?

There are four truisms with regard to special skills or gifts:

1. With all skills—whether hitting a curve ball, drawing a giraffe, playing the accordion, writing a novel, dancing the rumba, solving an equation, singing opera, playing a video game, swimming the butterfly, or repairing a heart valve—some of us are challenged, others are competent, and a small minority are truly gifted.
2. With all skills, there is a small but infinitely important difference between an accomplished amateur and a gifted professional.
3. With all gifts, great potential can be enhanced appreciably by prodigious effort and devoted practice.
4. With all special gifts, there are downsides as well as the more obvious upsides.

I propose that these truisms apply to the capacity to mentalize as well.

An example of the paradox of a downside to a special gift was right before my eyes for many years. It involved my oldest daughter, Elisa Eliot, who is now a professional actress and singer. Elisa is blessed with perfect pitch. As a very young child, Elisa refused to sing in public, including during the entirety of grade school. It was only later that Elisa confided to her mother and me how much it bothered her to hear people sing off key and how embarrassed she would be if she were to do so herself in public. As a result of her special gift, Elisa put a lot of pressure on herself and missed out on a lot of fun, as well.

As reviewed above, although most of us have intact abilities to mentalize, there are others whose impairments in mentalization, such as hypomentalism and hypermentalism, are associated with serious psychiatric disorders. I propose that there are also a very small number among us who are exceptional—gifted, if you will—in their aptitudes for mentalization. I have termed these people supermentalizers, defined as follows: At rare and exceptional levels, supermentalizers not only keep the *minds* of themselves and others in mind but also the *feelings* of themselves and others in their minds and feelings.

All of the aforementioned truisms that apply to special skills and gifts also apply to people who are *supermentalizers.*

Who Are Supermentalizers, and Where Can They Be Found?

The short answer is that, although rare and generally low-key, supermentalizers are represented in nearly all walks of life. Just as higher concentrations of people who are gifted with hand-eye coordination can be found at the highest levels of professional sports such as baseball and tennis, supermentalizers are more widely represented among the most successful professionals of all stripes. When channeled constructively, supermentalization can be an extraordinary asset, especially for those who make their livings by being simultaneously aware of what is on the minds and in the feelings of others and of themselves—such as poets, theologians, educators, and psychotherapists. Great leaders in many fields often have this special ability.

What Are Supermentalizers Like?

Although they may appear to be no different from other people, supermentalizers are different from most of us in many important ways. To understand this difference, you must imagine yourself as having the ability to read the minds and feelings of others, although all supermentalizers fall far short of accomplishing this completely. Nonetheless, they pick up a great deal from their interactions with others, far more than most people without their special abilities. And a lot of what supermentalizers perceive from unsuspecting others leaves them anxious and highly uncomfortable. Unless they are employing their skills constructively as professionals, most supermentalizers tell me that they would be far better off *not knowing* what they accurately pick up from unwitting others.

For example, I know a woman who is a talented and successful professional, shy and modest, strikingly beautiful, and a supermentalizer. She intensely dislikes attending social occasions—especially dinners—where she does not know the people with whom she will be interacting. For many years she was not aware of the reasons for her social discomfort. However, she did pick up, quite clearly, that many of the other women at these social occasions hated her. Modest and secure, she just did not understand why they hated her. Her response was to remain quiet and passive in social settings and, where possible, to avoid them altogether.

A second example is another close friend who is a gifted physician and supermentalizer who is the chairman of a department in a prestigious medical school. The members of the faculty at that medical school are notoriously competitive, giving rise to the ironic characterization "At John Doe Medical School, a friend is someone who stabs you in the stomach." This physician is painfully aware that many of his colleagues, while trying to appear friendly and respectful, envy, devalue, and wish the very worst for him. He once told me, "I spend my work days dumbing down what I perceive and feel. That's the most difficult part of my job."

Some Common Characteristics of Supermentalizers

Supermentalizers share many common characteristics. First of all, they have sharpened sensory perception and awareness. In other words, they have finely tuned hearing and are attentive listeners; they are careful, systematic observers; and, often, they are even supersensitive to tastes, smells, and how things feel. They are highly cognizant of the behavioral and emotional patterns of others and notice when these patterns change. For example, supermentalizers carefully monitor the body language, speech patterns, and mental associations of others. When they detect changes from the normal patterns, they are excellent at figuring out what has brought about these changes.

As exemplified by professional athletes, musicians, and artists—professions in which special talents tend to run in families—there are often several members of a given family who are supermentalizers. The nature of the communications among two individuals in the same family who are supermentalizers often approaches "extrasensory" or paranormal. When they are together, these individuals complete one another's sentences and do not need to be told what is on the other's mind, no matter how remote the thought or idea is from the topic of that moment. They find it to be useless to try to hide a problem or an apprehensive feeling from one another. Even when apart, they may think about similar subjects simultaneously. They can be so quick at sensing important, unforeseen family occurrences that it often seems that they know something has transpired before it actually happens. As with other senses—such as vision, hearing, or touch—supermentalism comes naturally and feels "natural" to those with this ability. They often take their special facility for granted and are surprised when they learn that others don't have this capacity.

The plot thickens, however, when there is just one supermentalizer in the family. That individual does, indeed, seem to be able to read the minds and feelings of his or her close relations, who find it spooky and irritating. Members of their family feel as if their boundaries are constantly being violated, as though they live in a house with glass walls and no doors. The problem is that supermentalizers can't help what they are so clearly perceiving any more than they can willfully turn on and off their vision or hearing without wearing blindfolds or earplugs. In the case of supermentalizers, however, blockade of their special sensibilities would require general anesthesia.

The interactions of supermentalizers with most people who are not in their immediate family are vastly different from how they relate to family members. Supermentalizers have learned from bitter experience not to acknowledge directly to others what they are perceiving, whether good or bad. In our communications with most others, there is an expectation of a mutuality of perceptions and reality testing, and when that is not achieved, uncomfortable dissonance develops. For example, when someone with supermentalizing ability accurately picks up that another person is not in the best of moods, there is a tendency for that person to deny the truth and resent the intrusion. Because of their awareness of this phenomenon, supermentalizers tend to hold back on most things and, therefore, appear to others as shy, reserved, withholding, or even snobbish.

Supermentalizers do not limit their special perceptive capacities to what others are thinking or feeling about them but also sense what others are feeling in general. This applies to human suffering. Supermentalizers, therefore, tend to be among the most empathic and compassionate of all people. As such, they are often at the forefront of recognizing and taking action to help others in need, even in circumstances that endanger their own safety and well-being.

Many also tend to be deeply affected emotionally by what they perceive and may themselves require the support and protection of others. In treatment, I try to help people who suffer from various ramifications of their supermentalizing facilities negotiate the line between social withdrawal and overexposure to the painful realities and tragedies of the human condition. For example, it might be too upsetting for a nurse who is a supermentalizer to work on a pediatric cancer unit, but he could serve quite ably on a geriatric medicine service where it can be less demoralizing and where the elderly respond so therapeutically to compassionate caregivers.

Finally, because supermentalizers are so finely attuned to the wishes and wants of others and because they have such refined empathic facility, many of them have problems with overpleasing others. Thus, although they arrive at overpleasing others by a different route from those who have low self-esteem and histories of trauma and/or impaired attachments, the results are practically indistinguishable. Thus, supermentalizers frequently manifest all 20 of the common features of people who are stuck in pleasing others, as summarized in Table 11–2.

What Are Some Examples of the Special Problems That Supermentalizers Have?

Subtle, mildly dysfunctional behavioral patterns are omnipresent in supermentalizers' daily lives, and most can be traced to their need to overplease. Let us consider, for example, their shopping patterns at department stores. Supermentalizers will waste time looking for items because they do not want to "bother" the store's personnel. They also deny all requests of salespeople to help them choose among potential purchases because they will feel great pressure to buy exactly what the salesperson is suggesting. In general, they have very low sales resistance because, if they demur from an acquisition, they can detect clearly the disappointment of the salesperson. No matter what the problem with an item or how recently it was purchased, supermentalizers are reticent to return purchases to department stores. Family members will fruitlessly explain to them that the department store has return policies expressly because they want to satisfy their customers. That does not matter to supermentalizers because they just cannot endure experiencing the displeasure of the personnel who work in the exchange department.

Going out to eat in restaurants is an ordeal for supermentalizers. If, for example, their waiter seems unhappy or overstressed for *any* reason—known or unknown—their meal will be ruined. It matters not how good the food is. They grit their teeth as the waiter reviews the specials of the day because they feel great pressure to go along with the suggestions, whether or not that choice seems appealing to them.

Supermentalizers would never dream of asking waiters for anything "extra," such as another serving of bread, some special seasoning, or even for their glass of water to be refilled. They would rather go hungry than mention that something is wrong with their food—even if someone else's choice is placed in front of them by mistake. They do not bother to tabulate the bill that is presented to them because they would never point out any mistake to the waiter. When dining with others, supermentalizers will *always* pick up the check—even if they have paid the last several times they have gone to dinner with the other diners. No matter how poor the service, they overtip ridiculously in order to avoid the disappointment or, heaven forbid, the resentment of their waiters. Given these self-imposed barriers, supermentalizers do whatever possible to avoid going out to eat. It is a torment. If, for some reason, they are compelled to go to a restaurant, they will go to one where they are familiar to the staff, and they will always order the same thing. Therefore, no one is disappointed. They feel it is a good thing when a waiter doesn't even bother to bring them a menu.

Supermentalism, Trauma, and Treatment

First 6 Months of Treatment

Let us now return to the case of Eleanor Lai. Not only was Eleanor a supermentalizer, with the innate gift of being exceptionally sensitive to the cognitions and feelings of others, but she also was primed during her childhood and young adulthood to monitor closely the moods of her mother to assay her personal safety. As discussed, her attentiveness to and perceptions of my frame of mind and reactions during all of our sessions were fine-tuned and highly accurate. She had little ability to tolerate my slightest dissonance or disagreement. It is no wonder, therefore, that she reacted so strongly to her peers who were threatened by her many assets.

Eleanor's superior talents at dance evoked the competitive enmity of her peers at the Houston High School for the Performing and Visual Arts, and her lithe beauty and academic brilliance aroused the retaliation—disguised as helpful concern—of her roommates at Harvard. Although Eleanor was usually naïve as to the true source of the disapproval of her peers (i.e., her exceptionalism), she was, nonetheless, especially aware of and vulnerable to their acerbic displeasure with her. In these situations, her level of anxiety welled so high that she was willing to do almost anything to mitigate her peers' displeasure with her. Ultimately, however, Eleanor's self-destruction was the only thing that would please these secretive conspirators, and she unconsciously, obediently obliged.

Eleanor's treatment advanced in stages. First, her devastating family situation was stabilized by establishing a protective legal and physical buffer between her and her abusive mother. Next, her weight was stabilized by her work in psychotherapy in close collaboration with her dietitian. Third, she began her reentry into the academic and dancing domains by returning as resident instructor at the Houston Ballet Academy, where she soon returned to a performance level that permitted her to practice with the professional members of the dance company.

During our treatment, her interactions and involvements with others steadily increased. She continued to work at her volunteer teaching job at the Houston middle school, and issues with her students and their parents and with her instructors and school administrators inevitably emerged. She returned to the Houston Ballet Academy as both a volunteer teacher and a company dancer. Predictably, Eleanor's many difficulties associated with her overpleasing came to the fore in this competitive environment. These all provided grist for the mill of our 4-days-per-week psychotherapy sessions, as we analyzed and worked to develop new skills at dealing with these problems and preventing their future occurrences.

Eighteenth Month of Treatment

Eleanor approached her psychotherapy as she would learning a new dance in ballet: openly, earnestly, and tenaciously. Intelligent and curious, Eleanor readily absorbed and applied the new concepts and behavioral changes that I suggested and progressed rapidly in treatment. Never before did she have the "luxury" of being able to concentrate on dancing nearly full time, and she attained new heights of technical accomplishment, which were recognized by the dance masters and administrative leaders at the Academy and in the company. Given her talent and love of dancing, she was confronted with considerable external and internal pressure to concentrate on dancing and to defer returning to Harvard for the foreseeable future.

Struggling with this classic approach-approach conflict, Eleanor and I decided to invite her father to one of our sessions to gain the benefit of his input, wisdom, and love.

Dr. Y.: It has been a long time since we have visited, Dr. Lai. I am delighted to meet with you again and to catch up on so many things.

Dr. Leonard Lai: So very much has happened. Most important, Eleanor is not going to die. I thank you with all of my heart, Professor Y.

Dr. Y.: Eleanor did all the hard work. As you know so well, Dr. Lai, you have a remarkable daughter.

Dr. Leonard Lai: My mother and father in China are great people. Eleanor is like them. We will go to China to visit them this summer. Eleanor has not seen her grandparents since she was very little baby. We are so excited.

Dr. Y.: Please catch me up on what has been going on with you, Dr. Lai.

Dr. Leonard Lai: I am now a happy man. I work full time in the medical school—75% research and 25% clinical work and teaching. I sold my company for very much money. Eleanor is now very rich person. But she is like her father. She doesn't care too much about money. Our family has been poor for thousands of years in China. Still very good people. Only one who cares about money is Ruth. She is now in jail for 7 years for fraud to American government. Ruth always called me a communist. She was wrong. I was never a communist. She is the communist. Communists love money but hate freedom. Ruth has much money and is not free.

Dr. Y.: Eleanor, why don't you tell your father why you invited him to join us today?

Eleanor Lai: I want your advice, Daddy. I don't know whether to return to Harvard next year or to concentrate on my dancing full time. Now that I am so much better, I think that either one would be great for my growth as a person.

Dr. Leonard Lai: I think it is better for you to be a scholar. Chinese people respect learning more than dancing. You must agree, Professor Y.? You love to learn too.

> **Dr. Y.:** I know what's right for me, Dr. Lai, but not what's better for Eleanor. You and she would know that better than I. But it might be possible for her to do both. Eleanor has the ability and drive to accomplish that at a high level.
>
> **Eleanor:** I know that you mentioned that a long time ago. But it seemed so unrealistic at the time, I was not paying much attention.... But I don't apologize!
>
> **Dr. Y.:** You could petition Harvard to let you return as a part-time student. I know that most universities make such exceptions for people with unusual talents in the arts or athletics. You certainly qualify for that, Eleanor. That would allow you to dance with the Boston Conservatory. If Harvard won't approve your petition, I know that Columbia and Barnard have a special program with Juilliard. I have had much experience at Columbia and am confident that they would love to have you join them.
>
> **Dr. Leonard Lai:** Best that you do what Professor Y. advises, Eleanor. We Chinese still respect our teachers.

Postscript

Eleanor's petition to Harvard to continue to pursue her degree as a part-time student was approved, and she also was accepted as a company dancer at the Boston Conservatory. Currently, she is flourishing in both worlds, although, for now, her dancing responsibilities are occupying most of her time. Her ultimate career goal is to become an educator, either in dance or in science. But that's not the big news.

Eleanor has a serious ongoing relationship with a graduate student at Harvard Business School. He is from China, and Eleanor did me the great honor of introducing him to me during a follow-up session on one of her visits to Houston. I found him to be very much like Eleanor and her father: modest, studious, and polite. In a very understated way and only because I inquired about his background and family, he informed me that his family owns of one of China's largest international construction companies. Their company, to which he is heir, specializes in building mammoth, complex projects including dams, highways, sports stadiums, oil refineries, nuclear reactors, and the like. Leonard later told me what he thought of the young man:

> **Dr. Leonard Lai:** I like Eleanor's boyfriend very much. We come from same type of people in China. My father also made big buildings in China—as a hand laborer.

Neither Leonard nor I have any idea about whether or not Ruth would approve of him. Eleanor said she doesn't care.

References

Allen JG, Fonagy, P, Bateman, AW: Mentalizing in Clinical Practice. American Psychiatric Publishing, Washington, DC, 2008

American Psychiatric Association: Diagnostic and Statistical Manual of Mental Disorders, 5th Edition. Washington, DC, American Psychiatric Association, 2013

Crespi B, Badcock C: Psychosis and autism as diametrical disorders of the social brain. Behav Brain Sci 31(3):241–320, 2008

Fonagy P, Target M, Gergely G: Atachment and borderline personality disorder: a theory and some evidence. Psychiatr Clin N Am 23:103–122, 2000

King-Casas B, Sharp C, Lomax-Bream L, et al: The rupture and repair of cooperation in borderline personality disorder. Science 321:806–810, 2008

Sharp C, Croudace TJ, Goodyer IM: Biased mentalizing in children aged 7–11: latent class confirmation of response styles to social scenarios and associations with psychopathology. Soc Dev 16:181–202, 2007

Sharp C, Pane H, Venta A, et al.: Theory of mind and emotion regulation difficulties in adolescents with borderline traits. J Am Acad Child Adolesc Psychiatry 50:563–573, 2011

Yudofsky, SC: Fatal Flaws: Navigating Destructive Relationships With People With Disorders of Personality and Character. American Psychiatric Publishing, Washington, DC, 2005

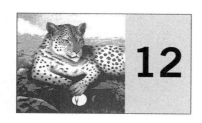

12

Stuck in Adolescence and Cyberspace, Part I (Discover): The Case of Lester Silber

When Autism Spectrum Disorder Is Complicated by Being Bullied

If I am not for myself, then who will be for me?
And if I am only for myself, then what am I?
And if not now, when?
—*Rabbi Hillel the Elder*

I am in blood stepped in so far that should I wade no more,
Returning were as tedious go o'er.
—*William Shakespeare*, Macbeth, *Act III, Scene 4*

"Who picked on you, Lester?"

Stuck in "My" Machines

i expend my life—
    what's left of me—
    awakening by Machines,
    listening to Machines,
    playing on Machines,
    measuring with Machines,
    working for Machines,
    courting on Machines,

counting on Machines

    racing in Machines,
    running on Machines,
    rushing to Machines,
    and, mostly,
    gazing at Machines
    for
    ways to touch you.

But they won't let me.

"Smile for the Picture!
Stand still,
or you'll be blurred!"

"Look at the Phone,
not at me, Silly!
At "my" Cell Phone!"

i expend my life—
what's left of me—
searching "my" Machines,
checking "my" Machines,
begging "my" Machines,

counting on "my" machines

    to help me find you;
    to help me know you;
    to let me hear you;
    to let me see you;
    to let me reach you;
    to let me

Be
with you

in a sound,
or
in a symbol
on a screen.

But you're not there,
even when you're here;

and i'm not here,
even when i touch you;

even when I *am* you.

Do "our" Machines come between us?
No, that could never be.

Must be our damn connection!

The Case of Lester Silber: D1 (Discover) Assessment Component

"Plain Vanilla" Problems

The call came from Mr. Jack Edelstein, a patient whom I had treated many years previously. A prominent commercial real estate developer, he is known in his field as "Jack the Hammer."

> **Mr. Jack Edelstein:** Good afternoon, Stuart. I know you are always busy, so I will get right to the point. I'm asking you for a favor. I would like you to treat the 24-year-old son of dear friends of mine and Janice. The father, Ken Silber, is an invaluable technical consultant to me for several of my businesses. The problem is that their son is a basket case, but he won't accept any help. His parents are worried to death about him. He's ruining their lives. Would you meet with the Silbers to give them some guidance?
>
> **Dr. Y.:** Of course I will, Jack. Just have them call my office. How are you and Janice?
>
> **Jack Edelstein:** I know you don't have time for niceties, Stuart. Neither do I. Let's both get back to work. And by the way....

Dr. Y.: Yes, Jack?

Jack Edelstein: Some shrink once told me that I don't express my appreciation enough. So, thank you, Stuart.

About a week later my sainted administrative assistant, Mrs. Hoffman, introduced me to Marsha and Kenneth Silber just as they were jumping to attention from their seats in the waiting area of my office. With his thinning gray hair parted ruler-straight, with the perfectly symmetrical Windsor knot of his Brooks Brothers tie lynched to his larynx, and with the Solingen steel–sharpened creases of his gray summer-weight suit knifing perilously toward his crotch, Mr. Silber could have modeled for a 1950 Norman Rockwell cover of *Accounting Today*. Mrs. Silber anxiously spewed forth more "Thank yous" on the short walk from the waiting room to my office than Jack the Hammer Edelstein bestows in a decade.

Mr. Kenneth Silber: Marsha and I are so grateful to you for seeing us. We are absolutely desperate about our son, Lester. It is a very, very long story, Doctor, which I will try to make short. He's 24 years old now and has been nearly dysfunctional for the past 6 years. We are afraid he is getting dangerously close to a dead end.

Dr. Y.: What exactly do you mean by "a dead end"?

Kenneth Silber: It's just a feeling that Marsha and I have had lately. We sense that he is getting desperate. For years we have been supporting him completely, and he does nothing. He used to have some loser friends he hung around with, but he doesn't even see them anymore. Now he just sits around and plays video games day and night. Mostly at night. He refuses even to try to get a job. He won't go see a psychiatrist for help, even though we've begged him to do so for years. He lives in a modest townhouse that we own. It's a pigsty. He looks and dresses like a homeless person.

A few months ago, some of our friends encouraged us to give Lester what they called "tough love." They said to cut off our support of him completely, so he would be forced to fend for himself. When we told him we would stop giving him any money unless he got a job or saw a counselor, he just said that he didn't care. We wanted to talk to you before stopping his money. We're afraid he might do something to himself.

Dr. Y.: Has he ever been suicidal or self-destructive in any way?

Kenneth Silber: Thankfully, not yet. But he is wasting years from his life being so unproductive. That's a kind of suicide, isn't it?

Although every person is unique and there are subtle—but important—differences in each psychiatric problem, Lester's troubles had familiar trappings. Representative examples of what other parents have told me over the years include the following:

- "Our kid was completely normal until he fell in with the wrong crowd during high school."
- "When he started smoking marijuana, everything changed. He changed. He lost all motivation. Don't let anybody ever tell you that marijuana is safe."
- "All he did in college was go to parties, drink, and hang out with his friends. We were shocked to learn that he didn't even show up at most of his classes in his second semester. No surprise that he failed out of school. Even though we have been told repeatedly by his teachers that he is extremely bright but an underachiever."
- "My son doesn't do anything productive these days. And all of his friends are just like him. All they do is drink beer, smoke pot, stay up all night, and spend most of their time on the Internet or playing video games on their computers."

Mrs. Marsha Silber: As you can probably tell, Doctor, I am a nervous wreck over this. The truth is that I haven't had much of a life for many years. All I do is worry about Lester. I can't make myself stop worrying. I worry about him when I go to sleep, and I wake up with a sick feeling in my stomach knowing that nothing has changed.

Lester's sister, Rebecca, is so upset with me. She is 4 years older than Lester and has pretty much given up on him. She has done everything right in her life, but she says I can't seem to get any pleasure from that. She says I never pay attention to what's going on in *her* life, only to Lester's problems. Tragically, she's probably right.

Mr. Kenneth Silber: Marsha and I just can't figure out what went wrong. Or what we did wrong in parenting Lester. We think he was always loved and supported. He grew up in the same home as his sister, Rebecca, and like Marsha says, she is doing great. The best we know, nothing traumatic ever happened to Lester, or to any of us. As a family, we're pretty much plain vanilla ice cream.

Dr. Y.: Let's not get ahead of ourselves. Before we speculate about causes, we need to identify exactly what the problems are. To accomplish that, I will need to meet with Lester, and he will have to cooperate. Did you invite Lester to join us at our meeting today?

Kenneth Silber: Yes. We practically begged him on our hands and knees to come with us today. He wouldn't hear of it. Yesterday, we were so desperate to get him to come with us to see you that we even considered asking Rabbi Berg to call Lester. Rabbi Berg is retired, but Lester looked up to him for many years before his bar mitzvah. We finally decided not to bother Rabbi Berg. Lester wouldn't have listened to him anyway. He stopped listening to good people many years ago. Doctor, do you think that we should try that "tough love" thing?"

Dr. Y.: Modifying the word "love" with angry-sounding adjectives will be confusing. The words "tough love" will carry mixed messages for both of you and for Lester. No matter how you rationalize it, you will feel guilty about exercising so-called "tough love." Lester will sense your guilt and mixed feelings and may try to manipulate you in self-destructive ways.

What we want to understand is how to motivate Lester to help himself. As paradoxical as it may sound, let's try to find a way for him to have *more* control, not *less* control. From what you tell me, he seems to be motivated to play video games. How motivated is he by these games?

Kenneth Silber: Very much so. I would say he's addicted to them. We rarely stop by his place without seeing him on his computer absorbed in playing these war games. He has told me that he is on a team of other players from all over the world, and they compete with other teams. He plays with a computer keyboard and stares at this gigantic flat-screen TV monitor where all the action takes place. There are expensive speakers all around the room, and they are turned up way loud. It looks and sounds like you are in a movie theater watching a battle scene from *Saving Private Ryan.*

The only thing Lester and I do together these days is to install or fix equipment for his video games. He used to be very good technically, but he got rusty. Sometimes, when his computer crashes he calls me to help him fix it. He makes it sound like there's some kind of emergency. Like he is having a heart attack, God forbid.

Dr. Y.: What do you think he would do if it were inconvenient for him to play his computer games?

Kenneth Silber: To put it mildly, he would be upset. What do you have in mind?

Dr. Y.: Lester is stuck, and he seems to have no motivation to pull himself out of the mire. We need to help motivate him to make some healthful choices. I assume that you pay the electric bills in your townhouse where he lives and plays his computer games. Why not give him *the choice* of accepting professional help or cutting off his electricity? That won't endanger him or even cause him too much discomfort in December in Houston. If he refuses my help, he will "only" have to go somewhere else to play. It will be inconvenient, and the game technology would be compromised. His choice, however. I think that you will feel far better about doing that than taking away his support for food and shelter.

Kenneth Silber: What should we say when he calls us and demands that we turn the electricity back on?

Dr. Y.: Before you cut off his electricity, meet with Lester in the townhouse and tell him that you love him deeply and unconditionally. In addition, tell him that you realize that are not helping him by supporting his current lifestyle. Worse, you both are anguished because you are afraid that you are harming him through your unconditional support. Let Lester know that you have had to learn that unconditional love and unconditional support are not one and the same.

Kenneth Silber: Then what?

Dr. Y.: Let him know that you will not turn his electricity off if he seeks professional help with me. That means that he must attend his therapy sessions at the frequency prescribed by his doctor and that he must participate in good faith. As long as he continues to work in his treatment, your support will be the same as always. The most important thing to communicate is that *the choice is entirely his, not yours.*

Mrs. Marsha Silber: Not having electricity seems like "tough love" to me.

Dr. Y.: Lester is 24 years old, and he is doing nothing to support himself—currently, or for the future. You are taking care of everything for him. Not providing electricity for him—*if he so chooses*—doesn't sound so "tough" to me.

Kenneth Silber: Boy, do I agree with you, Doctor! I think it's a great idea except for one detail. If he chooses to come to see you for treatment, won't he still be playing video games day and night?

Dr. Y.: Ideally, I would like to begin treatment *while* he is still playing the games. I want to learn directly from him what he is *getting* from these games, before we discuss what he is *missing* on their account. That process will sharpen our *discovery* of what he can't seem to derive from so-called "real life."

So I hope he chooses to see me right after you present him with his choices so that the electricity need not be turned off at all. As with many other types of addiction, it probably would be best if his withdrawal from video games is tapered—as opposed to being stopped abruptly—or "cold turkey" as it is called with drugs.

I am no authority on video games and would like to be prepared when Lester calls on me, as I am confident he will do at some point. Would you happen to know the video games that he plays most frequently?

Kenneth Silber: He plays only one game these days: World of Warcraft.

Dr. Y.: Please give me 2 weeks to begin to learn about this game and related games before offering Lester his choice.

Supervision

The continuing education of psychiatrists and other medical and mental health professionals is essential. For those psychiatrists who are certified, periodic recertification through standardized written testing is required to maintain certification. Most of us are aware that this process is a fairly good measure of our keeping up with the ever-advancing *knowledge base* of our field, but what about the *skill base* that is so essential for us to be at the top of our profession? What about the indispensible *art* of our craft? That cannot be measured by any written test of which I am aware.

Therefore, many of us seek out what we call supervision from the most gifted of our colleagues to assure ourselves that we are providing optimal care—knowledge, skill, and art—for our patients. We usually present a patient whom we are currently treating and for whom we believe we could use help in that patient's care. Most often, we schedule weekly hour-long meetings with our supervisor on an ongoing basis and pay the supervisor his or her regular clinical fee each time we meet.

Although I was aware that an ever-growing number of people were experiencing a vast array of psychiatric problems related to computer games, had read scientific papers and had attended scientific presentations related to these problems, I knew almost nothing about the computer games per se. I therefore sought out counsel from Mr. Ronald Bronner, a brilliant young computer scientist and engineer with training in neuroscience. Mr. Bronner understands the fundamental elements of how the games are created to attract, entertain, and hold the interest of players.

> **Mr. Ronald Bronner:** Are you telling me that you have never played a computer game, Dr. Y.? Not even a simple game on your cell phone?
>
> **Dr. Y.:** Yes.
>
> **Ronald Bronner:** Then it will not be sufficient for you just to read up on these games; you must learn to play them yourself. Only then can you really understand what your patients are experiencing.
>
> **Dr. Y.:** I have not been addicted to a drug or dependent on alcohol but still do my best to treat people with these problems.
>
> **Ronald Bronner:** Not a fair comparison. You know a great deal about the neurobiology of alcohol and drugs, and I assume that you have, at the very least, tried legal drugs like caffeine and alcohol. I also assume that you have taken a prescribed pain medication.
>
> I will set up a video game station in your home and will take you through a series of gaming experiences that you must have in order to understand what your patients are getting from their play—both the good and the bad things. There is just no way around it but through it, Dr. Y.

Exactly 2 weeks after our meeting, Mr. Kenneth Silber e-mailed me that he was about to present Lester with the choice of having electricity in his apartment or having treatment with me. The next day Lester called to schedule an appointment.

"It"

Although unable to find Lester's eyes through the uncut, oily black hair that clumped about his pallid forehead and cheeks like patches of tar on a white sand beach, I was confident that they were cast toward his torn, laceless sneakers. Without uttering a word or acknowledging the gesture, Lester slumped with obedient reluctance into the office chair toward which I had beckoned with open right hand and outstretched right arm. After a few minutes, I broke the silence.

> **Dr. Y.:** What's "it" stand for?

Lester started to look up toward me but, reconsidering in midmotion, looked back toward his sneakers.

> **Lester Silber:** Huh?
>
> **Dr. Y.:** I am referring to your World of Warcraft T-shirt.

Rivaling his hair and sneakers for unkempt, filthy raggedness was his bleached-out, blotchy, once-black T-shirt that proclaimed in confrontational red font, "Warriors do it with RAGE!" I was grateful that my video game supervision with Ronald Bronner was giving me some bearings in Lester's adoptive world.

A true "gamer," Lester mumbled a disinterested challenge:

> **Lester Silber:** Whatever you want it to mean, Doc. What would you like it to say?
> **Dr. Y.:** That's your call, Lester; it's your shirt. If I were wearing a T-shirt today, it would say, "We're on the same TEAM."

Responding in a tone dripping with disgust, Lester said,

> **Lester Silber:** Warriors don't pull the plug on their buds.
> **Dr. Y.:** That's the difference between tactics and strategy, Lester.
> **Lester:** Huh?
> **Dr. Y.:** Tactics occur below the shoulders, and strategy takes place above the shoulders. Pulling the plug on a bud might turn out to be the best thing a "bud" ever did for his friend. Better even than shooting some electronic enemy the instant it pops up on his screen. Besides, no plugs have been pulled. You still have your electricity.

Lester shifted uncomfortably in his chair. His body language revealed to me that he was angry with himself for venturing even this far into my unpredictable world: a world with unfair, inexact rules; a world that he couldn't control; a world into which he did not fit; a world that he despised.

Supersaturated with contempt, his rage was contagious. I struggled to keep my feelings in check. I tried to remain aware that before me was a pale, scrawny, physically defenseless young man, not some slimy night crawler for me to pull from its filthy dark hole to skewer on my psychiatric fishhook. I had to keep in mind that the picture that he was projecting to me and to the rest of the world mirrored how he believed that he had been treated. A reflection of how he would want me to treat him in order to confirm his victimized, defeatist, escapist world view. I elected to remain quiet for a while, and Lester chose to do the same. Finally, I pierced our membrane of silence with an exploratory probe.

Dr. Y.: Who picked on you, Lester?

For the first time, he couldn't keep himself from looking up at me. I didn't expect him to respond, so after a few more seconds of his silence, I continued.

> **Dr. Y.:** So far, Lester, you haven't told me a whole lot about your-self—just what I can see and sense. But that tells me more than you might imagine. It tells me that you were picked on in grade school; scapegoated in middle school; and, worst of all, pretty much ignored in high school and college. But there is a big problem with the world you have chosen to live in.
> **Lester Silber:** Yeah, what's my problem?
> **Dr. Y.:** Your problem, Lester, is that you are not *really* doing "it" with anyone. Not with "rage" or with anything else. Although I am pretty certain that what I said is correct, I don't expect you to agree with me…at least not yet. All that I would like you to do at this point is to answer my question.
> **Lester:** I forgot what you asked.
> **Dr. Y.:** Who picked on you?

After another prolonged silence, he spoke.

> **Lester Silber:** Everyone.
> **Dr. Y.:** What's your first memory of being picked on?
> **Lester:** Doesn't some doctor slap you when you come out of your mother?
> **Dr. Y.:** Who's the first person you remember who picked on you, Lester?
> **Lester:** Why would I care? That was forever ago.

Lester Silber's flair for pushing people away was rivaled only by his facility for not letting people get close to him. Although related, these "defensive devices" are not the same. Lester's principal tools of alienation that pushed people away were argument and condescension, while his disaffection, avoidance, disinterest, and hopelessness isolated him even further. These defensive devices were all manifested in his response, "Why would I care?" His illusion of power derived from his negative attitude and stance as embodied in that question. There are two sides to this illusion of power:

1. He saw no reason to lower himself to respond meaningfully to my query.

2. I needed to convince him that both the question and I were worthy of a response. In both cases, Lester holds all the cards. As always when a patient poses a question to me—even one for which he does not expect a response—I did my best to answer it.

> **Dr. Y.:** Because you are a human being and because it hurt you deeply when you were excluded and picked on.

Lester seemed puzzled by my response, and I sensed that he was searching his mind for a retort. None came to his mind. Surprisingly to me and, I believe, to him, he actually answered my question:

> **Lester Silber:** My best friend, Jimmy Comstock.

Family Business

This sliver-sized opening permitted me, for the moment, to sidestep Lester's peppering me with pop-up power struggles by asking questions about his friend, Jimmy Comstock. In answering the questions, he provided important background information about himself and his family.

As a child, Lester had lived in the middle class Houston suburb of West University, which is near Rice University, where his father was on the computer science faculty. When Lester was 5 years old, Mr. Silber left academia in order to start his own computer servicing business. Mrs. Silber also began to work nearly full time to manage the front office of their fledgling enterprise. As a result, Mr. Silber began to be away from home for much longer hours than he had previously, and when he was at home, he was preoccupied with work. As the business grew, Mrs. Silber also brought home the unfinished paperwork of the day, and this work frequently spilled over into their weekends.

Much later in his treatment, when Lester had begun to talk with me in full sentences and even in paragraphs, he said,

> **Lester Silber:** I remember that both Dad and Mom were around our house almost all of the time until I was 5 years old. After they started the business, they were rarely around and had little idea about what was going on with me. They were the only parents who didn't show up at Honors Day at school when I got some math prize or science award. Mom would say, "We would have loved to be there, Lester, but we were working so hard to make Rebecca's and your lives better."

Jimmy Comstock lived next door to Lester, and their mothers were close friends. Since the time that they were infants, they would play together almost every day—in their homes or in the parks nearby. Jimmy was bigger, stronger, more coordinated, and more outgoing than Lester.

> **Lester Silber:** I definitely was the follower, never the leader. I always did what Jimmy wanted to do. And like all the other kids in our neighborhood, all he wanted to do was play baseball.

In the era when Lester grew up in West University, there were many children in his age group who played together in the several beautiful, well-equipped parks near his home. Little League baseball was and remains the center of the recreational universe of many, if not most, West University boys.

> **Lester Silber:** Jimmy's dad would play pitch and catch with us. Both Jimmy and his father threw the ball really hard. They kept saying, "get in front of the ball, Lester; don't run away from it." Every time I tried to do that, it would bounce and hit me in the face. And then they would laugh at me.

(At the time that Lester recounted this "get in front of the ball; don't run away from it" story, I thought that this baseball experience would later serve as an excellent metaphor for how he had adapted to the pain in his world through withdrawal and avoidance.)

At age 5, both Lester and Jimmy were enrolled in West University's Tadpole Division of Little League.

> **Lester Silber:** I remember clearly the first day of baseball tryouts for the Tadpoles. I couldn't believe how many kids my age were there. Must have been over 50 kids there with their parents. And they all were much bigger than I and all seemed to know each other really well. Even worse, they all were great at baseball. Everybody except me. When they were choosing up teams that day, Jimmy shouted in front of everybody, "Don't choose Lester! He plays baseball like a girl." And Jimmy was my best friend. My *only* friend.
> **Dr. Y.:** Well you managed to "do it" somehow, Lester. You turned yourself into a baseball.
> **Lester:** Huh? I don't have a clue what you're talking about.
> **Dr. Y.:** As your T-shirt says: You "do it with RAGE." These days

when people see you coming, they want to get out of your way. Like a hard-liner to third base. It works for you at a huge cost. You don't get hit in the face much these days, but I'm guessing you don't get kissed there either.

Connections in Psychiatry

After Lester told me about his first day of Little League, I was no longer repelled by his appearance or attitude. I had connected with his oceanic reservoir of hurt that had been dammed up and damned shut by murky deposits of the silt and sludge of countless taunts and rejections.

As stated in Chapter 4, "Stuck in My Job," and Chapter 7, "Stuck in My Marriage," I strive to connect with my patients through their strengths and through my appreciation of what they value most about themselves. Not through their problems. I believe that I also must communicate an emotional understanding of their agony before they will permit me the privilege of helping them find pathways to healing.

From the horrendous time and regulatory demands of modern medicine to our personal prejudices to the armored defenses of Lester Silber, there are always barriers to establishing this emotional connection. But the connection must be made, or our patients won't grant us the privilege to help them. And patients are not fooled by caregivers who *act* concerned or *feign* compassion, even if these clinicians are otherwise competent.

Lester somehow realized that I had some sense of the pain and humiliation that he had experienced thus far in life. Like a street vendor displaying his wares, I laid out before Lester what would be my approach to his treatment. He didn't refuse.

Bullied and Stoned

As did his older sister Rebecca, Lester attended West University Elementary School from kindergarten through the fifth grade and West University Middle School through the eighth grade. The township of West University is proximate to Rice University and to the Texas Medical Center, which is the largest medical complex in the world (currently comprising 54 member institutions, including 2 large medical schools, 5,000 physicians, 15,000 nurses, 5,700 research scientists who work full time, and $3.4 billion in annual research funding). Reflecting these demographics, many of Lester's classmates at West University Elementary School were the children of scientists, academicians, and medical professionals. One would have expected this to be an ideal environment for a child who had special aptitudes for science and mathematics. Although Lester excelled in all of his subjects, he recalled being quite unhappy.

> **Lester Silber:** I was not able to make friends, so I spent most of my time alone. I dreaded going to recess because I was the worst at everything. Also, I was usually the smallest kid in my class. Even when I was in the fifth grade, people thought I looked like a second grader. This made me the brunt of a lot of jokes and constant bullying.
>
> **Dr. Y.:** Please share with me some specific examples.
>
> **Lester:** I hardly know where to start. I don't remember ever being called by my own name in school. In elementary school, everybody called me "Silber Putty," mainly because I was so soft, weak, and uncoordinated. In middle school I was called "Lesser Sister" because people thought that I was gay.
>
> I was teased constantly by the boys and was the object of endless pranks. I could rarely walk to class without someone coming up behind me and knocking all my books and papers out of my hands. Much younger kids would trip me in the hallways, push me down the stairways, and hit me hard in the arm and stomach when I walked to school. They thought it was cool to be able to beat up someone so much older.
>
> If I ever came close to making a friend, that kid would be taunted and called a "fag." No surprise that no one wanted to have anything to do with me. I was often the only kid in the class who was not invited to parties, unless their parents made them invite me. When I got to the parties no one would talk to me, and I would end up standing alone by myself. Funny, I hated not being invited to parties, and I hated going there on the few occasions when I was invited.
>
> The girls treated me a bit better: they ignored me completely. I think they noticed the trash cans in the classrooms more than they noticed me. At least trash cans were of some use to them.
>
> **Dr. Y.:** Did you notice *them?*
>
> **Lester:** If you're asking me if I am gay, Dr. Y., I'm not. Although many times I wished I were gay. I envied the gay guys. They had many more friends than I ever had and seemed to be having a lot more fun. They could protect themselves from the boys better than I could, and the girls actually seemed to like them. By the time that I was in college, it had become cool to be gay. But it never became cool to be me. That's one thing that never changes.

Lester discovered two islands where he felt safe and valued. He was treated kindly and supportively by his teachers at West University Elementary School, and he responded by being a diligent student. He had excellent handwriting and was hard working and well organized. Lester appreciated the objectivity and rationality of science and mathematics, subjects in which he always was at the top of his classes. He also loved technology—especially computers—and took many online courses to learn computer programming.

When Lester was not doing his class work, he usually retreated to his second island of safety. This island was populated by an international group of online friends who shared his passion for computer technology and Internet-related frontiers. Although he never met these individuals in person, he believed them to be close and genuine friends. Lester therefore spent many hours alone in his bedroom, which, with all the computers, wires, and spare parts, looked like the storeroom of an electronics laboratory.

Just before Lester was to enter the ninth grade, his family moved to a newer and bigger home in the nearby neighborhood of Bellaire, which enabled him to attend Bellaire High School. His new school had a far larger student body, was a more socioeconomically diverse school than West University Middle School, and enjoyed one of the highest academic rankings among the public schools in Texas.

> **Lester Silber:** I didn't know anyone in Bellaire High, and I thought that was a great thing. I thought that I might be able to escape my image as a total loser and maybe even make some new friends.
>
> At first I was shocked and terrified by how enormous the school was and how big some of the students were. They looked like grownups to me. I wasn't bullied at all at Bellaire, and I wasn't noticed either. I felt I had escaped my past of being a totally weird geek and being hated.
>
> Eventually, I got to know a few guys who were into computers in the same way that I am. Of course, they were also geeks and nerds like me. I was surprised when I found out that most of them smoked pot. It wasn't long until I tried some.
>
> **Dr. Y.:** Do you remember how you felt on that occasion?
>
> **Lester:** Oh yes. I liked it. I could relax better.
>
> **Dr. Y.:** Are you more comfortable around other people when you smoke?
>
> **Lester:** It's more that I just don't care. But I wouldn't say I am any more social when I'm stoned. But what I really like is to be stoned when I play video games.

Dr. Y.: Why is that?

Lester: I'm really not sure. I think it helps me get into games more. It makes them more real and fun.

After his first experience with marijuana in the ninth grade, Lester slowly but progressively increased his smoking, in tandem with the increased time he spent playing video games. By the 11th grade he was playing World of Warcraft as soon as he came home from school, often not stopping until the early hours of the next morning. There were times that he stayed up all night doing cyber battle. For the first time that year, his grades fell slightly in some subjects—but not in his mathematics, physics, or computer courses. He also spent less time with his small group of friends.

Up in Smoke

During his years at West University Elementary and Middle Schools, Lester was an exemplary student. He had diligently completed every school assignment on time and had earned nearly perfect scores on all of his standardized tests—including those in English, history, and Spanish, which were his weakest subjects. When, for the first time, his grades began to slip in his junior year of high school, Mr. and Mrs. Silber were summoned to a meeting with Lester's academic advisor, Mrs. Carla Earhart.

Mrs. Carla Earhart: Lester's English and Spanish teachers have reported to me that he does not seem to be motivated. He is not paying attention or participating in class. On one occasion in Spanish he actually fell asleep. There is such a difference from his previous levels of performance that we are all very concerned about him. We wanted you to know about this change as soon as possible so we can determine its causes. Do you know if there are any problems with him personally, or at home?

Mr. Kenneth Silber: No. In truth, I am stunned. To our knowledge, Lester has never had any problems at school or anywhere else. What do you think we should do?

Mrs. Earhart: I think it's best to start by talking to Lester. Both you and us. I will meet with him later this afternoon to share our concerns. Maybe he will tell us what the matter is.

Lester was not forthcoming with either Mrs. Earhart or his parents about how many hours he was playing video games or about his marijuana smoking. Rather, he told them that he was "feeling bored by school" but would try harder. When Mrs. Earhart asked Lester if he would like to meet with the school counselor, he declined. She also called his parents to discuss Lester's being evaluated by an "outside professional."

> **Mr. Kenneth Silber:** We're not ones to run to counselors at the first sign of a problem. Our friends tell us that their children's therapists often *caused* more problems than they solved. Lester's grades are still excellent in all his courses other than English and Spanish. He has promised us to try harder in school, and we are confident that everything will work out for the best.

Lester received the message that he must try harder and complete his assignments, but he continued to put in the minimum possible effort. Nonetheless, his grade point average slipped slightly that year, largely because of the B's that he received in English and Spanish. His parents reasoned that his true forte was science and mathematics and that he ultimately would be fine if he continued to excel in those areas.

Over that summer and in the beginning of the 12th grade at Bellaire High School, Lester increased his hours playing video games along with his smoking of marijuana. Toward the first grading period of Lester's senior year, Mrs. Earhart once more called in Mr. and Mrs. Silber for a conference about Lester.

> **Mrs. Carla Earhart:** Thank you for coming in again. I am afraid that Lester's effort and performance continue to fall. I met personally with all of his teachers before today's meeting with you. Uniformly, they believe that Lester is not engaged and is performing significantly below his potential.
>
> **Mr. Kenneth Silber:** Is he also underperforming in math and science?
>
> **Mrs. Earhart:** His aptitude is so high in these subjects that it is hard to gauge. He is still an A student in those courses, but his teachers don't believe that he is putting in any effort whatsoever. He does not participate in extracurricular activities in math or science and does not take advantage of his opportunities as an advanced placement senior to take college level courses at Rice or the University of Houston.
>
> **Kenneth Silber:** If he's getting A's, what's the problem?
>
> **Mrs. Earhart:** At this time, he is failing two of his required humanities courses—American History and American Literature.

Lester has not handed in a single assignment, and he has already been absent for 7 days of school.

There are two main points that we want to make today. First, Lester must pass *all* of his courses this year in order to be eligible to graduate from high school. Second, we are very concerned that he has personal problems that need to be addressed.

Kenneth Silber: Are you sure that you are not making too much of this? Lester has never once gotten into trouble. We agree that he might not be the traditional type of student, but neither was Bill Gates. He dropped out of Harvard during his first year there.

Mrs. Earhart: Very likely, Lester will never drop out of Harvard because he will not be accepted to Harvard. Unless he makes major changes very soon. He might have perfect scores on his college admissions tests, but schools like Harvard look at other things, as well. He has not participated in any extracurricular activities, nor will he get the strongest recommendations from his teachers if he continues his present level of effort. He simply is not meeting up to his potential.

Mrs. Marsha Silber: Ken, we should listen to what Mrs. Earhart recommends. She's the professional. What do you think we should do, Mrs. Earhart?

Mrs. Earhart: I believe that the place to start is to have our school counselor or an outside expert of your choosing evaluate Lester to determine if he has any personal problems that are interfering with his performance.

Kenneth Silber: Oh, here we go with the shrinks again. Like I said last time you hauled us in here, so many friends who sent their kids to shrinks say that they only made things worse. Shrinks turn everything into some kind of sickness, probably so they can charge big money for their services. Even worse, they put kids on drugs that not only don't help them but get the kids addicted. I have to say that I'm very skeptical about taking this approach.

Mrs. Earhart: That has not been our experience at all at Bellaire High School. We have found these consultations to be indispensible. With regard to Lester, I believe that it would be irresponsible not to have a professional evaluation at this point.

Marsha Silber: Please, please listen to her, Ken. I don't feel that Lester is doing his best. He has always been shy, but now he is even more isolated. He hardly talks with us and doesn't call his sister at college any more. He doesn't go to Shabbat services like he used to every week. He spends all of his time locked up alone in his room. Probably in front of his computer. I'm getting really worried about him.

Kenneth Silber: You've just described my best employees and most of the geniuses in Silicon Valley. These guys might be a bit different, but they are changing the world, while doing very well for themselves.

Mrs. Earhart: Even geniuses develop personal problems, Mr. Silber. I will set up an appointment for Lester with Dr. Davis, our school counselor. Let me know if you prefer to seek the consultation of an outside professional. I have a list of professionals in our community with whom we have worked before. But I will need the report of a licensed professional if you choose to go in that direction.

The dialogue of Mrs. Earhart and Mr. and Mrs. Silber is a distillation of my many subsequent interviews with Lester, his parents, his sister, several of his teachers, and the psychiatrist who saw him on one occasion. A different picture of Mr. Kenneth Silber emerges from how he presented himself in his initial encounter with me as a parent highly motivated to have his son in treatment. At that point in Lester's decline, I am certain that he was more prepared to trust a psychiatrist. Certainly, Mr. Silber's initial negative attitude influenced Lester's defiance as manifested in his behavior during our first session. Nonetheless, mental health professionals must always be open to perceptions and conclusions from others that vary from what we hear from our patients as well as from their families. Ideally, it is invaluable to secure as many points of view as possible in order to gain a broad, balanced depiction.

I welcome the participation of families in my treatment of patients. Historically, psychiatry has discouraged this approach as interfering with our establishing a therapeutic alliance with our patients. When I was a resident, my supervisors warned me that family involvement would "contaminate" my patient's transference to me. Beyond this generalization that has no basis in evidence, my supervisors did acknowledge the invaluable historical information and patient support that family members can bring to bear. Hermetically sealing psychiatric care has isolated our profession and has alienated psychiatrists from those who love and support our patients the most: their families. As a result, we, needlessly and deservedly, have lost public credibility that has been difficult to regain.

After Mr. and Mrs. Silber's meeting with Mrs. Earhart, Mr. Silber spoke with Lester.

Mr. Kenneth Silber: Your mother and I were called in to meet with your high school advisor for a second time. She tells us that you are missing classes and not turning in your assignments. She warned us that unless you get professional help, you might not graduate. Do you have anything to say about this, Lester?

Lester Silber: Nope. But I'll try harder.

Kenneth Silber: That's what you said last year after we were called in. But obviously it's not working out. As you know, Lester, I'm not big on psychological counseling, but we're being pushed into a corner. Mrs. Earhart issued a vague threat that you won't get good college recommendations from your teachers unless we take her advice. I'm going to set you up to see somebody. Probably one visit will be enough, just to say we followed through on her advice.

Mr. Silber next approached Dr. Isadore Berger, a child psychiatrist whom he knew from his synagogue.

Mr. Kenneth Silber: I was wondering if you would evaluate my son, Lester. He seems to be having some problems in school, and his school advisor thought we should get him checked out professionally.

Dr. Isadore Berger: I'm sorry to hear that, Ken. Lester's always been such a fine and bright young man. Lately, I've missed seeing him at synagogue services. He used to come almost all the time. Thank you for your confidence in me, but I'm going to have to decline. I'm retired now. I closed my office 6 months ago.

Kenneth Silber: Are you still licensed, Isadore?

Dr. Berger: Yes.

Kenneth Silber: Then I would like you to see him just once, as a special favor to us. Marsha and I don't want to send Lester to anyone whom we don't know well. And therefore don't know if we can trust.

Dr. Berger: All right, Ken. I will see Lester. But please understand that if he requires further care, we must refer him to someone else.

Kenneth Silber: I understand, but I really don't think it's serious enough to come to that. Thank you so very much, Isadore. This is a great relief for us.

As soon as his father told him that he was going to meet with Dr. Berger, Lester sought out advice from Trevor, one of his Internet friends who once told him that had been "sent to" several psychiatrists.

Trevor: You just won the lottery, Lester. I'll tell you how to play this.

Lester Silber: But I don't want to see a psychiatrist. I won't know what to say to him.

Trevor: Most important is what you *don't* say. First thing, do your parents know that you smoke?

Lester: No way. I don't think they even suspect.

Trevor: Perfect. Then the first rule is you *never* admit to the doctor that you smoke pot or take any drugs. Coming clean on that won't go anywhere that's any good. So when the doctor asks you if you have ever tried marijuana, say "Never. That would be nuts." The psychiatrist will ask you tons of questions about your childhood, about your parents and your sister. Just tell him everything was perfect. That your family left you alone and never once bugged you. Then he'll ask you a bunch of questions about how you feel: if you ever wanted to kill yourself and shit like that. Just say that everything is great. Otherwise he'll put you on some antidepressant that will fuck up your head. Trust me on that one, Lester.

Where this can be a good deal is if you can get him to give you some Adderall. I actually think speed is great, and you might too. But that doesn't matter. If you don't like Adderall, you can always sell it or trade it for pot. I promise you, it's better than money. Everybody loves the stuff. When I'm playing Warcraft on Adderall, I rule!

Lester: Why would the doctor give me Adderall?

Trevor: Because you are going to Google and memorize all of the symptoms of attention-deficit disorder and make like you got every one of them. You'll tell the shrink that ADD is the real problem why you are fucking up in school—because you can't pay attention in class. That way, he found something and did something. And everybody congratulates themselves and stops bugging you.

Lester followed most of Trevor's advice during his meeting with Dr. Berger. Essentially, he denied smoking marijuana or having any emotional symptoms or family problems. However, Lester did *not* lie about having attention-deficit disorder in order to get drugs. He always liked Dr. Berger, and he would not have felt good about manipulating him.

After he met with Lester, Dr. Berger asked Mr. and Mrs. Silber to meet with him in person.

Mr. Kenneth Silber: Well, Isadore, is Lester OK?

Dr. Isadore Berger: I really can't tell, Ken. He didn't open up to me at all. According to him, everything is fine. When I asked him about his problems in school, he minimized them. When I asked him about what he would like to do in the future, he said he hadn't given much thought to that. I came away thinking he might be trying to hide something from me. Or from himself.

Kenneth Silber: I think you're reading too much into this. Things *really aren't that bad.* His real interest is computer science, and he does very well in his math, science, and computer courses. He just doesn't care that much about the humanities. I don't think there's any more to it than that.

Mrs. Marsha Silber: If anything is going on or bothering him, what would you suspect it could be?

Dr. Berger: It could be a lot of things, Marsha. He didn't seem to have much motivation or to be excited about his future. That can happen when young people are depressed or when they have a dependency problem.

Kenneth Silber: Dependency on what?

Dr. Berger: The most common dependencies for teenagers these days would be alcohol or marijuana.

Kenneth Silber: No way! He doesn't even like to drink. On Passover he won't even sip his wine. Marijuana is out of the question. Lester has never done anything like that in his life.

Dr. Berger: Perhaps. But you wouldn't be the first parent fooled by his adolescent child.

One other consideration has to do with his personality. He didn't seem that comfortable communicating with me. He answers were monosyllabic, without any effort to elaborate or carry on the conversation. When I asked if he had anything he would like to share with me or ask me, he simply replied, "no." Even though we had known each other from synagogue, he showed no interest in me or the others with whom he used to be involved. He doesn't do much physically and didn't express any interest in sports or girls.

Kenneth Silber: What are you getting at, Isadore?

Dr. Berger: Specifically, it is possible that he has avoidant personality disorder. Although the diagnosis of a personality disorder officially can't be made until the patient is 18 years old, Lester has many of the features of avoidant personality disorder. He doesn't seem to want to get close to his peers, is socially awkward, avoids getting involved in social activities, and seems to feel inferior.

Kenneth Silber: It sounds like you are saying he is shy. We know that. What I am going to do now is to make sure that Lester passes his senior year of high school and keeps on track to getting accepted to a good college. Thank you, Isadore. You've been a big help.

With Lester's permission, I spoke with Dr. Berger 6 years later. Dr. Berger was well aware that Lester was not forthcoming with him and that his father was not open to Dr. Berger's conclusions or recommendations: "Essentially, they both blew me off entirely, Stuart. I hope they are now ready to participate. Good luck with that."

World of Academic Warcraft

High School Struggles

Mr. Silber had tried to persuade Dr. Berger to write a "whitewashed" psychiatric report to Lester's high school advisor. He asked him to conclude that Lester did not suffer from a psychiatric disorder and that he would not require further professional help. Dr. Berger refused to comply.

Instead, Mr. Silber had his lawyer write the principal of Bellaire High School a letter. I asked the Silbers if they had saved a copy of that letter, which they shared with me. In the letter, the attorney made the following arguments and points:

1. Lester had no "record" at Bellaire or West University Elementary and Middle School of problems with his deportment or violations of school rules, regulations, or guidelines.
2. Lester had a consistent record of superior academic performance, with only recent problems involving a decline of grades in two courses.
3. Any putative physical and mental health issues of Lester's therefore had no adverse effects on Bellaire students, faculty, staff, or the school environment.
4. Until Lester turned 18, medical decisions regarding him were the responsibility of his legal guardians—in this case, his parents—and were not the prerogative of any municipal school system.
5. Lester and his family had the legal right to gain access to Lester's official high school records and other communications to colleges made by Bellaire faculty and staff. Mr. and Mrs. Silber would exercise that right of disclosure and reserve the right to

take legal action for damages related to any "hearsay specula-
tions" about Lester's physical and/or mental health.

Lester Silber: Dad then hired a tutor to sit with me at home for
2 hours every day. She made sure I completed all of my Spanish and English assignments and studied for my quizzes and
tests. Having a tutor forced me to do the work, which was
easy, and spend less time playing video games. My grades shot
back up to A's in all my courses.

In his senior year, on the advice of his father, Lester applied to
Rice University's and the University of Texas' engineering schools in
computer sciences. Given his high grade point average and nearly
perfect scores on his standardized aptitude tests, he was accepted to
the advanced placement programs of both. Both Lester and his parents agreed that he should attend the University of Texas (UT) in order to leave Houston and get a "fresh start."

Brief Life of a Longhorn

Lester made a Herculean effort to "turn over a new leaf" at UT.

Lester Silber: I knew that I had been spending far too much time
playing video games and smoking pot and was determined to
change that in college.
Dr. Y.: How did you plan to do that?
Lester: I didn't have a plan. I just thought that I could make myself
stop. It turned out to be harder for me to stop playing computer games than the pot smoking. I used my computer all day
long for school, so I had to fight my temptation to play games
nearly every minute of the day.
Dr. Y.: Did you make friends at UT?
Lester: No. Lots of the engineering students joined fraternities.
Most of the others were also interested in going to football
games, meeting girls, and drinking beer. I didn't feel comfortable doing those things. I always feel out of place. The classes
and tests were easy for me, so I finished my work in no time
flat. The rest of the time I had nothing to do.

Unfortunately, once more Lester set forth on his bold quest as a
"lone warrior" with no defined plan, no involvement of his family,
no organized exploration or utilization of college services or resources, and no support from a mental health professional.

As I learned in my tutorial with Mr. Bronner, many video games begin with an unarmed, nearly naked novice who is "plucked down" into a dangerous, distant, weird world to fend for himself. Once more, the seductive hype and hope that video games would parallel real life proved tragically illusory for Lester. He could not begin to fend for himself in this strange, foreign, complex, new universe of his university.

> **Lester Silber:** I held out for almost two semesters. No video games and no pot. I got straight A's the first semester. But around March of my freshman year, I crashed. First, I started playing World of Warcraft again. I found playing World of Warcraft wasn't much fun without pot, so I went back to smoking when I played. Soon, I was playing and smoking as much as ever. Maybe even more.

By March of his freshman year, Lester was playing video games nearly all of the time. He would play all night and sleep much of the day. He had stopped attending classes. Consequently, he received incompletes in all of his second semester courses and was placed on academic probation.

Crashing in Austin

Lester was honest with his parents about his abuse of marijuana and video game playing. Nonetheless, he was able to convince them to allow him to stay in Austin for the summer semester in order to take two computer science classes. Because his dormitory was closed for the summer, he decided to rent a room in a rundown house leased by a former UT graduate student who had been selling him marijuana. Four other former university students lived there as well.

Lester made another concerted effort to stop smoking and playing video games, but, once more, he was unsuccessful. Living in a house populated by several other renters and many visitors who openly smoked marijuana much of the day and night rapidly softened his resolve. Within 2 weeks, he had returned to smoking regularly and playing video games. He didn't keep up with the courses' written assignments and stopped attending classes before midterms.

> **Lester Silber:** I told my parents that I was bored by college and that I wanted to drop out and get a job in Austin.

Dr. Y.: How did they respond?

Lester: My mother was very upset, but my father understood. Some of his best employees are geeks who had dropped out of college.

Dr. Y.: Did you try to find work?

Lester: Not really. I mainly hung out in the house with the five other guys who were living there. I had a lot in common with some of them. They all smoked and played video games, and two were really good at math and computer sciences like me. But nobody went to school or had real jobs.

Dr. Y.: How did you spend your days?

Lester: Slept mostly during the daytime. All the action was at night. People would come by to buy grass and other stuff and then stick around to hang out. Everybody would get high.

Dr. Y.: What did you enjoy about living there?

Lester: I liked hanging out with people who never put me down. But I hated the noise. Heavy metal and rap music that was blaring all night. And strangers were always walking into my room when I was trying to concentrate on my video game.

Dr. Y.: Did you meet any women?

Lester: There were lots of women around. But they were always stoned, and most were hooked on hard drugs. I never had much to say to them.

Just before the new year, the Austin police raided the house. The six residents, including Lester, as well several others who were present at the time, were arrested and charged with drug trafficking and drug possession. Significant amounts of cocaine, methamphetamine, marijuana, heroin, prescription narcotics, and prescription stimulants were found and confiscated from the house. In addition, materials for processing and packaging drugs, bags of cash, and paraphernalia for drug use were also discovered and taken as evidence.

Mr. Silber posted Lester's bail and hired a defense attorney in Austin to defend him against very serious charges. Lester moved back to Houston to live in the family-owned townhouse and, ostensibly, to look for a job. Initially, the police and prosecutors had great difficulty believing that Lester could live amidst so much illegal drug activity without being significantly involved. After about a year of intense legal negotiations, he was given a suspended sentence for drug possession, which would be expunged from his record if he had no further drug convictions over the next 5 years. The legal fees cost Lester's family more than $100,000.

Dr. Y.: How did you feel about your parents having to pay so much money to your lawyers?

Lester Silber: OK, I guess. I told them not to hire the lawyers. I never sold any drugs. Besides, I didn't really care if they convicted me on something.

Dr. Y.: But prison terms in Texas are notoriously long for people convicted of drug trafficking.

Lester: If they wanted to put me in jail for something I never did, it's not my fault.

Lester Silber's DSM-5 Diagnosis

Diagnosis

Lester was diagnosed with the following DSM-5 disorders (American Psychiatric Association 2013):

1. Autism spectrum disorder 299.00 (F84.0), level 1, requiring support; without known medical or genetic condition or environmental factor; without accompanying intellectual or language impairment
2. Cannabis use disorder, severe 304.30 (F12.20)
3. In addition, Lester met the criteria for Internet gaming disorder, severe, which is listed in DSM-5 as a condition for further study.

Discussion of Diagnosis

Asperger's Disorder/Autism Spectrum Disorder

Clinical Presentations

The fifth edition of the American Psychiatric Association's *Diagnostic and Statistical Manual of Mental Disorders* (DSM-5; American Psychiatric Association 2013) classifies Asperger's disorder as an autism spectrum disorder (ASD). Asperger's disorder is among the least severe conditions on this spectrum. People with ASD exhibit dysfunctions of communication and social interactions as well as restricted, repetitive patterns of interests, activities, and behaviors. Importantly, in the less severe cases, there are usually no significant delays in language or cognitive development. People with ASD can be highly intelligent.

The first signs and symptoms of these conditions usually are detected in the second year of life with delays in social interactions with caregivers and delays in verbal communications. For example, the toddlers do not respond with smiling when smiled at by their mothers, nor do they sustain eye contact with their mothers while being nursed or during bottle feedings. They often do not seem to be comforted by familiar voices or the touches of familiar people, nor do they respond warmly to being cuddled. They fail to imitate parental movements or expressions and do not frequently reach out to be picked up or carried. They do not point at objects they want to have, wave bye-bye, imitate noises, or use words by age 16 months, as compared with other children of that age.

As children with ASD grow older, they develop unusual and repetitive play patterns such as carrying around toys without playing with them. They will repeat, seemingly endlessly, the same movements or gestures, will become preoccupied with parts of objects, and do not like to depart from their most familiar life routines. They show little interest in having friends and fail to recognize and respond to social cues of young peers, such as when their peers are upset with their behaviors. An example might be that they evidence displeasure when *other* children take away their toys but don't seem to understand why a peer would become angry when they take their playthings. They have difficulty making or keeping friends because they have little interest in sharing enjoyable activities with them. They seem incapable of understanding the "gives and takes" of conventional relationships or expressing empathy.

Prior to meeting with Lester, I had treated several adults with ASD, most often those with strong scientific aptitudes and accomplishments. In our first session, my suspicions were raised that Lester had a milder form of this condition, or what formerly was termed by DSM as Asperger's disorder, now classified in DSM-5 as autism spectrum disorder. Among the clues that I observed in our initial meeting were the following:

- Despite the welcoming greeting and helpful, upbeat demeanor that I did my best to maintain throughout our session, Lester did not appear friendly. Rather, he seemed disinterested and dismissive.

- Lester rarely looked me directly in the eye.
- Lester was not spontaneous, forthcoming, or expansive in our discussion. Nor did he bring up unrequested information. He would respond to open-ended questions with one-word answers or brief phrases. For example, when I asked him "Please tell me about your parents," Lester replied, "They're OK."
- Lester did not appear engaged or interested whatsoever in me or my feelings.
- Lester was not gracious, nor did he engage in social niceties: no "thank you," "please," "if it's not too much trouble," or other expressions of appreciation.
- Lester saw the world in "blacks and whites," with no sense of the subtleties, conflicts, and complexities involved in his own feelings, thoughts, and motivations or those of others.
- Lester was cognitively concrete, quantitative, and not abstract. This led to his difficulties with "thinking psychologically." For example, when I asked him if he had any idea why he was bullied throughout elementary school and middle school, he said, "Because they were bigger than me." When I asked him what seemed to be the problems that he was having in his English and foreign language courses, he replied, "I'm getting low grades."
- Lester had difficulties discerning "the big picture" with regard to his personal goals, aspirations, and future life. When I asked him what he would like his life to be like in 5 or 10 years, he replied, "I don't know. I have never thought about it." I inferred that Lester did not know *how to go about* thinking about his future—any more so than many of us would know how to approach a complex problem in theoretical physics, with which Lester would be facile.

For the DSM-5 diagnostic criteria for autism spectrum disorder, see Box 12–1.

Box 12–1.   DSM-5 Diagnostic Criteria for Autism Spectrum Disorder

299.00 (F84.0)

A. Persistent deficits in social communication and social interaction across multiple contexts, as manifested by the following, currently or by history (examples are illustrative, not exhaustive; see text):

   1. Deficits in social-emotional reciprocity, ranging, for example, from abnormal social approach and failure of normal back-and-forth conversa-

tion; to reduced sharing of interests, emotions, or affect; to failure to initiate or respond to social interactions.

2. Deficits in nonverbal communicative behaviors used for social interaction, ranging, for example, from poorly integrated verbal and nonverbal communication; to abnormalities in eye contact and body language or deficits in understanding and use of gestures; to a total lack of facial expressions and nonverbal communication.

3. Deficits in developing, maintaining, and understanding relationships, ranging, for example, from difficulties adjusting behavior to suit various social contexts; to difficulties in sharing imaginative play or in making friends; to absence of interest in peers.

Specify current severity:

> **Severity is based on social communication impairments and restricted, repetitive patterns of behavior** (see Table 2 [DSM-5, p. 52]).

B. Restricted, repetitive patterns of behavior, interests, or activities, as manifested by at least two of the following, currently or by history (examples are illustrative, not exhaustive; see text):

1. Stereotyped or repetitive motor movements, use of objects, or speech (e.g., simple motor stereotypies, lining up toys or flipping objects, echolalia, idiosyncratic phrases).

2. Insistence on sameness, inflexible adherence to routines, or ritualized patterns of verbal or nonverbal behavior (e.g., extreme distress at small changes, difficulties with transitions, rigid thinking patterns, greeting rituals, need to take same route or eat same food every day).

3. Highly restricted, fixated interests that are abnormal in intensity or focus (e.g., strong attachment to or preoccupation with unusual objects, excessively circumscribed or perseverative interests).

4. Hyper- or hyporeactivity to sensory input or unusual interest in sensory aspects of the environment (e.g., apparent indifference to pain/temperature, adverse response to specific sounds or textures, excessive smelling or touching of objects, visual fascination with lights or movement).

Specify current severity:

> **Severity is based on social communication impairments and restricted, repetitive patterns of behavior**.

C. Symptoms must be present in the early developmental period (but may not become fully manifest until social demands exceed limited capacities, or may be masked by learned strategies in later life).

D. Symptoms cause clinically significant impairment in social, occupational, or other important areas of current functioning.

E. These disturbances are not better explained by intellectual disability (intellectual developmental disorder) or global developmental delay. Intellectual disability and autism spectrum disorder frequently co-occur; to make comorbid diagnoses of autism spectrum disorder and intellectual disability, social communication should be below that expected for general developmental level.

Note: Individuals with a well-established DSM-IV diagnosis of autistic disorder, Asperger's disorder, or pervasive developmental disorder not otherwise specified should be given the diagnosis of autism spectrum disorder. Individuals who have marked deficits in social communication, but whose symptoms do not otherwise meet criteria for autism spectrum disorder, should be evaluated for social (pragmatic) communication disorder.

Specify if:

With or without accompanying intellectual impairment

With or without accompanying language impairment

Associated with a known medical or genetic condition or environmental factor (Coding note: Use additional code to identify the associated medical or genetic condition.)

Associated with another neurodevelopmental, mental, or behavioral disorder (Coding note: Use additional code[s] to identify the associated neurodevelopmental, mental, or behavioral disorder[s].)

With catatonia (refer to the criteria for catatonia associated with another mental disorder, [DSM-5] pp. 119–120, for definition) **(Coding note:** Use additional code 293.89 [F06.1] catatonia associated with autism spectrum disorder to indicate the presence of the comorbid catatonia.)

Source. Reprinted from the *Diagnostic and Statistical Manual of Mental Disorders,* 5th Edition. Washington, DC, American Psychiatric Association, 2013. Used with permission. Copyright © American Psychiatric Association.

Alexithymia

The term *alexithymia* refers to a condition in which a person has severe limitations in being aware of and, therefore, being able to identify and describe his or her emotions and those of others. Human emotions have many, far-reaching purposes related to survival. Emotions regulate our capacities to thrive in social systems, to communicate usefully with others, and to make rapid and "correct" decisions. Additionally, emotions alert us to pay attention to those factors in our lives that require prioritization by directing our conscious minds to focus our behavior on what is important and to keep us from being distracted by what is trivial. Finally, our emotions guide what we do and do not place in our memory banks.

A fundamental problem for people with alexithymia is their inability to distinguish the bodily feelings associated with emotional arousal from the cognitive sources of these feelings. For example, they will find themselves in situations where they perceive from their somatic sensations that they are angry but won't necessarily understand *why* they are angry. With limited ability to gauge the intensity or discern the sources of their emotions, they are unable to calibrate their responses accordingly. They therefore are prone to overreacting to relatively minor "irritations" that affect them personally—such as someone cutting ahead of them in a cafeteria line—and underreacting or reacting dispassionately or inappropriately in social situations involving others. When trying to console a friend who told him he lost his beloved grandfather, Lester said, "People die when they get old. Your grandfather wouldn't be the first person in history not to live forever." Because their responses evoke such untoward reactions from others, people with alexithymia learn, early on, that it is better to withdraw from social interactions than to suffer the bewildering, often punishing responses of others.

When people first encounter someone with alexithymia, they often experience him or her as being detached, disinterested, unfriendly, and somewhat weird. Later, as they get to know the person with alexithymia better, they may also find him or her to be superficial, unempathic, unemotional, self-centered, rigid, unimaginative, unintuitive, and difficult to deal with. Therefore, a vicious social cycle occurs wherein both parties withdraw and the person with alexithymia becomes isolated.

Alexithymia can be either a *state* or a *trait* phenomenon. If this condition is caused by an underlying brain-based dysfunction—most likely from disturbances in the neuroanatomic and/or neurophysiological pathways that process emotions—it is considered a trait type of disturbance. On the other hand, if the alexithymia is a reaction to a traumatic experience that overwhelms the person's sense of safety and long-term security, it is considered a *state* phenomenon. These distinctions are often made in medicine to determine prognosis and to guide treatment. However, because brain-based alexithymia will affect social experience as well as that individual's interpretation of social experience and because social experience will affect brain neurobiology, state or trait distinctions currently have limited value in the treatment of people with this condition.

Taking a History: Psychiatry as Torture

As I have emphasized throughout this book, the act of securing a psychiatric history is therapeutic for the patient. Never is this principle more relevant than for someone with Asperger's disorder or who has related disorders involving alexithymia. However, if the clinician endeavors to take a psychiatric history in a conventional fashion, it will become torture for the patient and the professional and will discourage the patient from engaging in further treatment. A core problem of people with these conditions is their difficulties in connecting and correlating past events with their *emotional* reactions to those experiences. They are able to describe events factually but are unable to ascribe *significance* or *importance* to those events. Thus, a mental health professional taking a psychological history from a person with Asperger's disorder feels that the patient is offering minute, insignificant details about an endless succession of events that illuminate very little that is relevant to his or her psychological problems or psychiatric disorders. It would take literally the patient's lifetime up to that point to obtain a psychiatric history in this fashion.

The only ways around this problem for the mental health professional are

1. To enlist family members and significant others in taking the psychiatric history
2. To "teach" the patient how to mentalize while the history is being taken[1]

I always do both under these circumstances.

Discussion of Diagnosis of Autism Spectrum Disorder With Patient and Family

Treatment of patients with any type of illness—especially psychiatric illnesses—*should* involve using their assets to deal with their medical challenges. Lester Silber is blessed with a brilliant technical and analytical mind. In addition, he is innately objective and dispassionate. Therefore, after discussing with him my impression that he met diagnostic criteria for autism spectrum disorder, I presented Lester with several seminal scientific papers on the neurobiology and characteristic features of the condition and how psychiatry goes about making this diagnosis. The following dialogue took place after he had reviewed this material.

---

[1]Please refer to Chapter 11, "Stuck in Pleasing Others, Part II (Decide and Discipline)," for an extensive discussion of mentalization.

Dr. Y.: Well, Lester, what do you think?

Lester Silber: It is obvious that I have a mild type of autism. I find that quite interesting. I do have problems with how psychiatry goes about making a diagnosis, however. You guys have real problems with the sensitivity and specificity of your diagnostics. Too much overlap. No doubt the brain is so complicated that you don't have technology to do any better. You need to find hard markers. Do you agree?

Dr. Y.: I agree fully, Lester. I also would like to take the opportunity to say that you have a rare and remarkable gift for science. I would like to see you put it to use someday.

Thereafter, I invited Mr. and Mrs. Silber to join us for a session in order to communicate to them *our* diagnostic impressions.

Dr. Y.: Thank you for joining us today. I don't expect you to be surprised by Lester's diagnoses of marijuana and video game dependence. I also believe strongly that he has a mild form of autism spectrum disorder, formerly called Asperger's disorder, which is a very mild form of autism.

Mr. Kenneth Silber: Let's hold on right now. With all due respect, I think you are getting carried away. That's my problem with psychiatry. You guys never leave well enough alone. Let's get back to reality here and deal with the real problems—the video games and pot smoking. That's what we signed up for.

Dr. Y.: I understand fully why you would react so strongly. I would like to discuss with you my reasons for coming to this conclusion and share with you some scientific literature on autism. I also would like to ask you a few questions.

Kenneth Silber: Let's start with the questions.

Dr. Y.: OK. Autism is a hereditary condition. As you know, that means it tends to run in families. Do you know of anyone in either of your families who was diagnosed with autism?

Mrs. Marsha Silber: Ken, maybe you should tell him about your Uncle David.

Kenneth Silber: Let's stay on topic, Marsha. This is about Lester, not my Uncle David.

Dr. Y.: If I may ask, who is Uncle David?

Kenneth Silber: My father's younger brother. He had severe autism. He had to be put in an institution when he was about 20. He became too violent to manage. I barely knew him. This is a family tragedy, and I don't buy that it has anything to do with Lester. His problem is that he is not aggressive enough.

Lester Silber: Please read the literature, Dad. I did, and I am convinced I have autism. It explains a lot of things to me.

Cannabis Use Disorder

For the first time with the most recent edition of DSM, the current level of the severity of substance use disorders is determined and coded. If a patient fulfills at least six of the DSM-5 criteria, he or she is diagnosed to be at the "severe" level, which applied to Lester. Specifically, he craved smoking, particularly when he was playing video games; was unsuccessful in his several attempts to stop smoking marijuana; did not meet his school or personal obligations when smoking; experienced reduced motivation for social interactions while smoking; gradually increased the amount he smoked in order to obtain the wanted effects; and found that he developed headaches and became anxious and irritable on stopping.

Lester rarely smoked marijuana when he wasn't playing video games. Even the most superficial search of the Internet reveals many references to the belief that people play video games better when they are "on weed." There are assertions on the Internet that, just like with jazz- and blues-playing musicians, many expert video game players and professionals will play only "when they're baked."

This state-dependent phenomenon is not uncommon for most other types of substance use disorder. For example, many college students drink alcohol exclusively on those days of the week when they and their classmates frequent bars—usually on Thursday, Friday, and Saturday nights. The problem is that on the days that they *do* drink, they binge, and they are at greatly increased risk of getting into serious trouble—physically, emotionally, and/or legally.

Another example of state-dependent substance use disorder is that of Orthodox Jewish cigarette smokers. According to traditional Jewish law, they are not permitted to light fires on the Sabbath or on Holy Days. For this reason, there are occasions when they do not smoke for three successive days and nights. When I have asked heavy smokers who are Orthodox Jews how they handle their craving and the withdrawal effects of nicotine, they reply, "Oh, I don't have the slightest desire to smoke on the Sabbath or holidays, nor do I have nicotine hangovers. However, when I leave synagogue after the Sabbath or Holy Day is over, I light right up—often without even thinking about it." Not only does this illustrate the powerful effect of the environment on substance use and abuse but also the potency of the brain and mind to influence biologically based drives, symptoms, and behaviors.

For the DSM-5 diagnostic criteria for cannabis use disorder (American Psychiatric Association 2013), see Box 12–2.

Box 12–2.   DSM-5 Diagnostic Criteria for Cannabis Use Disorder

---

A. A problematic pattern of cannabis use leading to clinically significant impairment or distress, as manifested by at least two of the following, occurring within a 12-month period:

1. Cannabis is often taken in larger amounts or over a longer period than was intended.
2. There is a persistent desire or unsuccessful efforts to cut down or control cannabis use.
3. A great deal of time is spent in activities necessary to obtain cannabis, use cannabis, or recover from its effects.
4. Craving, or a strong desire or urge to use cannabis.
5. Recurrent cannabis use resulting in a failure to fulfill major role obligations at work, school, or home.
6. Continued cannabis use despite having persistent or recurrent social or interpersonal problems caused or exacerbated by the effects of cannabis.
7. Important social, occupational, or recreational activities are given up or reduced because of cannabis use.
8. Recurrent cannabis use in situations in which it is physically hazardous.
9. Cannabis use is continued despite knowledge of having a persistent or recurrent physical or psychological problem that is likely to have been caused or exacerbated by cannabis.
10. Tolerance, as defined by either of the following:
    a. A need for markedly increased amounts of cannabis to achieve intoxication or desired effect.
    b. Markedly diminished effect with continued use of the same amount of cannabis.
11. Withdrawal, as manifested by either of the following:
    a. The characteristic withdrawal syndrome for cannabis (refer to Criteria A and B of the criteria set for cannabis withdrawal, [DSM-5] pp. 517–518).
    b. Cannabis (or a closely related substance) is taken to relieve or avoid withdrawal symptoms.

Specify if:

In early remission: After full criteria for cannabis use disorder were previously met, none of the criteria for cannabis use disorder have been met for at least 3 months but for less than 12 months (with the exception that Criterion A4, "Craving, or a strong desire or urge to use cannabis," may be met).

In sustained remission: After full criteria for cannabis use disorder were previously met, none of the criteria for cannabis use disorder have been met at any time during a period of 12 months or longer (with the exception that Criterion A4, "Craving, or a strong desire or urge to use cannabis," may be present).

Specify if:

In a controlled environment: This additional specifier is used if the individual is in an environment where access to cannabis is restricted.

Code based on current severity: Note for ICD-10-CM codes: If a cannabis intoxication, cannabis withdrawal, or another cannabis-induced mental disorder is also present, do not use the codes below for cannabis use disorder. Instead, the comorbid cannabis use disorder is indicated in the 4th character of the cannabis-induced disorder code (see the coding note for cannabis intoxication, cannabis withdrawal, or a specific cannabis-induced mental disorder). For example, if there is comorbid cannabis-induced anxiety disorder and cannabis use disorder, only the cannabis-induced anxiety disorder code is given, with the 4th character indicating whether the comorbid cannabis use disorder is mild, moderate, or severe: F12.180 for mild cannabis use disorder with cannabis-induced anxiety disorder or F12.280 for a moderate or severe cannabis use disorder with cannabis-induced anxiety disorder.

Specify current severity:

305.20 (F12.10) **Mild:** Presence of 2–3 symptoms.

304.30 (F12.20) **Moderate:** Presence of 4–5 symptoms.

304.30 (F12.20) **Severe:** Presence of 6 or more symptoms.

Source. Reprinted from the *Diagnostic and Statistical Manual of Mental Disorders,* 5th Edition. Washington, DC, American Psychiatric Association, 2013. Used with permission. Copyright © American Psychiatric Association.

Internet Gaming Disorder

Internet gaming disorder is not yet an official diagnosis but is listed in a special section of DSM-5 detailing "conditions for further study" (American Psychiatric Association 2013, pp. 795–798). I strongly believe that the high *prevalence*, clinical *symptomatologies*, levels of *disability*, and *brain centers* involved for people with video game dependencies closely parallel other use disorders that presently are included in DSM-5. The reason that the American Psychiatric Association Task Force on DSM-5 did not include Internet gaming disorder as an "official" diagnosis is that more scientifically verifiable data are required to substantiate a new diagnosis.

One recent study that I believe is especially relevant to Lester found that boys with autism spectrum disorders spent nearly twice as much time playing video games than their peers with "typical development" (Mazurek and Engelhardt 2013). A greater percentage of boys with ASD preferred role-playing video games, which is associated with a "higher problematic video game use than those who did not" (Mazurek and Engelhardt 2013, p. 264).

For the proposed DSM-5 criteria for Internet gaming disorder, see Box 12–3.

Box 12–3.   DSM-5 Proposed Criteria for Internet Gaming Disorder

---

A. Persistent and recurrent use of the Internet to engage in games, often with other players, leading to clinically significant impairment or distress as indicated by five (or more) of the following in a 12-month period:

1. Preoccupation with Internet games. (The individual thinks about previous gaming activity or anticipates playing the next game; Internet gaming becomes the dominant activity in daily life).
   Note: This disorder is distinct from Internet gambling, which is included under gambling disorder.
2. Withdrawal symptoms when Internet gaming is taken away. (These symptoms are typically described as irritability, anxiety, or sadness, but there are no physical signs of pharmacological withdrawal.)
3. Tolerance—the need to spend increasing amounts of time engaged in Internet games.
4. Unsuccessful attempts to control the participation in Internet games.
5. Loss of interests in previous hobbies and entertainment as a result of, and with the exception of, Internet games.
6. Continued excessive use of Internet games despite knowledge of psychosocial problems.
7. Has deceived family members, therapists, or others regarding the amount of Internet gaming.
8. Use of Internet games to escape or relieve a negative mood (e.g., feelings of helplessness, guilt, anxiety).
9. Has jeopardized or lost a significant relationship, job, or educational or career opportunity because of participation in Internet games.

Note: Only nongambling Internet games are included in this disorder. Use of the Internet for required activities in a business or profession is not included; nor is the disorder intended to include other recreational or social Internet use. Similarly, sexual Internet sites are excluded.

Specify current severity:

Internet gaming disorder can be mild, moderate, or severe depending on the degree of disruption of normal activities. Individuals with less severe Internet gaming disorder may exhibit fewer symptoms and less disruption of their lives. Those with severe Internet gaming disorder will have more hours spent on the computer and more severe loss of relationships or career or school opportunities.

Brave New World of Video Games

Video Game Standard Time

At the conclusion of Lester's first session with me, we determined that he would start out by seeing me twice per week. As per usual in establishing a schedule for a new patient, the discussion was revealing.

> **Dr. Y.:** What days and times are available for you?
> **Lester Silber:** I usually don't get up before 1:00 in the afternoon, and I must be back at my townhouse by about 5:30.
> **Dr. Y.:** Why is that?
> **Lester:** I start playing World of Warcraft at 5:30 P.M. every day and pretty much don't stop before 6:00 A.M. I stop later on some days if I'm in a crazy raid. Most of my team is from Korea, other parts of Asia, and Europe. That's the best time for us to play.
> **Dr. Y.:** How would 3:00 P.M. on Tuesdays and Fridays work for you?
> **Lester:** I can make that happen, but I have to be back in my house by 5:00 P.M.

Lester met his part of the bargain. He arrived promptly for each of his biweekly appointments and did his best to participate. Without his acknowledging that he had any reason to see me other than to keep his electricity on, Lester's participation was limited to his answering, as best as he was able, the questions that I posed. Because his current life revolved around and, for the most part, was limited to his playing World of Warcraft, many of my questions related to his history and "relationship" with video games.

> **Dr. Y.:** How did you get started playing video games?
> **Lester Silber:** I have been playing video games since I was a little kid. My dad introduced me to them when I was about 5 years old after he bought a Sony PlayStation. I would play games with him and with the few other kids in the neighborhood who would play with me.

Lester went on to say that he played both "kids' games" and "grown-ups' games" since he was 5 years old. Even though he most often played alone and even though video games became his favorite recreational pastime, the games did not interfere with his schoolwork until the 10th grade.

> **Lester Silber:** Although I always loved playing video games, I always had the discipline to stop until I started smoking pot. At first, the only time I smoked pot was when I played World of Warcraft or StarCraft online with other players and in teams. I don't know exactly why, but I think it is because I feel more relaxed and less worried about making mistakes when I am stoned.
>
> **Dr. Y.:** Do you think that you started smoking at school for the same reasons?
>
> **Lester:** Things don't bother me as much when I'm stoned.
>
> **Dr. Y.:** Do you mean "people" or "things" don't bother you so much?
>
> **Lester:** "People," for sure. I stop caring what they think about me.

My Introduction to Video Games

As discussed previously, because I knew almost nothing about video games, I sought out supervision from Mr. Ronald Bronner, an expert in both neuroscience and computer science. One purpose of this supervision was for me to gain an experiential overview of the different types of video games in order to learn the different ways in which vulnerable people might become dependent on them. The following is a summary of the introductory video game tutorial that Mr. Bronner prescribed for me. First, Mr. Bronner believed that I should have an overview of the types of games.

Overview of Types of Video Games

Twitch Games

Twitch games, commonly found on mobile platforms, utilize rapid-reward circuitry stimulation. Playing these types of games results in brain-motor pathways being involved in what is termed *procedural memory* until mastery is achieved. Procedural memory is required for the performance of automatic motor and cognitive behaviors that have been learned, such as riding a bicycle, tying shoes, or driving a car. Such memory is established by repeating complex activities many times until the cognitive and motor pathways required for those actions work automatically. Satisfaction with high performance is associated with a pleasing meditative or "flow state."

People who are highly anxious and have obsessions are vulnerable to becoming dependent on this type of game as a form of soothing escapism, at the expense of failing to address the underlying sources of their problems. Interestingly, people with attention-deficit/hyperactivity disorder, whose attention span is usually compromised, can perform well on these tasks with total attention and focus for protracted periods of time. Super Hexagon was the twitch game chosen by Mr. Bronner for me to play.

Real-Time Strategy Games

Real-time strategy games require fast reflexes, intuitive decision making, and strategic planning, all operating simultaneously. The brain's capacity for multitasking is challenged and developed by this game genre. The construct of these games mirrors competitive sports, and dependency comes from the associated pleasures of both mastery and escapism. As per all sports—whether as a participant or a viewer—one can avoid responsibilities and problems through overindulgence as participants and fanaticism as viewers. Not surprisingly, several of the video games in this category have developed into competitive professional sports in which a handful of game players are superstars who gain wealth and notoriety, just as can happen in football, baseball, and basketball. The game selected to introduce me to real-time strategy games was Epic StarCraft II, and, as a spectator, I also viewed on YouTube the play of Mike "Husky" Lamond, a well-known expert in this game.

Normal Strategy Games

Unlike real-time strategy games, performance on normal strategy games is not time-sensitive. The games, which have evolved from traditional countertop board games, often have some level of historical realism. With regard to people becoming dependent on playing these games, Mr. Bronner said the following: "Essentially, these games are like chess to the nth power. These games are, in many ways, more dangerous than real-time strategy games because vulnerable people with obsessive-compulsive disorder can burn huge amounts of time analyzing a given move." The games After-Action Report from Gary Grigsby's War in the East and Panzer General were selected by my supervisor for purposes of demonstration.

First-Person Shooters

First-person shooter games usually have a single-player component and a multiplayer component. Traditionally, the single-player component has the player take the role of a lone combatant (often a "space marine") fighting against a near-limitless horde of zombies/Nazis/demons by using an arsenal of progressively more powerful and technologically more advanced weaponry. Often, this category of game involves explicit graphics depicting large amounts of gore, blood, and terror. Although my instruction did not involve my playing a game in this category of games, I watched Mr. Bronner deftly play Call of Duty and was also shown videos about the player classes in the game Team Fortress.

Simulation Games

Simulation games mimic so-called "real life" tasks, challenges, and activities. These types of games can serve the bridging purposes of entertainment, practice, learning, and even solving vexing social or scientific problems. Serious educators have long understood that important learning and mastery goals can be achieved by making a game of the "work" of acquiring new skills and knowledge. From learning to fly new prototypes of aircraft to practicing for delicate cardiovascular or brain surgical procedures, realistic simulations can be edifying and exciting.

People who are, by nature, more literal and concrete than abstract and people who have problems discerning the so-called real from unreal (e.g., people with delusions or hallucinations) may be particularly vulnerable to this type of game. In addition, all of us have been in situations where we complement reality through comparison to a simulacrum or simulation: "She is as pretty as a picture," "That lake should be on a postcard," "Dancing with him was like being in a movie," etc. Mr. Bronner reminded me of the following: "When the Apollo astronauts were asked about what the moon landing was like, they responded, 'It was beautiful, just like our drills.'"

Examples of simulation games include the city building game genre, such as SimCity, and a wide range of mathematical, scientific, medical, sociological, and architectural types of puzzle-solving and construction-based games.

Role-Playing Games

Role-playing games allow players to transport themselves mentally and spiritually into a detailed, epic virtual universe constructed by game designers. Not only are these games excellent for escapism but they also permit the player to think, act, and, most dangerously, *feel* like a hero. Players are also given the option to behave in a devious and dastardly fashion, but this is a much less popular gamer choice. Usually, the player leads a small squad of heroes, who may become virtual friends (or lovers!) through the course of the adventure.

People with impaired self-esteem or who are not fulfilled adequately in their personal lives (e.g., in school, jobs, love relationships) are particularly vulnerable to becoming dependent on these types of games. I observed Mr. Bronner's adept play of Mass Effect, which is one of the best among these types of game. Interestingly to me, the originators of Mass Effect were two physicians.

Massively Multiplayer Online Role-Playing Games

Massively multiplayer online role-playing games will be described in great detail through the following consideration of World of Warcraft, the game on which Lester Silber was dependent.

World of Warcraft

I confess that as a mental health professional, I was shaken by what I encountered when I first read about and became a casual player of the video game World of Warcraft. As I will detail later, the potential of this type of game to attract, entrap, and harm people with certain specific psychiatric problems and psychological vulnerabilities is far reaching.

Game Essentials

The rudiments of this game, which is among the world's most popular, with more than 8 million subscribers, is well described in its beginner's guide Web site, which is titled "What is World of Warcraft?" The following are what I took away as the highlights from this description.

The general category of this type of game is called a *massively multiplayer online role-playing game*. What that means is that World of Warcraft can accommodate thousands of players interacting with each other while they are playing this game in real time. Each player can have a specific identity, as defined by the explicit skill set, abilities, and other identifying qualities of the character the player chooses. The game's beginner's guide gives the following example: "Mages are powerful spellcasters who use magic to inflict damage on their enemies from afar but are very vulnerable to attacks. These traits define the role of the mage: hang back, do a ton of damage, and hope to kill the monsters before they kill you."

Role-playing means that the individual player becomes a specific character in the game's fantasy world, which is shared, potentially, by thousands of other players. The guide also states, "Much of the game's advanced content is geared towards groups of players working together to explore dangerous dungeons and defeat powerful monsters."

The entire game takes place in an unbelievably elaborate, interactive fantasy universe where noble good guys are aligned to fight and gain dominance over cunning and evil bad guys. The game player adopts the role of a fantasy hero, or a persistent online persona, who accumulates, over playing time and through intense effort, mental, physical, and material powers to pursue his or her lofty goal. Thus, the player, through his or her fantasy identity, creates his or her own unique personality, temperament, physical look and prowess, and history.

The graphics and sound features are artistically outstanding and somewhat realistic, in an idealized way. Finally, in World of Warcraft, you pay to play. Beyond the subscription fee, there are options to purchase special expansions of the game that can become quite costly to an involved player as well as sustain that person's ongoing interest in playing the game.

Preliminary Conclusions

As I learned more about World of Warcraft and similar video games, my concern about its addictive potential for certain people with special psychiatric vulnerabilities became progressively heightened. In Chapter 13, "Stuck in Adolescence and Cyberspace, Part II (Decide and Discipline)," I will review the current scientific thought about whether or not dependencies on video games should be conceptualized as an addiction and/or a specific mental disorder.

My initial impressions of the dangers of this game to Lester Silber (and others with certain psychiatric vulnerabilities) are summarized as follows:

- Lester tried to build up his low self-esteem through identification with an imaginary heroic character, as opposed to actualizing his potential in the real world.

- His game identity progressively melded with and replaced his real-life personal identity.
- He came to believe that he was on a mission to accomplish something important in a game, at the expense of having realistic goals and plans in his real life.
- He perceived that the rules of the game are clear and fair, in contrast to what he experienced as the confusion and unfairness of real life.
- He could measure his personal accomplishments using the various reinforcements built into the game—tokens, honor points, levels, treasure repositories, etc.—instead of substantive achievements in real life.
- He devoted endless hours to gaining skills, power, and expertise at playing a game, which he feared that he would "lose" and "waste" if he were to expend time and effort to advance in the real world.
- The game has an addictive quality for Lester: in order to excel, he has to play more and more. If he were to play less, he would lose his edge and the resulting "high" from superior performance.
- He developed "pseudorelationships" with other players of the game instead of making and sustaining relationships and friendships in real life.
- He felt loyalty and obligations to the game players on his team and would be reluctant to "let them down" by expending more time and effort on other interests and relationships in the real world.
- He felt omnipotent and godlike in the game, not only by creating his own imago (i.e., "himself") but also by overcoming the "evils" in this fantasy world. This power and drama were hard to match in his real life.
- He experienced fewer lasting consequences of failure in the fantasy world of the game than he did in real life.
- He was neither confronted nor challenged by time limits in the game as he was in real life.

References

American Psychiatric Association: Diagnostic and Statistical Manual of Mental Disorders, 5th Edition. Washington, DC, American Psychiatric Association, 2013

Mazurek MO, Engelhardt CR: Video game use in boys with autism spectrum disorder, ADHD, or typical development. Pediatrics 132:260–266, 2013

Stuck in Adolescence and Cyberspace, Part II (Decide and Discipline): The Case of Lester Silber

The stone which the builders rejected, has become
the main cornerstone (of the temple)
—*Psalms, ascribed to David, King of Judah*

This above all: to thine own self be true,
And it must follow, as the day the night,
Thou canst not be false to any man.
—*William Shakespeare*, Hamlet, *Act I, Scene 3*

"You think rationally. Most people don't."

D1 (Discovery) and D2 (Decision) Components

Overview

As a result of his autism spectrum disorder (ASD), Lester had not learned mentalization skills and therefore was unable to comprehend or fulfill the expectations and needs of other people.[1] Consequently, he was ostracized and bullied by his peers, which evoked his confusion, anger, misogyny, and misanthropy. He responded by withdrawing from people and from engaging in the group activities of everyday life. He filled that void with a total immersion in violent

---

[1]Please see Chapter 11, "Stuck in Pleasing Others, Part II (Decide and Discipline)," for a review of mentalization.

role-playing video games, which provided Lester with illusory engagement, feelings of potency, an outlet for aggressive feelings, and pseudo relevance in a fantasy cyberworld.

A "chicken and egg" challenge emerged as I set about crafting Lester's treatment plan:

- It would be necessary for Lester to give up video games and marijuana in order to learn how and to have the time to engage with other people and, thereby, reap the rewards of meaningful human connection; however,
- Without believing that engagement with others could be safe, rewarding, or even possible, he had no incentive to "trade away" what currently gave him pleasure and purpose—the video games and marijuana.

In my view, the most viable solution to this problem would be a *corrective emotional experience* through psychotherapy. In treatment Lester first would learn how to interact meaningfully and rewardingly with his doctor and then would apply his new knowledge and skills to relationships with others and to activities in real life. No small order for either of us.

Given Lester's dearth of interpersonal and social experiences and skills, the boundaries among the *discovery, decision*, and *discipline* components of the Fatal Pauses 3-D Method of Getting Unstuck were more blended than is usual. In particular, Lester's treatment component would closely coincide with the discovery component. And, as I would learn later, Lester could exhibit a remarkable capacity for discipline.

Key Features of Lester Silber's Being Stuck in Pause

1. *How Lester was stuck:* Dependent on video games and marijuana
2. *Goals for change:* Replace video games and marijuana with human interactions and social activities
3. *Central, unresolved conflict* (approach-avoidance): Craves human connection; dislikes and is fearful of people
4. *Hallmarks of Lester's being stuck*: Amotivation, nonproductivity, social withdrawal, demoralization, irritability, frustration, confusion, low self-esteem

5. *Binary problem/solution*: Wants to play video games and smoke marijuana but fears and distrusts interactions and connections with others/stop playing video games and smoking marijuana and learn how to relate and connect with others
6. *Critical decision points*: No smoking or playing video games (the Power of No); engage in psychotherapy and return to college (the Power of Go)
7. *Corollary factors required to achieve resolution:* Reengage with family; make efforts to make new friends and date young women; and engage in structured social activities by taking college courses, resuming part-time employment, attending religious services, etc.
8. *Resolution:* Engage in biweekly psychotherapy to learn how to relate to others; taper off of video games and marijuana

The Power of Go and the Power of No

When a patient is dependent on a mind-altering substance such as marijuana, psychiatrists prefer to stage treatment by first withdrawing the individual from the drug and thereafter addressing the multifarious factors that led to and sustain the dependency. Our thinking is that a person whose brain is being poisoned must stop using the toxin before his or her brain is capable of recognizing and repairing the sources of the problem. Ideally, a similar approach should be taken with patients with nondrug addictions such as gambling and video game dependence. Understandably, if a person is spending most of his or her waking hours gambling in casinos, poring over racing forms, or ruminating about losses, his or her time and mind are not available to focus on treatment. The ideal, however, is not always practical or possible, as was the case with Lester.

As indicated above, Lester had little incentive to replace the structured and highly stimulating world of video games for relationships with people—whom he did not understand and could not control and whom his life experience had taught him not to trust. I would liken his situation to that of Ms. Anita Anthony (Chapters 5 and 6, "Stuck in My Body"), who required psychotherapy to understand the sources and defensive roles of her overeating before she was able to change her calorie-intensive diet. For Lester, therefore, the Power of Go preceded the Power of No, which meant that he would have to show up twice a week to engage seriously in psychiatric treatment before he stopped smoking marijuana and playing video games.

In the process of replacing the void left from discontinuing Lester's life-orienting, time-consuming, and mind-enslaving patterns of Internet gaming and cannabis use disorders, the Power of Go would be required for his reengagement in life in a variety of realms to include 1) initiating a regular exercise and diet regimen in order to gain and maintain a healthy and attractive body; 2) participating in structured activities outside his townhouse, such as attending synagogue; 3) writing and submitting applications and taking the aptitude and achievement tests necessary to reapply to engineering school; 4) working part time in his parents' computer-servicing business in order to promote socialization and provide structure to his day; and 5) extending the requisite effort to make friends—male and female—of his own age.

Treatment

Insight-Oriented Psychotherapy

Many mental health professionals maintain that *insight-oriented psychotherapy* (also called *psychodynamic psychotherapy*) is contraindicated for people who have ASD and alexithymia, even for those with the milder forms. They believe that such treatment is inherently ineffective, agonizingly frustrating for both the patient and the therapist, and may interfere with or replace other more beneficial treatments, such as cognitive-behavioral therapy. I could not disagree more. I believe that insight-oriented psychotherapy is effective, stimulating, and essential for these patients to achieve their full potentials. It is true that people with ASD are not "psychologically minded," but those on the milder end of the spectrum can learn to become so. Insight-oriented psychotherapy helps the patient learn how to mentalize, and it can be combined successfully with other therapeutic approaches—including cognitive-behavioral therapy, interpersonal therapy, and medications. I also believe insight-oriented psychotherapy is respectful of patients who deserve to understand, experience, and remediate the fundamental reasons that they and their families have suffered so greatly.

Just like within the fashion industry, there are certain people who do *not* do well with "off-the-rack" treatments. Insight-oriented psychotherapy can be effective for a patient with ASD only if it is specially tailored by the clinician to meet the specific problems and needs of that individual. Clinicians must be flexible, intuitive, and inventive in modifying this invaluable type of psychotherapy to accommodate the unique needs and special challenges of their patients. In the section that follows, I will present the ways that insight-oriented psychotherapy is traditionally practiced and how it should be modified for the benefit of people like Lester, who had a milder form of ASD, and for other adult patients who exhibit alexithymia but do not have ASD.

Traditional Insight-Oriented Psychotherapy

To encourage patients to determine for themselves what issues and problems are most relevant to them, the therapist usually obtains a psychological history by asking open-ended questions such as "What is your father like?" The therapist notes and addresses those areas that the patient selects and emphasizes in his or her response from among the vast array of historical possibilities. As discussed above, this approach with a patient with ASD will lead to a blinding blizzard of details that obscures relevant information about key conflicts and their causalities.

Insight-Oriented Psychotherapy Modified for Patients With ASD

The clinician must be far more active, specific, and directive in the acquisition of historical information from patients with ASD. I liken this process to that of an angler who is fishing for the first time in a remote, vast, deep lake. First the fisherman will gain general information about the types of fish that populate that region in order to select the appropriate baits and lures. That step would correspond to the clinician knowing as much as possible about the neurobiological and psychosocial aspects of the illness *before* treating patients with ASD. This will guide the clinician's questions on the basis of the types of life problems that people with ASD are likely to encounter.

Next the fisherman will ask people who are local to the region for tips and help about "how to fish" that specific lake—i.e., where in the lake to fish, what time of day is most productive, how deep to place the bait, reliable techniques for attracting the fish to the bait, etc. This corresponds to the clinician's involving family members, teachers, former clinicians, reliable friends, etc., to help provide information about the life and specific problems of the patient with ASD.

Finally, and most importantly, the fisherman will bring to bear the skills and artistry to interpret, adapt to, and influence what occurs both in and out of the water while fishing. Is the wind blowing too hard to fish in this spot? Will that fallen tree shelter the bait fish that will attract the bigger fish? Do I detect a ripple of interest around my lure on that last cast? Should I retrieve the lure more slowly, perhaps even let it sink to the bottom like an injured minnow? Did I try to set the hook too firmly for the fish's delicate lips? Will the line break if I try to pull the fish into the boat too rapidly? What will I do with the fish once it is in the boat? Is the fish worth keeping? Did I spook other fish when I reeled in this one? Should I move to another spot on the lake?

In preparing for and taking my psychiatric history with Lester, I did the following:

- I thoroughly reviewed the latest scientific literature about autism spectrum disorders—especially about innovations in assessment and treatment.
- I contacted and spoke directly with experts in the field about Lester for guidance about what to look for and best practices in treatment.
- I met with Lester's parents and his sister on numerous occasions—always with Lester in the room—to gain historical information about Lester and his family, to form my own impressions about his family members, to learn how they affected Lester, to inform them about my sense of Lester's problems and what was occurring in his treatment, and to solicit their impressions about my approach to his treatment and Lester's progress.
- I contacted by phone his previous psychiatrist, Dr. Isadore Berger; his counselor at Bellaire High School; his rabbi; and two of his high school teachers who had special relationships with him.
- On the basis of what I was learning, what Lester told me, and what I observed in treatment, I asked Lester numerous progressively more focused and informed questions.

- Most importantly, during *all* of my interactions with Lester, I did my best to explain to him precisely what I was doing and why I was doing it. This process served to teach Lester *how to mentalize.*

It was Dr. Berger who told me about the result of an open-ended question he posed during his only meeting with Lester:

Dr. Isadore Berger: Please tell me about your father.
Lester Silber: He's OK.
Dr. Berger: Just OK?
Lester: Yes.
Dr. Berger: Is there anything more that you would like to tell me about your father?
Lester: No. I can't think of anything.

Although Dr. Berger suspected that Lester had depression and was abusing alcohol or marijuana, he did not gather much specific historical information about Lester, nor did Lester learn a great deal about himself from their interchange. This does not mean, however, that Lester was incapable of a lengthier, more detailed response. As will be shown, if Lester were asked to recount specific events without his having to ascribe importance to those events, his descriptive memory would prove exceptional.

The following is a representative example of how I pieced together a psychiatric history from Lester, an approach that I also use when treating other patients with ASD. I purposely began by asking relatively open ended question about his father in order to test my suspicion that this approach would prove unfruitful. Thereafter, I became increasingly more directive.

Dr. Y.: How did your father treat you when you were a little boy?
Lester Silber: He was nice to me.
Dr. Y.: What exactly do you mean when you say your father was nice?
Lester: He didn't hit me.
Dr. Y.: Did anyone in your family ever hit you when you were a little boy?
Lester: No.
Dr. Y.: Did anyone else ever hit you when you were a little boy?
Lester: Yes.
Dr. Y.: Who hit you when you were a little boy?
Lester: My friends in school.

Dr. Y.: Lester, I want you to remember a specific incident in which a friend hit you when you were a little boy. Then please tell me as much as you can recall about what happened.

Lester: This happened when I was in the first grade. It was 3:22 P.M., and I was walking home from school. Because it was fall, October 23 to be precise, the live oak trees in front of the school had dropped a lot of acorns on the ground. Three of the biggest kids in my class were hiding behind the trees waiting for me. They had stockpiled a bunch of big acorns, and when I walked by they started throwing them at me. The first few hit me in the face and head and stung very bad. I started to run, and they chased after me. I kept getting hit with acorns in the back of my head and neck and on my bare arms and legs. I was wearing my favorite shirt— a white Sesame Street T-shirt with a picture of the Cookie Monster on it. And my green shorts. Finally, I tripped, and they all stood around me and laughed. I turned over on my stomach and tried to protect my face with the sidewalk, which was full of dust, dirt, leaves, and empty acorn shells. The squirrels had gotten to most of them already. Then Tommy Casey gave me a spanking on my bottom, and they all laughed even harder at me. They were out of acorns, so after a few minutes they ran away.

Dr. Y.: What were you feeling?

Lester: I don't remember.

Dr. Y.: Were you afraid?

Lester: I don't know.

Dr. Y.: I would suspect that you were. That was why you were running away. Later, we will talk a lot about what "being afraid" feels like and how to know when you are afraid. But I have another question about your feelings. Were you angry?

Lester: I don't remember.

Dr. Y.: Do you know what anger feels like?

Lester: When I was little, I would scream, kick the floor, and sometimes hit myself when I was angry.

Dr. Y.: That sounds like a temper tantrum, which is one of the extreme forms of anger that you direct at yourself or at objects. When you feel that type of anger, you usually are frustrated because you're not getting your way. Everybody has degrees of anger, some of which are less intense than a tantrum, and some more intense. We will also spend a lot of time, Lester, learning about anger.

Clearly, this is an arduous, time-intensive process for both patients and clinicians. It is work, made more difficult because so many of the goals and positive reinforcements are not realized for many years (so different from the immediate reinforcements of video games). Patience is required from the patient, from his or her family, and from the therapist. Therefore, early in treatment it is essential that the clinician informs both the patient and the family of the arduousness and the long time frame of the treatment process. Otherwise, patients and their families will become dissatisfied, demoralized, and disengaged.

For Lester, these real-life payoffs would be the satisfaction of having warm, meaningful relationships and the fulfillment of work-related success. I was teaching Lester about mental facilities that come "naturally" to most of us through intact brains and "fortunate" socialization.

Additionally, I wanted to express immediately to Lester how sad I felt *as* he told me what he went through. And I wanted to comfort him. However, I was concerned that my expressions might distract Lester from learning about his own feelings. Learning about compassion and empathy would have to wait until much later. He had to understand and feel better about himself first. And that would take time.

The advantage of an insight-oriented psychotherapeutic approach for patients with ASD is that while they are providing their personal psychiatric histories, they are simultaneously learning how to ascribe nuance to their feelings and, thereby, significance to past and current life events. As in all therapy of this type, the primary learning for Lester would be through the analysis of his ongoing relationship with me, where the variables could be controlled—as opposed to all other life experiences.

Insight

Traditional Insight-Oriented Psychotherapy

The powerful influence of psychoanalysis on the practice of psychotherapy and general psychiatry over the first two-thirds of the twentieth century shaped psychotherapists' current concept of what *insight* means. In his classic textbook *Psychodynamic Psychiatry in Clinical Practice* master psychoanalytic clinician and educator Glen Gabbard, M.D., wrote,

> The ultimate goals of psychoanalysis and those treatments weighted toward the expressive end of the continuum involve the acquisition

of insight, which may be defined as the capacity to understand the unconscious meanings and origins of one's symptoms and behavior. Although Freud never used the term *insight*, he did define the goal of analysis as making conscious what is unconscious, which is certainly a significant aspect of insight. (Gabbard 1994, p. 91)

Thus, today, most mental health professionals who practice insight-oriented psychotherapy continue to equate *insight* with a patient's new understandings of how unconscious conflicts, drives, and emotions affect their present feelings, behaviors, and choices. Additionally, insight reveals how patients' unconscious processes influence their psychological symptoms and psychiatric disorders. For example, insight would comprise a patient's new understanding of how she unconsciously transfers her negative feelings for an authoritarian father to important male authority figures in her current life and how this leads to problems in her relationships with such individuals.

In the mental status examination, a standardized process of evaluation of all psychiatric patients and a required component of their medical records, insight has two distinct but interrelated components:

1. The extent to which patients comprehend and appreciate how their psychiatric disorders influence their relationships, behavior, and critical life decisions. For example, patients with manic euphoria often exhibit poor recognition of their impaired judgment with regard to how they dress, spend money, regulate their language, and treat other people. Their poor insight invariably leads to their getting into big trouble.

2. The degree to which patients realize and accept that they require treatment for their psychiatric problems. For example, even though a person has wreaked havoc with his family, his friends, his boss at work, and a police officer as a result of his mania, this individual might still feel euphoric and omnipotent and resist accepting any help from a mental health professional to treat the underlying illness. In fact, people with mania usually feel that *they* are uniquely sane in an insane universe and that it is everyone else who needs *their* help. This is termed *poor insight*.

Both forms of insight are necessary for and can be acquired by people with the milder forms of ASD.

Insight-Oriented Psychotherapy Modified for Patients With ASD

The thinking of people with ASD is concrete and literal, which makes their gaining insight into psychological causalities of their problems difficult—but not impossible—to come by. Again, the psychotherapist must be more active and directive in using insight-oriented psychotherapy in treating people with Asperger's disorder than he or she would be in caring for patients without this condition.

> **Lester Silber:** The only reason I came to see you today is because my parents made me. They said if I didn't come they would turn off my electricity.
>
> **Dr. Y.:** So how do you feel about me?
>
> **Lester:** You're fine.
>
> **Dr. Y.:** What do you mean by "fine"?
>
> **Lester:** Just that. You're fine.
>
> **Dr. Y.:** Does that mean that you like me?
>
> **Lester:** I guess so.
>
> **Dr. Y.:** What do you like about me?
>
> **Lester:** You think rationally. Most people don't.
>
> **Dr. Y.:** Do you like the way that I treat you?
>
> **Lester:** I guess so.
>
> **Dr. Y.:** I will try to treat you with the utmost respect, Lester. I will count on you to tell me when you believe or feel that I don't. Aren't you angry with me for having to make the choice to come see me or, otherwise, have the electricity shut off in your apartment?
>
> **Lester:** It's not an apartment. It is a townhouse. I'm not mad at you. I know you're trying to help me. I get it that you can't help me if I don't come to see you.
>
> **Dr. Y.:** You are correct. I am trying to help you, Lester. Nonetheless, it is possible to have mixed feelings. Do you believe that you need my help?
>
> **Lester:** No. I don't believe that I need any help. I feel fine. I just want to be left alone.
>
> **Dr. Y.:** You can feel angry at a person whom you still like. These two feelings are not mutually exclusive. And I understand and am comfortable with your feeling about me in *both* ways.

Agency and Autonomy

Traditional Insight-Oriented Psychotherapy

A primary goal of insight-oriented psychotherapy is to help the patient develop greater agency and autonomy. In insight-oriented psychotherapy, clinicians take special care not to be overly directive or prescriptive, which can engender a patient's dependency on the therapist. Improved autonomy and self-agency are usually among the goals of insight-oriented psychotherapy. Clinicians try to assume an empathic, nonjudgmental therapeutic stance through a variety of techniques that enhance the clarity and relevance of information without being overly directive. As summarized by Dr. Gabbard, clinicians accomplish this delicate balancing act with the following techniques: *interpretation* of what a patient has told them, sharing with them their *observations* of what the patient has revealed, *clarification* of the information that a patient has provided, *encouragement to elaborate* on relevant subjects, and *validation* of the patient's observation insights (Gabbard 2009, pp. 52–56). The therapist's offering specific advice to the patient is generally discouraged, although there are acceptable exceptions.

Insight-Oriented Psychotherapy Modified for Patients With ASD

To retrieve historical information from patients with ASD and to help them change their dysfunctional behaviors, therapists must be active and directive. In addition to using all of the techniques described in the previous paragraph, clinicians must help their patients learn how to mentalize and think psychologically. This form of psychoeducation is best explained by example, as demonstrated in the following two exchanges that took place after Lester had been in treatment with me for more than a year.

The first example involved our discussion of Lester's having been socked in the nose by a classmate in the third grade. Lester had never understood why he was hit by Larry Benjamin, who had just received a failing grade on a mathematics quiz. The incident took place in the lunchroom at a table with five other students.

> **Larry Benjamin:** I just don't understand why I keep getting such terrible grades in math.
> **Lester Silber:** It's because you're stupid in math, Larry.

Lester's and my discussion of this "ancient" incident was as follows:

> **Dr. Y.:** Do you recall what you were thinking when you responded to Larry in that way?
>
> **Lester Silber:** Sure. He asked me a question, and I gave him an honest answer. I don't lie to people. He *is* stupid in math. He had trouble following anything that was going on in class.
>
> **Dr. Y.:** How do you think Larry felt when you told him he was stupid in front of so many of his friends?
>
> **Lester:** How would I know how he was feeling? I didn't ask him, so he didn't tell me.
>
> **Dr. Y.:** I think he did tell you when he socked you in the nose. Another way of figuring out what he felt is by examining how you felt when you were in a similar situation.
>
> **Lester:** Impossible. I never failed a math test in my life.
>
> **Dr. Y.:** But you did strike out a lot when you played Little League.
>
> **Lester:** More than "a lot." *Every* time that I was at bat.
>
> **Dr. Y.:** Did your teammates ever make remarks about your batting that embarrassed you?
>
> **Lester:** Lots of times.
>
> **Dr. Y.:** Please share with me one or two of these times.
>
> **Lester:** If there were already two outs before I was about to bat, they would say, "Let's get our gloves on and start walking. In three pitches we're back on the field." Or somebody would say to one of the kids whose father is a doctor, "I'm glad your dad is here; if Lester even fouls a ball, I'm going to have a heart attack." Or somebody else would say, "Too bad your baby sister can't pinch-hit for Lester. She's much more likely to get a hit."
>
> **Dr. Y.:** I know you were not trying to make fun of Larry Benjamin when you called him stupid in math. Even though he was not strong in that subject, I believe that he felt the same way that you did when your Little League teammates made those insensitive remarks about you. The problem was that neither you nor your teammates thought about how the *other* person would feel before they made their comments. The bottom line, Lester, is that it's important for you to think about how the *other* person might feel *before* you make a comment about them.
>
> **Lester:** *Every* time?
>
> **Dr. Y.:** Yes. *Every* time!
>
> **Lester:** That's a lot of work.
>
> **Dr. Y.:** Yes, it's a lot of *hard* work. But it will become easier with lots of practice, and your effort will pay great dividends.

As reviewed in Chapter 11, mentalizing involves keeping simultaneously *your own mind in mind* and *the minds of others in mind*. A second example of how I used a directive and active approach in insight-oriented psychotherapy was to help Lester learn how to examine his own thoughts and feelings.

> **Dr. Y.:** How did you feel when the fathers of all the other kids came to their Little League games but your father never did?
>
> **Lester Silber:** Dad told me that he had to be at work to support our family.
>
> **Dr. Y.:** That's a factual memory, Lester. Not a feeling.
>
> **Lester:** I don't remember how I felt, so I must have felt fine.
>
> **Dr. Y.:** That's one possibility, but I would like to suggest other possibilities. You are a very observant and rational person, Lester. You observed that most of the fathers of the other kids also had jobs and that they also had to support their families. Maybe you thought that your father didn't come to games because he was embarrassed about how poorly you played baseball.
>
> **Lester:** I was the worst player in the entire league. Why would he show up to watch me strike out and never, ever catch the ball?
>
> **Dr. Y.:** Because he loves you, no matter whether you perform well or poorly in a baseball game.
>
> **Lester:** I don't follow what you are getting at, Dr. Y.
>
> **Dr. Y.:** It is possible that you felt undeserving of your father's love because you were not good in baseball.
>
> **Lester:** Oh, I get it now. Like in elementary arithmetic, "if equals are added to equals, the results are equal."
>
> **Dr. Y.:** Now I'm not following you, Lester.
>
> **Lester:** The other guys' fathers came to all their games. I assumed it was because their fathers were more proud of them because they were so good at baseball. I do remember thinking at the time that Dad would show up if I could learn how to hit home runs. But there was no chance of me doing that. I never once got to first base. Do you think he should have come anyway?
>
> **Dr. Y.:** Yes. But let me add that I'm not practicing what I preach. I didn't go to many of my own children's events at school. I was always at work. But I love them deeply. Just like your dad loves and cares about you. Still, I didn't show up enough, and I know they noticed and didn't like it. I am sorry for that to this very day.

This is a complex interchange, and, in many ways, it is atypical for the conduct of "usual" insight-oriented psychotherapy. More traditional psychotherapists would fault me for "telling your patient how he felt or should feel" and for "interfering with the transference between you and your patient by revealing far too much about your personal life and feelings." That certainly would be true if I were treating a patient without ASD who was more psychologically minded.

Most traditional psychotherapists would have to be taught theoretical physics in a *very* different way from that which was required for Lester. He had mastered advanced, graduate school level concepts in mathematics and physics when he was in the fifth grade. My point is that psychotherapy (and education) should be shaped by and fitted to the needs and abilities of patients, not the other way around—a common, guild-like, and unfortunate practice in my field that I term *Procrustean psychotherapy.*

It is not too far of a stretch that Lester would have concluded that his father did not attend any of his Little League games because he played the game so poorly. He certainly was getting similar messages from his peers and their fathers, who made fun of him and didn't want him on their teams for that reason. It was important for Lester to understand, from his father's perspective and from my own personal experience, that everything is not exclusively "black and white." Fathers can make mistakes by not showing up, yet they still love their children very much.

Ultimately, Lester's feeling worthy of being loved and his being able to have some sense of what goes on in the minds of others would be required for him to have deeper connections with other people. Additionally, his having a more realistic, granular view of me as a well-intended but far-from-perfect person was essential for bringing about his change and growth.

- If he could like me with all my flaws, he could like himself as an imperfect being.
- If he came to trust me, an example of another "imperfect authority figure," he could learn to take advantage of his own intellectual gifts to gain and accept authority and power for himself.
- If he would learn to accept and love his "imperfect self," he could make deeper connections with others—who also would not be perfect.

Early on in Lester's treatment I knew that the lure of *deeper connections with others* would have to become Lester's primary reason to risk trading his virtual world of video games for the less safe, less controllable world of other people.

Lester Silber: When I went to Austin, I really tried to stay off of video games and pot—once and for all. I was certain that I would succeed. Why do you think that I didn't, Dr. Y.?

Dr. Y.: For better and worse, Lester, we humans are social animals. In Austin, you needed in your life, but didn't have, three things: *commitment, relevance,* and *connection.* And you still don't have them. Our work in treatment will focus on your learning to understand these three ephemeral, but nonetheless essential, needs and how to go about fulfilling them for yourself.

Lester: I really don't get what you are talking about, Dr. Y. But if you believe it's important, I'll work on it.

D3 (Discipline): Giving up Marijuana and Video Games

"AMJ": Adios, Mary Jane

Without question, Lester Silber had a different brain from most people, and that was the primary source of his psychiatric symptoms and disabilities. Nonetheless, the longer he was in treatment the more I appreciated the formidability of his cerebral assets. Among these were the gifts of rational thought, logic, intellectual precision, cognitive focus, and memory for details. As treatment progressed and his trust of me deepened, I increasingly enlisted and deployed his intellectual assets to counter his psychosocial problems. As discussed, his review of the scientific literature of ASD led him to understand and readily accept that he had a mild version of the disorder.

After about 4 months of treatment, I believed that Lester was sufficiently engaged in and supported by his therapy to begin to address directly his marijuana abuse and video game dependency. Once more I shared with him what I considered to be the least biased and best designed scientific papers on the effects, side effects, and safety of marijuana. By our next session he had read the papers and drawn conclusions.

Lester Silber: I read the papers on cannabis. Your field, Dr. Y., has a long way to go before it's a true science.

Dr. Y.: What do you mean specifically?

Lester: Far too many variables to control to achieve 100% accurate conclusions.

Dr. Y.: That's the nature of doing research involving humans—we are more than our molecules and less controllable than robots. "Perfection" is not possible in human behavioral research.

Lester (*with dry irony*): I know, and it's too bad about that. I could never work in your field. It would drive me crazy. Still, it's very clear that weed fucks up the brain. Stands to reason. If THC [tetrahydrocannabinol, the psychoactive component of cannabis] had evolutionary value, we wouldn't have to smoke the stuff. Our livers would make it for us.

Dr. Y.: Agreed. So what conclusions did you draw from the journal articles about your use of marijuana?

Lester: Just like I said: it's bad for the brain. I stopped smoking pot 2 days ago.

Dr. Y.: Did you experience any withdrawal effects?

Lester: Nothing physical. But it's not as much fun playing World of Warcraft when I'm not stoned, and I'm not as good at it.

Dr. Y.: I believe that you made an intelligent decision, Lester. Even though you may not enjoy the video games as much, you should find that you will have more energy and motivation to do and, perhaps, enjoy *other* things.

TREATMENT PRINCIPLE 12

The patient's strengths and assets should always be in the forefront of psychiatric care. Not only should these resources form the basis of the alliance between the patient and clinician but also they must be mobilized and directed to effect therapeutic change.

Relinquishing Video Games: An "Essential Taper"

A fundamental premise of the Fatal Pauses 3-D Method of Getting Unstuck is to reduce the conflicts that underlie being stuck to binary "yes" or "no" choices with no gray areas that undermine decisions to take action. In this chapter, I have also made the case that mental health professionals must eschew theoretical dogma and show flexibility in treating *all* patients—especially those who have ASD.

In treating Lester, I discovered that he is blessed not only with daunting intellectual gifts but also with remarkable tenacity and work ethic. These assets are not unusual for people with milder forms of ASD. As Lester increasingly began to trust me, I developed a paradoxical concern for a professional: that he would follow my recommendations *too closely and too soon*. His own input and judgment were imperative about whether or not he were *ready* to make a life change as all-encompassing (for him) as stopping video games, no matter how positive that change would ultimately prove to be.

> **Lester Silber:** I know you are not a big fan of my playing video games all the time, Dr. Y. Do you think I should stop?
> **Dr. Y.:** I believe that is a decision that we should make together.
> **Lester:** I read the articles that you gave me on how video games can have similar effects on the brain that drugs do. I don't want any part of that.
> **Dr. Y.:** Like many drugs that we become dependent on, it might be best to taper the video games. And to extend the metaphor, Lester, we often have to replace the abused substance with something safer.
> **Lester:** Explain, please.
> **Dr. Y.:** For example, when detoxifying someone from chronic alcohol dependence, we switch him or her to tapering doses of a benzodiazepine to prevent delirium tremens and other withdrawal effects. What do you think about your systematically reducing the time that you play World of Warcraft and replacing the time with playing StarCraft and with new activities outside your townhouse?
> **Lester:** You did your homework, Dr. Y. I like StarCraft a lot, but I don't get hooked on it like I do on Warcraft. I'll bring the taper schedule to my next session.

Although the dialogue above might seem unrealistic for most people with a significant substance use disorder, it is prototypical for a patient with ASD. Our discussion is an example of taking advantage of Lester's brain differences that cause problems in other areas. Although Lester's superrationality, concrete thinking, and tendency to view the world in blacks and whites did not serve him well in interpersonal relationships, these qualities could be directed constructively in his treatment. If a rational, scientifically corroborated case could be made to change a behavior, no matter how ingrained, Lester would make the change. In other words, his *decision* and *discipline* capacities are "off the chart."

True to his word, Lester drew up and followed a taper regimen for video games that reduced his playing time by an average of 8.3% per month over 12 months, which meant that he would stop playing altogether in exactly 1 year. I countered by encouraging Lester to begin the process of reapplying to engineering schools, and he agreed.

> **Lester Silber:** What college would accept me? You know that I will tell the truth about my drug abuse and arrest.
>
> **Dr. Y.:** The truth will also show that you are gifted in physics, math, and engineering and that there are sound medical reasons for the difficulties that you have experienced. You can count on me to help you with your application and to write the medical letter to the engineering school.

Because of their precision, perfectionism, and black-and-white thinking, Lester and many other people with milder forms of ASD tend to be overly modest. If they do not achieve perfection, they believe that they have failed. For Lester, a 97% on a physics examination was an indication that he did not understand the subject matter: "Engineers can't afford to be a whopping 3% off target," he reasoned. For this reason and because of how they are mistreated by their peers, most people with ASD have low self-esteem.

Lester wrote the initial draft of his application to engineering school. Predictably, he emphasized his deficiencies without alluding whatsoever to his abilities and accomplishments. Helping him rewrite his application letter afforded me the opportunity to analyze with him the high costs to his self-esteem associated with his perfectionism as well as to compliment him on his superior intellectual gifts and character traits.

Not surprisingly, Lester was readily accepted to pursue a B.S. in computer engineering at the Cullen College of Engineering at the University of Houston (Cullen Engineering). He also kept to his taper protocol.

What Women Want

Painfully shy, insecure, and generally distrustful of people, Lester had almost no dating experience. In taking his sexual history, I learned that he was also entirely devoid of a fantasy life. Rather, similar to his practice in so many other critical realms of his life, he sublimated his sexual drives through computer-related activities. Lester's understanding of sexual behavior and his sexual experience came almost entirely from two Internet-based sources: 1) video pornography from free Web sites such as Pornhub, of which he was a regular viewer, and

2) video games. He did not engage in the myriad of fee-based real-time interactive sexual sites. I was careful not to make the technical error of communicating to Lester that sexuality was too sensitive of a subject for us to address directly in his treatment.

> **Dr. Y.:** What type of Internet pornography interests you, Lester?
> **Lester Silber:** I don't understand what you're asking me.
> **Dr. Y.:** Describe what happens in some of your favorite videos.

By posing directed questions, I learned that Lester was especially aroused by pornography in which older women would assume sexually assertive roles with younger, more passive men. This preference reflected Lester's conflicted relationship with his dispassionate father and his much closer bond to his warmer, more nurturing, and emotionally responsive mother. Passivity and immaturity would permit Lester, unconsciously, to feel less "responsible" for his sexuality and, therefore, less vulnerable to the competitive retaliation of his father. Although his lack of initiative and sexual passivity might "work" for him in cyberspace, it would retard any real-life opportunities. Although psychodynamic interpretations of this type would be too abstract and theoretical to be of benefit to Lester, they helped to confirm what I had hypothesized to be his central sexual conflicts and guide my approach to preparing him to understand and relate respectfully and responsibly to eligible young women.

The Internet-based video pornography that Lester regularly viewed usually consisted of 15- to 20-minute segments, approximately 98% of which were dedicated to explicit sexual activity between or among the actors. In almost every segment, the characters were portrayed as meeting one another for the first time at the beginning of the scenarios. Said another way, the establishment of the relationships in the scenarios that led up to sexual activities generally took about as much time, but with far less engagement, than ordering and receiving French fries in the drive-through lane of a McDonald's restaurant. As revealed in the following interchange, that pattern formed Lester's expectations in real-life heterosexual relationships.

> **Dr. Y.:** Lester, what do you want in a relationship with a woman?
> **Lester Silber:** Sex.
> **Dr. Y.:** And what do you think a woman might want from a relationship with you?

Lester: How would I know? I'm not a woman.
Dr. Y.: What do you imagine a woman would want in a relationship with you?
Lester: I would guess sex and money.
Dr. Y.: A positive physical relationship and financial security are, at some point, important to most young women. They are also interested in being understood, respected, valued, and treated as equals, which takes some time and effort to convey.

As stated, Lester's other source for conceptualizing who women are and what women want came from their depictions in video games. Most of the role-playing video games that he played involve violence perpetrated by and against dangerous and attractive women. Women are also objectified as "rewards" for heroes who have been successful in conquests. We therefore devoted the full year in which Lester was tapering from video games to preparing him for mature and respectful involvements with young women. To "learn by dating" would have carried a high potential for Lester to misunderstand, disrespect, and mistreat women, who would, understandably, respond by rejecting him.

Basic Training and the Power of Go

As discussed in this chapter, several of the tenets of psychotherapy that derive from theories and practices that were established in the early twentieth century do not work well for patients with ASD, like Lester. Among these is the proscription of psychotherapists from being too directive in the lives of their patients. During the year that Lester was tapering his video game play—with my strong encouragement, direction, and support—he began to reengage in semistructured activities outside of his townhouse. He returned to attending synagogue on a regular basis, did part-time work in his father's computer servicing business, and volunteered at Texas Children's Hospital to teach computer use to children with developmental disorders involving learning and cognition.

I routinely "prescribe" a specially tailored diet and exercise regimen to almost all of the patients whom I treat. Seldom have these recommendations been more needed than they were by Lester. He had not exercised at all since the 10th grade, when 2 hours a week of gym were required during the school year. Uncoordinated and having experienced so much ridicule on playgrounds and ball fields by his peers, Lester staunchly resisted my initial efforts to motivate him to work out. Compounding matters, most of his meals over the many years of his video game dependency consisted primarily of salty snack foods extracted hurriedly from family-size Mylar bags next to his computer.

> **Lester Silber:** You can't imagine how uncoordinated I am, Dr. Y. It's hopeless for me to do anything physical.
>
> **Dr. Y.:** You're right, Lester. I don't believe it. First of all, being physically fit does not require athleticism. It is a matter of routinized, systematic conditioning that you, of all people, should be good at. Second, you play video games at an incredibly high level, and that entails quick reflexes and good hand-eye coordination. Just as you trained yourself to be able to do this well, you can be trained to succeed at many physical activities.
>
> **Lester:** What do you suggest?
>
> **Dr. Y.:** First join the Jewish Community Center and hire a personal trainer. Begin with fitness training that increases your strength, aerobic conditioning, and balance. Then take yoga classes, bicycle spinning classes, and lessons in running and swimming technique. If you put in a fraction of the time and effort that you did for video games, you can become accomplished in all of these sports. And you will become strong and physically fit. You also will look and feel great.
>
> **Lester:** Makes some sense. I'll try.

As an added bonus, each experience provided many fertile examples from which Lester could learn in psychotherapy about how to relate better with people individually and in group settings.

Back to Life

Having a Fit

At my further encouragement, Lester took some advanced placement tests before entering Cullen Engineering in the fall. As a result, he placed out of all of the introductory prerequisite courses for his degree, and that encompassed much of the curriculum of his freshman and sophomore years. Professor Edwin Milstein, the undergraduate dean of Cullen Engineering, asked Lester to meet with him before the beginning of the academic year.

> **Dean Edwin Milstein:** Lester, at this point do you have any areas of computer science that are of special interest to you?

Lester Silber: Not really.

Dean Milstein: Given that you have tested out of more than half of your degree requirements, I want to make two suggestions. First, I advise you to take postgraduate level courses in your areas of strength, and, second, I want you to work on a project in the research lab of one of our faculty. Since you have no special interests at this point, I suggest that you work in the lab of Professor Michael Zhang. He studies mathematical models of computer security.

Lester: OK. I'm interested in hacking.

It appeared to me that Dean Milstein had read and heeded my letter of support that accompanied Lester's application to Cullen Engineering:

> I write this letter from the perspective gained from nearly 40 years of being on the faculty of three excellent research-oriented medical schools and being an active teacher of exceptional students in these institutions. Based on this perspective and experience, I would rate Lester Silber as having the intellectual and academic potential that would place him in the top 1% of this outstanding group of students.
>
> With the benefit of mentorship of carefully selected faculty, Lester has the potential to make transformational contributions to mathematics and computer sciences. Additionally, I have full confidence that his previous psychiatric problems are now being addressed and will no longer interfere with his academic progress or citizenship.

Professor Zhang proved to be the brilliant and caring mentor that Lester needed and deserved. Within 2 years under Professor Zhang's tutelage, Lester was functioning at the level of a junior faculty member. More importantly, for the first time in his life, he felt accepted, appreciated, and engaged. He loved the work and Professor Zhang. Lester accumulated sufficient credits to complete his B.S. degree in 2 years, and he promptly entered the Ph.D. program in computer science engineering at Cullen Engineering.

As a graduate student with Professor Zhang as his faculty advisor, Lester wrote several groundbreaking papers in prestigious basic science journals and received hefty federal research grants supporting the testing of his novel mathematical models for securing large and complex computer systems. The creative, innovative solutions that he formulated and tested and the relevance of Lester's work did not escape wide notice. The theoretical concepts that he developed were adopted for use by other academic disciplines, including structural biology.

As he approached the completion of his Ph.D. degree, Lester was intensively recruited by preeminent universities, giant international corporations, and many agencies of the federal government. He chose to remain in Houston to join the faculty of the University of Houston. He became a tenured full professor in 4 years and co-founded with Professor Zhang a start-up software development and consultation company to "harden" computer networks against sophisticated hacking. With Lester as president and CEO and Professor Zhang as scientific director, their company currently is based in Houston and has branches in Palo Alto, California; Cambridge, Massachusetts; Cambridge, England; Taiwan; and Haifa, Israel.

Having a Fan

To paraphrase Tolstoy from *Anna Karenina*, functional brains are, for the most part, alike, but those that are dysfunctional are dissimilar in their own unique ways. Lester Silber's brain is different from those of most of us. With his intellectual gifts and penchant for hard work, through psychotherapy and with the support and mentorship of the faculty of the University of Houston, Lester's return to academics and his establishing a pioneering and rapidly growing business, for the most part, went smoothly. However, his efforts to meet and form meaningful relationships with women were fraught with false starts, frustration, and feelings of rejection and humiliation. His brain seemed to be working against him, against the women with whom he tried to engage, and against my efforts to help him in this domain. He scoured the Internet for methods of attracting and courting women, and he favored reductionist, misogynous models over those that I and his family espoused.

A central theme to which Lester held with vice-like obstinacy was that *all women* wished to be dominated by powerful alpha males, while simultaneously viewing himself as a weak and passive beta male, or a woman's choice by default after she had been abandoned by a succession of alpha males. Lester rejected outright my psychodynamic interpretations of the patently defensive origins of this view; he discounted the many examples of what I had been told in my clinical and professional (i.e., academic-based) experience by strong, highly intelligent women; and he minimized the value of my analyses of what had gone awry in his real-life choices of and in his interactions with women in his many unsuccessful forays. After being rejected, he would say, "Of course women want nothing to do with me once they realize how weak I am." Gentle, modest, loyal, and generous by nature, Lester persisted in trying to recast himself into a macho video game–type hero with the ultimate result of either angering or frightening away a seemingly endless succession of otherwise eligible women. He discounted my oft-repeated advice from Shakespeare's Polonius, "This above all: to thine own self be true," as pathetically romantic and uncharacteristically naïve.

About a year after Lester received his Ph.D. degree, he was invited to present a paper on applied mathematics at a conference that was held in Paris, France. After his talk, Esther Rabinovich, a graduate student in computer sciences from the Technion Institute of Technology in Haifa, Israel, approached Lester. He was taken aback by her familiarity with and grasp of his work. Lester also believed her to be the most beautiful woman he had ever seen. Two months after he returned to Houston, Lester received an invitation from the chairman of the Computer Sciences College of the Technion Institute of Technology to come to Israel for 2 weeks as a visiting professor. The invitation prompted the following discussion in his next treatment session:

> **Lester Silber:** I don't think that I will accept the invitation.
> **Dr. Y.:** How did you arrive at that determination?
> **Lester:** My work is all preliminary. It's a long way from being perfect.
> **Dr. Y.:** My, my, my, Lester. I can't recall your ever being so immodest.
> **Lester:** How so? You should know by now, engineers require perfection.
> **Dr. Y.:** As we both know, the Technion is an elite research institution in applied mathematics and computer sciences. I would think, Lester, that you would accept their faculty's assessment of whose work is important in their field. Also, your accepting their invitation for a visiting professorship is a great opportunity for you to get to know Esther better. You were quite taken by her.
> **Lester:** Yes, but no way would she ever have any interest in me. We've run that failed experiment many times, with the same result.

> **Dr. Y.:** There you go again, Lester. From what you have told me about her, I believe that Esther is perfectly capable of making up her own mind. Most Sabras are.

With a great deal of encouragement on my part, Lester relented and accepted the invitation. Esther met Lester at the Tel Aviv airport and served as his guide and host for the 2-week visit. She introduced Lester to a group of brilliant young Israeli scientists and entrepreneurs in applied mathematics and computer sciences, and, to Lester's astonishment, their commonality in science and mathematics formed a foundation for lasting friendships. For the first time in his life, Lester had a circle of welcoming friends. Also for the first time, he was a member of a team for which he was perfectly capable of batting clean-up.

Romance budded between Lester and Esther while he was in Israel. Although I would have liked to believe that Lester's many years of intensive psychotherapy may have helped, somewhat, to prepare the soil for their relationship, it was Esther's special qualities that made it all possible. She saw through the many layers of defense that Lester had built up over his life as a consequence of being bullied and socially ostracized to the bedrock of his gentle temperament and generous nature. Esther's first-rate scientific mind seemed to matter most to Lester, but from a distance, I most admired her psychological insight.

Full Disclosure

Esther spent the following summer as a visiting research fellow at Rice University, and for the next 6 months she and Lester communicated over the Internet through Skype. On the basis of Esther's brief visit and substantial academic record, Rice University made a strong recruitment offer to her to join their faculty. Rice was not alone recognizing Esther's talents and scientific potential, as Cal Tech, MIT, and Stanford also entered the recruitment fray. In his treatment, Lester reported Esther's future employment opportunities in his characteristic, matter-of-fact fashion, and that prompted the following discussion in our treatment sessions:

> **Dr. Y.:** How old is Esther?
> **Lester Silber:** Almost 28 years old. Why do you ask?

Dr. Y.: I believe that the long-term implications of her relationship with *you* will strongly influence where she chooses to work when she graduates this spring.

Lester: I don't agree. Esther is a rational person. She will make that decision based entirely on the best place for her to do science.

Dr. Y.: You have been enthralled by Esther for 18 months. During that time you have not indicated any interest in seeing any other woman. Have you thought about whether or not you would want to marry her?

Lester: What's the point of that? No way would she want to marry me.

Dr. Y.: Why don't we first determine what you want? If you decide that you would like to marry Esther, then you can ask her. I don't believe that she will have a problem telling you what she would like to do or not to do.

Lester: I can't do that. I would be dishonest without first having full disclosure about my autism spectrum disorder. Obviously, I carry the genes for this condition, which could be transferred to her children.

Dr. Y.: What would you consider to be "full disclosure," Lester?

Lester: Esther's consulting someone who knows both the genetics of ASD and my phenotype. You're in the best position to do that.

Dr. Y.: It would be my great privilege if Esther would like me to do so. But, as you know, Lester, I am not exactly impartial toward you.

Lester: Then you should know that I'm not *that* stupid. I do love Esther, after all. And, as you are always telling me, Dr. Y., she's perfectly capable of factoring in your bias.

Within 2 months Esther returned to Houston for a follow-up visit at Rice University and to be with Lester. He steadfastly refused to broach the subject of marriage until after she met with me to discuss the potential ramifications of his autism spectrum disorder. Esther did not hesitate to accept Lester's invitation to join him in his next psychotherapy session.

Dr. Y.: Welcome, Esther. Lester has told me many wonderful things about you.

Esther Rabinovich: Really? That is great to hear. He is not big on complimenting me.

Dr. Y.: Even less so in complimenting himself, as I'm sure you have noticed. During the 6 years we have worked together I apply the "coefficient of Lester," which is a multiplier, to get an ac-

curate measure of how he feels about others. Your measure is
off the charts, Esther.

Esther: Before I entered the Technion, I served in the army. Although Lester frequently uses combat terms, at heart, he is quite different from other men who I have known. He is modest, gentle, does not exaggerate.

Dr. Y.: Lester is, indeed, different from most other people. Did he tell you that he has a mild form of autism spectrum disorder?

Esther: That was almost the first thing he told me about himself. But he never once mentioned the pioneering papers that he has written or the many international science prizes he has won for his research.

Dr. Y.: I am absolutely delighted to have the chance to meet with you, Esther. Nonetheless, the main reason Lester invited you to join us today is to provide you the opportunity to ask me any questions that you might have about his autism spectrum disorder.

Esther: I have read about his condition, and I asked my brother about it. He is a doctor who practices and teaches at Hadassah Hospital in Jerusalem. But I don't understand why Lester brought me here to see you.

Dr. Y.: Lester?

Lester Silber: So that Dr. Y. could answer your questions about my autism.

Dr. Y.: Esther knows that part, Lester. But why should that be important to her?

Lester: Because I love you, Esther. And I would like you to think about marrying me.

Esther: Then we don't need Dr. Y., and I don't need to think about it. *You* have answered all my questions, Lester. And my answer to yours is "Yes."

Six months later Esther and Lester were married in the Chagall Chapel of Hadassah Hospital. With the approval of Lester's parents, I accepted Lester and Esther's gracious invitation to attend the wedding in Israel, along with my wife, Dr. Beth. Professor Michael Zhang also was there, and he advised me as follows:

Professor Michael Zhang: Be sure to take a bunch of pictures of the wedding party. At least half of Lester's groomsmen and Esther's bridesmaids will someday win Nobel Prizes in Physics or Mathematics. And my bet is that Lester will be the first.

About a year after they were married, Esther gave birth to their son, Avraham Yosef. At this point he shows no evidence whatsoever of having autism spectrum disorder. And my bet is that Avraham Yosef will be pretty damn good at math and physics.

References

Gabbard GO: Psychodynamic Psychiatry in Clinical Practice: The DSM-IV Edition. Washington DC, American Psychiatric Press, 1994

Gabbard GO: Textbook of Psychotherapeutic Treatments. Washington, DC, American Psychiatric Publishing, 2009

Stuck in Success: The Case of Reverend Maynard Henden

The righteous will spring up like a palm tree,
shall grow tall like a cedar in Lebanon…
He shall still shoot forth in old age,
shall be full of sap and green.
—*David, King of Judah, Psalm 92*

So teach us to number our days
that we may gain a heart of wisdom.
—*David, King of Judah, Psalm 90*

"With all of his brains and wisdom, Maynard doesn't
seem to grasp the passage of time."

The Case of Reverend Maynard Henden: D1 (Discover) Assessment Component

Pastoral Counseling

Before driving home from the office, I was perusing my phone messages when one note in particular caught my eye:

> The Reverend Maynard Henden from Dallas called at 3:00 P.M. to inquire whether or not you do "pastoral counseling." His cell phone # is….

Although my usual practice is to return afternoon phone calls after dinner (it was about 8:30 P.M.), I wanted to get right back to Reverend Henden. I had met him on one occasion in the early 1980s, but we had not been in touch over the ensuing decades. Nonetheless, I kept up with his illustrious career as a pioneer in spiritual counseling for hospitalized patients, especially those with terminal illnesses. At the time of the call, he also was the president of an eminent university in Dallas.

So I delayed my trip home to return his call:

> **Reverend Maynard Henden:** Hello, this is Maynard Henden speaking.
>
> **Dr. Y.:** Hello, this is Stuart Yudofsky returning your call from Houston. Are you recommending pastoral counseling for me, someone you know, or yourself?
>
> **Reverend Henden:** None of the above. I believe that I have an absolutely and completely blessed life. It is my wife, Elizabeth, who is recommending that I get a psychiatric consultation. Given my current position, we thought that I should do this outside of Dallas. So do you have time to take me on?
>
> **Dr. Y.:** Certainly, it will be a privilege. As you probably know from your vocation, Reverend Henden, too many blessings can also pose problems. Would you like Elizabeth to join us at our first meeting?
>
> **Reverend Henden:** Yes. I think that she would be helpful to us both.
>
> **Dr. Y.:** Lord knows, I can use all the help that I can get.

The High Cost of Success, Part I

Three weeks later the couple traveled to Houston for the consultation. The Reverend and Mrs. Henden planted the flag at the pinnacle of positive first impressions. Tall, thin, and lithe, with glistening tributaries of silver gently mixing into the casual currents of their flaxen hair, the couple could have been mistaken for brother and sister.

Reverend Henden beamed beneficently as I greeted them in my office waiting room. Mrs. Henden was much more reserved. She examined me with the critical eye and reservations of a judge in the Westminster Kennel Club Show who was about to put through its paces an unworthy representative of an unworthy breed that, somehow, had made the finals.

For a reasonable sum at most moderate-price department stores, one can purchase the off-the-rack dark blue blazer, the Dockers press-free khaki slacks, and the light blue dress shirt with its button-down collar that Reverend Henden wore open about his neck. However, his overall presentation would be the envy of any NFL team owner posed in the front row of his loge with the expectation of being on camera at halftime. With Reverend Henden, it's "the man," both inside and out, who "makes the clothes." And Mrs. Henden was his perfect match in attire and effect. She is the type of woman whom men would notice no matter what she was wearing and whom their wives, despite their envy, would like. Not that she would care what others thought of her. Seeing her in the autumn of her life, one would be hard pressed to imagine that she could have been any more radiant and desirable in her spring.

Dr. Y.: I am happy to see you again, Reverend Henden, after so, so many years.

Mrs. Elizabeth Henden (*surprised*): Again?

Reverend Maynard Henden: I wasn't sure you'd remember me, Dr. Yudofsky. Elizabeth wouldn't have known that we met at Columbia-Presbyterian Hospital in the early 1980s in a multidisciplinary conference for a person with Kaposi's sarcoma, a type of cancer that results from AIDS. Dr. Yudofsky discussed the neuropsychiatric care of the patient, and I had presented on the spiritual dimensions of the case. Do I recall that correctly?

Dr. Y.: Admirably so. Reverend Henden spoke about the importance of treating someone with a terminal disease *not* as a medical problem but as a human being going through the natural process of dying. I presented some new data showing that the HIV virus could also infect the brain and how the patient's mental status would be affected by that. It seemed to most people attending the conference that we were in polar disagreement about the treatment approach, so I asked Reverend Henden if he could join me for coffee to discuss the patient further.

Reverend Henden: We found out that our approaches were absolutely compatible and that we had a lot in common.

Mrs. Henden: If I can interrupt this walk down memory lane, let's get down to why we came here to see you. I'll start. First and foremost, Maynard is a wonderful person, university president, minister, father, and husband. And I know, Dr. Y., that you are cognizant—as am I—of how I ordered these qualities. Judging by how he spends his time and mental energy, these are the exact order of his priorities. He is beloved by everyone in Dallas. And even though he is rarely around us, our three children and I love and respect him beyond all measure.

Reverend Henden (*interrupting mischievously*): Well, that about covers it. Time to hit the road back to Dallas.

Mrs. Henden (*impatiently*): No, that does not quite cover it. Your main problems, Maynard, are your strengths. You're both a good and a brilliant person. You are *too* good, and almost everyone you know gets that. And they take advantage of you. In effect, you have two full-time jobs. Beyond your colossal administrative responsibilities at the university, you've never stopped being a minister. You're often the first person people call when they're troubled or in trouble.

Reverend Henden: Isn't that what psychiatrists call an *idealized transference*, Dr. Y.?

Dr. Y.: Only if it is *not* true. Freud is rumored to have said, "Sometimes a cigar is just a cigar."

Mrs. Henden (*scoldingly*): Be serious—both of you! You are a busy man, Dr. Y., and we did not come all this way for joking around. I have known Maynard since he was 23 years old, when he had just started Divinity School at Duke. He has been working like a dog his every waking minute since that time. He never says "No" to anyone. He hardly ever takes a day off from work.

A university president's work is never done. Countless meetings; budgets; speeches; dinners with faculty, students, or board members almost every night; recruiting; and raising money. To compound all of that, he still does some ministerial duties. From officiating at weddings and funerals for close friends and supporters of the university to midnight hospital visits and vigils to getting calls at any time day or night when someone's child is in serious trouble with drugs or the police, he never stops.

Maynard loves his work and his calling, but his children and I think that the hours and stress are starting to take a toll on him. He looks tired to us. On rare occasions he gets irritable, and that is not like him at all. We think that the stress comes from doing so much administrative work that he truly dislikes. Also, the endless fund-raising and the university politics are wearing him down. He has to wake up at 4:00 A.M. every morning in order to have a single hour in the day to exercise, read, and write in peace, and these are the things he loves doing the most. He hasn't played a round of golf in over a year.

With all of his brains and wisdom, Maynard doesn't seem to grasp the passage of time. Our three boys have grown up and have jobs on the East Coast. Two of our sons live in New York City, and one lives in Boston. We rarely visit them. The wife of our oldest son is now pregnant. I can tell you both one thing for certain: I plan to be an integral part of the lives of our children and grandchildren. I have had it with Maynard's being there for everybody else but us.

Dr. Y.: What do you mean, exactly?

Mrs. Henden: I mean that I'm going to live near my children. With or without Maynard, I'm going to be in the lives of our children and grandchildren. And if that means having a home in New York City or Boston, I will get one. For several years Maynard has talked about cutting back, but, if anything, he is busier than ever. He needs to make a decision to change what he's been doing since I first met him, nearly 40 years ago.

Reverend Henden: Elizabeth is right. I am a victim of my many blessings. The university grows and grows, and with that growth come ever more administrative responsibilities. I'm 65 years old, and the university's board of trustees just had me sign a 5-year renewal of my contract. We're planning a billion dollar capital campaign for major expansions in our graduate schools and to develop international campuses. Our board says that they need me for stable leadership and fund-raising during that time. The new campuses will let us expand all of our educational and charitable missions. We will help so many people, if we can pull it off.

Mrs. Henden: Well, there you have it, Dr. Y. Despite all the tragedy that Maynard sees every single day of his life, he still believes that he will stay healthy and live forever. Meanwhile, he's missing out on so much of our family joy and fun, and we miss him. I've grown tired of waiting for him to see the light. I've grown tired of waiting around for him, altogether. Maybe you can do something with him. I haven't been able to.

Maynard Henden: Early Years

Maynard Henden was born in Beaumont, a quintessentially blue-collar town in eastern Texas. Like most of his friends, Maynard's father worked in one of the petrochemical industries that blotch Beaumont's wetlands with an acne of buildings, tanks, and towers that steam and flame their perennial sky with beige belches from lofty turrets and that infect the townfolk with dreams and delusions of fighting, football, and fast cars.

But Maynard and his father, Tom, were not like most other people in Beaumont. Tom Henden was the son of an impoverished sharecropper in a microscopic hamlet 40 miles northwest of Laredo, Texas. Attending the University of Texas at Austin on a football scholarship, Tom severely injured his knee during his freshman year and was unable to remain on the team thereafter. He earned his collegiate room and board by serving as the student manager for the varsity golf team and graduated with a degree in chemical engineering and a passion for golf. Tom married his high school sweetheart, whose father was the minister in the Methodist church in their small hometown.

By day, Tom Henden worked as a supervisor in a plant that manufactured benzene and other solvents, and in his off times, he played golf at the local public course. An ardent student of the sport, he began instructing Maynard in the fundamentals of golf when his son was 4 years old. The antithesis of the alchemy of Beaumont's petrochemical factories that transform ingredients from nature into synthetic poisons to all things living, Maynard's athleticism, hard work, and intelligence combined to make him what others mislabeled "a natural" in what must be among the most unnatural of all human pursuits: golf. By age 12, his game had surpassed that of his father, and in his junior year of high school, Maynard was the Texas state high school individual golf champion.

Also in Maynard's junior year of high school, tragedy struck in the Henden family. Stealthily sifting into pores and bronchioles, the benzene and other toxic solvents produced by the factory where Tom Henden worked drifted through his bloodstream to settle in and marinate his urinary bladder. Like so many others before him in his industry, Mr. Henden suffered a premature death—at age 47—from bladder cancer.

Devastated, Maynard, an only child, turned for solace to his warm and empathic mother, to his maternal grandfather who had retired from the ministry, and to his church. For 6 months he could not bear to pick up a golf club because it would wedge open the still-fresh wound of the loss of his father. Instead, he developed a passion for reading novels and poetry, where he searched for solace and existential meaning following the loss of his father. Maynard changed his life goal of becoming a professional golfer to being a minister, like his grandfather. Thereafter, golf became a means to that end.

Valedictorian of his high school class in Beaumont, Maynard received an academic scholarship to Duke University, where he double-majored in theology and in English literature. During his junior year he was bestowed the unusual honor of being named both to Phi Beta Kappa and captain of the Duke golf team. He viewed these distinctions as a Heaven-sent tribute to his father.

Also near the end of Maynard's junior year at Duke, Gaynor Bradford, chairman of the honors program in English, asked to meet with him.

Professor Gaynor Bradford: Have you thought about what you would like to do following your senior year of college?

Maynard Henden: Yes, sir. I plan to attend divinity school and hope to become a minister.

Professor Bradford: I would like to propose something else for your consideration. You are one of only two undergraduates at Duke whom the faculty would like to nominate for a Rhodes scholarship. It's a highly competitive process, but we believe that you will be a strong candidate. Not only are you an All-American in golf, but you're also very talented in English. We believe that you should take graduate studies at Oxford University in English literature and in creative writing.

Maynard: I am honored, but I respectfully must decline. My calling is to serve the Lord, and I believe that I can do that best in the ministry. It's all that I ever really wanted to do.

Professor Bradford: I hear what you are saying, Maynard, but I also want to make myself perfectly clear. What I am saying goes far beyond the Rhodes scholarship. You have a rare gift for writing, a talent that does not come along that often. Many in the English Department—and I am included—believe that your creative writing is the best that we have seen in all our years at Duke. Why don't you defer your decision to go to divinity school until after you apply for the Rhodes? Being a great writer and a theologian are not mutually exclusive. I think of the Jesuit priest Gerard Manley Hopkins, who, by the way, was a graduate of Balliol College, Oxford.

Maynard: You are too kind. But people my age are dying in droves in Vietnam. I can't delay my responsibility to my country or to my Maker. My plan's to go to the seminary and do my service obligation as a military chaplain. Perhaps it's true that I can write, but I don't have much to say. If all goes well after years of being a minister, I might have something worthy to write about.

In his senior year, Maynard applied to only one graduate school: the Duke Divinity School, which is one of 13 seminaries that are funded by the United Methodist Church. He was accepted and entered the school the following fall semester.

Elizabeth Poole: Early Years

The oldest of four children, Elizabeth was born and grew up in Charlotte, North Carolina. She deeply admired and identified with her father, Dr. Meredith Poole, a distinguished head and neck surgeon on the Medical School Faculty of the University of North Carolina's Charlotte Campus. In their work, recreation, and community service, the Poole family was a unit. They did nearly everything together. For example, with her mother and three brothers, Elizabeth delighted in accompanying Dr. Poole on annual summer trips to impoverished regions in Central America, where he would operate on the disfiguring facial abnormalities of scores of young children. As the oldest child, Elizabeth was chosen to assist her father in the surgeries and then join her mother and brothers in the preoperative and postoperative care. Elizabeth was the only daughter, and it was evident to all that she was Dr. Poole's shining light.

The Poole children were also outstanding athletes in a diverse array of sports. As a family, they would attend one another's sporting events—whether locally or out of town. Like her father, Elizabeth was comfortable with leadership, but never in the service of her own advancement or aggrandizement. Whether she was presiding over her younger brothers, drafting the closing arguments for the debating society, or directing the student governing body of her high school, remarkably, Elizabeth was never resented for her confidence and competence. Not that she cared that much about what others thought of her: she was more interested in living up to the standards and values of her parents and doing well according to the mandates of her Maker. The net result was that Elizabeth was perceived by others as being fearless. She always spoke her mind.

Although recruited by premier universities throughout the country for both her academic achievements and her prowess in tennis, Elizabeth chose Duke for its educational excellence and in order to be near her family in North Carolina. A history and government major, she continued to excel in the classroom and on the tennis court. Because she took a demanding course load and continued her active involvement with her family, Elizabeth had little time for social activities during college. She did not join a sorority and rarely even found the time to attend the home games of the fabled Duke basketball team. Not that she wasn't continuously being asked out by the boldest among potential suitors, but she knew her mind. Few could meet her measure.

For most of her life, Elizabeth had thought that she would become a physician like her father. Accordingly, in her first year at Duke she took standard premed requirements, including inorganic chemistry, biology, and calculus. Although she received good grades in these subjects, they did not interest her. Her father advised her not to get discouraged.

> **Dr. Meredith Poole:** Practicing medicine is nothing like taking premed science courses. You should hang in there, Elizabeth. Trust me, you'll make a great doctor.

Notwithstanding how much she loved and admired her father, Elizabeth knew her own mind, and eventually she realized that she did not want to be a physician. Instead, she thought about becoming an attorney—an advocate for those in our society without the power or resources to improve their lots in life. She aspired to help people like the impoverished children with cleft palates whom her father treated in Central America. She thought that she might someday want to serve others by influencing public policy or by serving in government. Ultimately, Elizabeth took a double major in history and political science and prepared for the admission tests to law school.

Although she was phenomenally busy with her academic work and varsity tennis, Elizabeth did find the time to attend church regularly. She worshiped at the Goodson Chapel of the Duke Divinity School, but she never met Maynard. Elizabeth attended services to pray, not to find dates. Two years behind Maynard at Duke, she did not lay eyes on him until her senior year. At that time, he was in his first year at the seminary. But they did not meet in church. She first saw him at a Duke community service event in which varsity athletes had volunteered to teach their respective sports to groups of children with disabilities from Durham.

> **Dr. Y.:** Do you remember what you were feeling the first time that you met Maynard?
>
> **Elizabeth Henden:** Let me tell you about it. When I first saw Maynard, he was engrossed in teaching some special needs kids how to hit a golf ball. He didn't notice me. There was an aura of gentleness and acceptance about him that put the kids at ease. They were all laughing hysterically and having so much fun hitting the golf balls in every direction but down the fairway. I could tell that Maynard didn't even notice their disabilities; he didn't care how well they hit the ball. He just wanted them to have a good time. And, for the magical moments that they were with him, the kids forgot that they were disabled.

As you can probably tell, Dr. Y., I am careful and deliberate by nature. Just like my dad the surgeon. I am not one to jump to
conclusions without having a lot of information. At the time,
I knew nothing about Maynard other than what I had seen and
learned during the 5 minutes I was watching him teach those
kids. Even so, I said to myself, "There's the man that you're
going to marry!" Yes, Dr. Y., I remember exactly how I was
feeling. I was madly in love. Does that answer your question?

Elizabeth made it a point to find out about Maynard through
mutual friends on the golf team and at the Goodson Chapel.

When they finally met some time later, he was as smitten with
her as she was with him.

Reverend Maynard Henden: I could barely breathe when I first
saw Elizabeth. To me, she was then, and still is after over 40
years, the most beautiful woman I've ever seen. She's always
saying that she chose me, that I was a sitting duck. But it's only
half true. Even though her assertiveness is much more obvious
than mine, the truth is that we are very much alike, Dr. Y. I
also go after what I want.

Dr. Y.: That brings up Elizabeth's point. Now that you are 65, do
you know what you want to do with the rest of your life?

Reverend Henden: Elizabeth is right. I have never once thought
about it. I just keep working each day without much thought
about what I want to do later in my life. Even though I minister to people who are dying, I think *I* can go on forever. I guess
I do need some help with that.

Elizabeth and Maynard

Fathers

Elizabeth and Maynard met for the first time on a Sunday morning
after church services, and they spent the rest of the day talking. They
both were shocked that they shared so many similar values and aspirations. Marveling that they were so much alike—bright, attractive,
intelligent, athletic, clean-cut, and generous of spirit—their friends
jokingly began calling them "Ken and Barbie." Thereafter, Maynard
and Elizabeth never dated anyone else.

When Elizabeth went home to visit her family, she told them that
she had "met someone special," but she delayed bringing Maynard
home to meet them.

Reverend Maynard Henden: We dated for about 9 months before I met her parents. To this day, I don't understand why she waited so long. My mother made a special trip to Durham to meet Elizabeth only 2 weeks after we first met, and, of course, they just adored each other. Why do you think that she waited so long, Dr. Y.?

Dr. Y.: I will only be speculating, but I do have some ideas. Before she met you, the most important person in Elizabeth's life was her father. He is her role model, and she idealizes him. You reap the benefits of her positive feelings for her father, which she has, in part, transferred on to you.

Reverend Henden: Oh, I know what you're getting at: She was afraid that I would disappoint him. That I wouldn't meet his standards for the man he would want for his daughter. I can understand that. He *is* a great man and does set the bar awfully high. Certainly too high for someone like me to clear.

Dr. Y.: I have come to the opposite conclusion, Reverend Henden. Because Elizabeth and her father are so close and because you are such a superior person, unconsciously she might have feared that he would be jealous of you. As if she had jilted him.

Reverend Henden: Oh please, Dr. Y. That's quite a stretch.

Dr. Y.: I have known a lot of surgeons in my time, and I have never known one who was not supercompetitive.

Fathers and Sons: The High Cost of Success, Part II

Dr. Y.: Did Dr. Poole play golf?

Reverend Maynard Henden: Yes, he loves all sports. When he was younger, he played both golf and tennis quite a bit. He played tennis in college, and it was the main sport in the Poole household. Why do you ask?

Dr. Y.: Did you play golf with him?

Reverend Henden: Now that you mention it, we never did. We played quite a bit of tennis though.

Dr. Y.: How did you do?

Reverend Henden: We played about even, until he got older and I got a bit better. He was amazingly good for his age. At first, Elizabeth and her brothers would beat me most of the time, until I got better from playing so much. After that we didn't play very much as a family. Probably because we all got so busy in our own lives.

Dr. Y.: Did anyone in the Poole family ever play golf with you?

Reverend Henden: Only Elizabeth. In Dallas we occasionally play on the same team in some charity tournaments. But Dr. Y., why are we talking about golf?

Dr. Y.: We both know what would have happened if any of the Pooles had played golf with you. Not only is everyone in the family highly competitive, but they stick together—even when it comes to you.

Reverend Henden: Dr. Y., several times you have told me that my sole task in psychotherapy is to be *present* in my treatment: to say whatever I am thinking, feeling, or experiencing when I'm with you in therapy. Well, here goes....

While we have been talking about the Pooles and playing tennis and golf, I have been thinking about my own father. And about how deeply I miss him. It makes me very uncomfortable.

Dr. Y.: Your dad was happy when you started to beat him in golf. The Pooles couldn't deal with that. You and your dad were entirely on the same team, and you miss that. You miss him.

Reverend Henden: It's totally unrelated, but the other crazy thing that I have been thinking is that I want you to stop calling me "Reverend Henden." That also makes me uncomfortable.

Dr. Y.: It's probably not all that unrelated. But, certainly, I'll call you President Henden or, if you prefer, Professor Henden. Or would you like that I call you Dr. Henden? I *am* aware that you have a Ph.D.

Reverend Henden: You know what I'm getting at, Dr. Y. Please call me "Maynard."

Dr. Y.: I'll be happy to do so, but only if you call me "Stuart."

Maynard: I'll try, but that might make me even more anxious, Dr. Y.

Stuart: You mean "Stuart," don't you, Maynard?

The above interchange might seem like irrelevant psychobabble to many readers, but it has far-reaching psychological importance for Maynard. At the time of Tom Henden's sudden death, 16-year-old Maynard was just starting to show his extraordinary prowess in both golf and academics. He also had grown taller than his father and was strikingly handsome. It was abundantly clear that Maynard would supersede his father in many spheres that are conventionally important to men—including golf, about which Tom was so passionate.

Unconsciously, Maynard believed that there was some magical association between his mounting prowess and the sudden death of his father, and thereafter, he was uncomfortable being a powerful man. Unconsciously, he found a "compromise" wherein he would allow himself to deploy his exceptional intellectual and athletic gifts to achieve success—only if it were accompanied by self-deprivation and service to humanity. Similarly, Maynard also had great difficulty permitting himself to have fun or to derive pleasure outside of his work. By toiling tirelessly for those in the greatest need and by depriving himself of enjoyment outside of his work, he also believed that he could magically prevent other sudden catastrophes—possibly even affecting Elizabeth or their children. The bottom line is that for Maynard, an enjoyable, relaxed retirement would feel dangerous and was terrifying.

I have long believed that tennis is among the most aggressive and patently competitive of all sports. Like boxing, it is not usually a team sport, and you face your adversary. (I would liken doubles tennis to tag-team wrestling, and if you listen closely to the dialogue among the participants and attend to their grunts and exclamations, you might be inclined to agree.) Unrecognized and untreated, the subtle, unexplored competitiveness between Maynard and Elizabeth would come to the fore if he were to retire and they were to spend far more one-on-one time together.

TREATMENT PRINCIPLE 13

The psychodynamics of personality do not change just because a person makes major situational or behavioral alterations in his or her life—such as finding a new job, moving to a different locale, giving up alcohol, or retiring to spend more time with the family. With important change, however, the "steady-state" of interpersonal relationships can be significantly disrupted. These interpersonal stresses are best anticipated and addressed in treatment before retirement in order to obviate shattered expectations and disastrous unintended consequences.

Maynard's request that I call him by his first name instead of by his professional title paradoxically made him feel safer by reducing his authority and, therefore, potency. Of course, I would never be complicit in his self-deprecation, nor would I be disrespectful to him. However, by both of us calling the other by his first name, we would level the playing field and share the work of treatment as equals. We would be on the same team, just like Maynard and his dad had been before Tom Henden died.

Father and Daughter

It was not love at first sight for Dr. Poole when he first met Maynard at the Poole family home in Charlotte.

Maynard Henden: From the moment I entered their palatial, antebellum home, I felt uncomfortable. Even though it was a Sunday afternoon, Dr. Poole was wearing an elegant black velvet sports coat and a designer-type of tie with the brand as a part of the fabric design. I was in my khakis and a generic polo shirt without any label on the outside. I never paid any attention to the label on the inside, either. My guess is that it would have been "Kmart." I found myself thinking two things: First, thank Heavens that I had decided against wearing my jeans or workout sweats, which would have been much more comfortable on the drive from Durham to Charlotte. Second, I immediately sensed that I was being judged by Dr. Poole on the basis of standards that I knew nothing about. For the first time in my life, I felt self-conscious and insecure about the clothes that I was wearing. I felt that I was auditioning for a part that should be cast with an entirely different character type.

Stuart Yudofsky: Who would play that role?

Maynard: Cary Grant—in a smoking jacket that didn't come from Kmart. From what Elizabeth had told me about her father, I was prepared for an entirely different person. She had emphasized her dad's devotion to his profession and his wonderful charitable work with the children in Central America.

Stuart: What else surprised you about Dr. Poole?

Maynard: His values. Both he and his wife, Margaret, hailed from old southern families—primarily Virginia and North Carolina. I learned later that the considerable wealth on both sides of their families dates back many generations, almost to the founding of our nation. He is a very formal person and seems to have rules for everything. I felt that Dr. Poole was judgmental about people who did not know or follow his rules. Like me. As you know, Stuart, I come from a blue-collar family in Beaumont, Texas. We did not have much money or belong to country clubs. In fact, the year after my father died, we had to go on welfare for a while. We didn't know about the different types of clothes that people are expected to wear for dinner as opposed to lunch. For a few years, we were happy to have enough money to buy something to eat for lunch and dinner. But we still were respectful and respectable people. From the very beginning—and even to this day—I felt that Dr. Poole thought I was respectful but not respectable.

Stuart: On what basis?

Maynard: It all boils down to money. Of course, I had no family money, and my career prospects as a minister weren't very good in that regard. I am embarrassed to say, Stuart, that I have never thought much about money—especially when it comes to making major life choices—such as my calling.

Stuart: What about Elizabeth?

Maynard: As you know, she idealizes her father. She was largely oblivious to Dr. Poole's reservations about my not being able to take care of her in the opulent manner that she was accustomed to since her childhood. Now that I think about it, Stuart, although Elizabeth is a lot like her father when it comes to personality, she favors her mother when it comes to her values. I don't think that she cares much about money, either.

Stuart: So how do you go about dealing with her family?

Maynard: As you know, I avoid confrontation whenever possible. I keep a low profile so that Elizabeth won't be put in a position to have to take sides between her father and me. For all of these years, I have acted as if I never noticed Dr. Poole's disapproval of me. But believe me, I notice. Still, after more than 40 years of my being married to his daughter and being the father to three of his beloved grandsons, his jury is still out on me.

Mothers' Love

Stuart Yudofsky: We have focused so much on Elizabeth's father; what's her mother like?

Maynard Henden: I adore Margaret Poole. She's very much like my own mother. Margaret has a nurturing, charitable, and loving soul. She is very spiritual, all about her family, the community, and the underdogs of this world. She is also highly intelligent. Elizabeth once told me that her mother got higher grades at the University of Virginia than Dr. Poole did. I think Margaret might have graduated first in her class at UVA, but she is so modest that she would never mention it. Although she dresses for the "grand dame" role to placate Dr. Poole, I think she could care less about these trappings. Best of all, she's not the least bit judgmental. I feel that she truly loves me as much as her own sons. I know that I love her as much as I do my own mother.

Stuart: My, my, my…Elizabeth *is* a lot like her father.

Maynard: How so, Stuart?

Stuart: Elizabeth married her mother.

Maynard: Thank you for the compliment, Stuart. I'll try to live up to it.

Starting Life Together

Elizabeth and Maynard exclusively dated one another from the time that they first met when she was in her junior year of college and he was in his first year of divinity school. Prior to meeting Maynard, Elizabeth had intended to apply to law schools in the northeast. Afterward, she decided to apply only to Duke Law School, a tacit recognition that the couple would marry someday. That day was during the June of Elizabeth's second year of law school.

Dr. Poole encouraged Elizabeth to become a corporate attorney in a prestigious southern law firm—preferably in Atlanta, Richmond, or Charlotte—but Elizabeth had other ideas. Her passion was to help children who were displaced by international conflicts, such as were then occurring in Vietnam and Cambodia and throughout Africa. Elizabeth hoped to help these children by working in a nonprofit organization that influenced public policy on a global basis. Through contacts at Duke Law School, she identified what she thought would be her dream job—working in New York City for the United Nations Children's Fund (UNICEF).

> **Dr. Meredith Poole:** Maynard, I worry about you and Elizabeth setting up shop in New York City. It's so impractical. Neither of you knows anyone in New York, and it's one of the most expensive places in the world to live. On the other hand, Margaret and I know tons of people in Charlotte and Atlanta who could help you both get started. Elizabeth could get a high-paying job in a big law firm in either city. Both would be much better places than New York to put down roots. I don't know how anyone can afford to raise a family in New York. I talked to Elizabeth about my reservations, but she wouldn't listen to me. Maybe you can get through to her.

> **Maynard Henden:** Thank you for your wisdom and advice. You make many excellent points that we need to think through. I will bring them all up with Elizabeth. You know better than I do, Dr. Poole, that she has a mind of her own. Right now Elizabeth has her heart set on working for UNICEF.

> **Dr. Poole:** Maybe so. But she's not being practical or realistic. You and Elizabeth should start thinking very soon about having your own children. She's almost 25, and her biological clock is ticking away fast. From the way I look at it, New York City is no place to raise kids. It's expensive, and it's dangerous. It's nearly impossible for kids to go outside to play—unless they have an

armed guard. Also, you better know that New York is crazy expensive. Elizabeth will have to make reservations 2 weeks in advance to play a game of tennis. Even then, she will have to play inside some tent, and it will cost her $50 an hour. I don't know where you'd go to play golf, Maynard. I bet you'd have to leave the damn state to do that, and the green fees for one round will cost you more than you both will earn in a month. The public schools are so dangerous that you'll have to send the kids to private schools, which also cost a fortune. New York just doesn't make *any* sense to me and Elizabeth's mom, or to most other Americans, for that matter.

Mental health professionals tend to emphasize the influences of the more difficult and dysfunctional parent on the personality characteristics of our patients. We also tend to focus more on our patients' problems and disabilities than on their assets and strengths. The defining aspects of Elizabeth's personality could be traced to *both* parents. She exhibited the assertiveness and strong-mindedness of her father and the admirable societal values, compassion, and nurturing qualities of her mother.

Both of her parents especially loved children and prioritized spending time together as a family, as did Elizabeth. The time and physical demands of Dr. Poole's surgical subspecialty of reconstructive head and neck surgery are notoriously high. Most physicians in his subspecialty have little time or energy for anything other than their profession. However, by the thoughtful planning of his schedule and militaristic time management, Dr. Poole was reliably involved in the lives of his wife and children. And he was not just with them in spirit; he showed up in person.

Although Maynard had planned to join the army as a military chaplain to serve his country during the Vietnam conflict, the war had ended just prior to his completion of his master's degree from divinity school. Identical to his experience as an undergraduate student at Duke, the faculty at the Divinity School was so impressed by his intellect and academic performance that they encouraged him to pursue the pathway they had chosen for themselves.

Professor Clarence Foshee: As you probably deduced from all the awards that you received when you got your master's degree, you have been a remarkable Divinity School student. The faculty would like you to stay on with us for your Ph.D.

> We have only two full scholarships for the doctor of philoso-
> phy in religion, and we would like to offer you one right here
> and now. You don't even have to go through the formal appli-
> cation process.
> **Maynard Henden:** I am honored, but that probably won't be pos-
> sible. My wife, Elizabeth, has her heart set on our moving to
> New York City. She wants to work for the United Nations or
> the International Red Cross.
> **Professor Foshee:** Well, how about this? Until Elizabeth gradu-
> ates, why not begin your Ph.D. here? If you decide to move to
> New York City the next year, I am confident that you can
> transfer to the Union Theological Seminary, which also has a
> strong graduate studies program.

Although it had never been his plan to pursue a doctorate degree
in religion, Maynard was becoming increasingly interested in the incipient field of pastoral counseling of hospitalized patients. He had
already established several key working relationships with cancer
doctors at Duke University Hospital, and Professor Foshee's generous proposition enabled him to develop this interest further. One
year later, the couple moved to New York.

New York, New York: Making It There

Maynard Henden

As Professor Foshee had advised, Maynard entered the second year
of his Ph.D. graduate school training at Union Theological Seminary in their special joint-degree program with Columbia University.
Through the Columbia association, he was able to work as a chaplain
intern on the cancer services at Columbia Presbyterian Hospital. At
Columbia Presbyterian he applied his novel models of spiritual counseling to patients who were hospitalized with life-threatening or terminal illnesses. Revolutionary for its time, Maynard's model involved
training spiritual counselors both in the classrooms of divinity
schools and at the bedsides of teaching hospitals. The goal of the
model is for clergymen of all denominations to gain the specialized
education, experience, and credentials to become an integral component of the medical team that is caring for the hospitalized patients.

Maynard wrote his doctoral dissertation on his spiritual counseling model, and it was so well received that he was invited by his

sponsoring institutions—Columbia Presbyterian and the Union Theological Seminary—to join their faculties. Taking advantage of his strong background in writing, Maynard expanded his dissertation into a textbook on spiritual counseling in the general hospital setting, which is now in its sixth edition and is a classic in the field.

> **Maynard Henden:** When I was offered positions on the faculties of the Seminary and Columbia, I knew that whatever decision I would make would be a turning point in my life. I had studied theology in the first place to be a small-town minister like my grandfather. In the most intimate and important ways, he was involved in the lives of just about everyone in his church and his parish. I knew that an academic career would take me in another direction.
>
> **Stuart Yudofsky:** How did you come to your decision?
>
> **Maynard:** I never decided. I rationalized that I could do both. Somehow, I would make my ministerial work the center of my academic career. And, in different ways throughout my career, I've always managed to do that—even as president of a large university.
>
> **Stuart:** At what cost?
>
> **Maynard:** You know that answer, Stuart. Elizabeth made that clear in our first meeting: at the cost of my not being there for my family.

Maynard's academic and ministerial work focused on integrating spiritual healing and medical practice. He was at the forefront of the introduction into American medicine of palliative and hospice care for patients with terminal illnesses. He wrote compellingly on the deleterious consequences of conceptualizing end-of-life experiences as *pathological* processes that must be "fixed," somehow, by medical interventions. He posited that dying patients, their families, and their doctors feel, somehow, that they have failed when a person dies. We all will die. Therefore, Maynard advocated reframing dying as a natural, inevitable process that affords opportunities to grow as a person and connect in new, important ways with family members and friends.

In 1982, the Centers for Disease Control and Prevention first named the conditions caused by the HIV virus *acquired immune deficiency syndrome (AIDS)*. At the time, there was widespread stigmatization of people with this illness, the vast proportion of whom were males who had "acquired" the condition through homosexual practices or through intravenous substance use. Effective treatments had not been developed for people with AIDS. As a result of the stigmatization, many among the great numbers of people who were dying of AIDS were dying alone and unsupported by their families and friends. Maynard formed spiritual outreach programs in support of people dying of AIDS throughout New York City and personally led daily and Sunday religious services at a new church in Greenwich Village that was opened by gay men with AIDS.

Maynard approached his spiritual interventions in a highly disciplined, academic fashion. He formulated theses that he studied by comparing the outcomes of those who participated in his carefully designed and monitored programs with control groups who did not receive these interventions. He applied for and received sizeable National Institutes of Health and other federal research funding for his work and broadly published his results in prestigious medical, theological, and social science journals. As a result, Maynard's academic career soared, as did his reputation as being a pioneer in the integration of spirituality and medicine. He was awarded a full professorship with tenure by Columbia before he was 40 years old.

Elizabeth Henden

Elizabeth's position at the United Nations (UN) was working with an international team of attorneys who supported the many, varied programs of UNICEF. At first, her work centered on helping to place the legion of parentless Cambodian and Vietnamese children into families in developed nations. She particularly enjoyed traveling to refugee centers in East Asia to visit with the children. Her tireless work ethic, her attention to detail, and her productivity were soon recognized and appreciated by her superiors in the legal division at UNICEF. At the UN, Elizabeth was widely regarded as an up-and-comer, and she was promoted to higher levels of leadership and responsibility.

However, Elizabeth's direct contact with children in her work made her long to become a mother. As her father had predicted, she became uncomfortably aware of the ticking of her biological clock. She loved her job, but at age 29, after 3 years of working at the UN, she reasoned as follows:

> **Elizabeth Henden:** I was truly torn. I loved my job but also longed to be a mother and start our own family. All of my good

friends from childhood, Duke, and in New York seemed to be having babies. I got to the point that I couldn't even look at a pregnant woman without breaking into tears. Maynard and I looked carefully into adopting a displaced orphan from the many with whom I fell in love on my trips to refugee camps throughout the far East. Given my responsibilities at the UN, however, it was an obvious conflict of interest. I was deliriously happy when I finally became pregnant.

Elizabeth planned to take a 3-month leave of absence from her job after the birth of their baby and then return to work full time at the career that she loved. However, she did not anticipate the strength of the bond to her baby, and she could not bear any separation from him. Reasoning that she could return to work part time when their son entered prekindergarten, she changed her mind about returning to the UN. With the births of their two other sons over the succeeding 5 years, Elizabeth never went back to work.

Although Dr. Poole's prediction about Elizabeth's not being able to be a working mother in New York City proved correct, he was wrong about the Hendens being unable to afford to raise a family there. For several reasons, finances did not turn out to be an insurmountable problem for Maynard and Elizabeth. First, they always lived within their means, so their finances balanced even after Elizabeth relinquished her job on the birth of their first child. Second, their children did not attend private schools. Instead, they were admitted through competitive testing to excellent public magnet schools in Manhattan. Third, in his calculations, Dr. Poole had neglected to take into account Elizabeth's trust funds from her wealthy grandparents on both sides of her family. These funds, which were substantial, became available to Elizabeth on her 30th birthday. Additionally, the combination of Maynard's academic salary and the royalties from professional textbooks and his best-selling self-help books on spirituality and hopefulness in death and dying generated good incomes. Fourth, the apartment that they rented soon after arriving in New York was converted into a condominium, which increased its value remarkably over the years. Their apartment was located in a great neighborhood near a park, and they loved living there. With Elizabeth's trust fund money, they were able to purchase the adjacent condominium and combine it with their own to make a wonderful urban home for their family of five. In summary, although they were by no means among the wealthiest New Yorkers, Maynard and Elizabeth loved living in New York and did so comfortably.

The High Cost of Success, Part III

As the years passed by, Maynard became an increasingly productive and respected administrator, educator, and researcher at Columbia and at the Union Theological Seminary, where he was also highly regarded as a minister and theologian. In both institutions he became the chairman of growing departments and centers involving spiritual counseling in medical settings. He also became an internationally renowned "thought leader" in the field of thanatology, which is the scientific study of death and dying. This is a highly interdisciplinary academic enterprise that takes into consideration biological, psychological, sociological, and spiritual perspectives of end-of-life phenomena. As a pioneer in recognizing and championing the psychospiritual needs of people with AIDS, Maynard became somewhat of an international celebrity—with countless invitations to write papers, contribute book chapters, appear on scientific panels, comment to news media, and be a featured guest on public radio and television. In order not to be distracted from his responsibilities in New York, Maynard was selective in his acceptances. Nonetheless, not only did he work long hours every day—including nights and weekends—but he traveled extensively.

Maynard was invited to be a visiting professor on a wide range of topics at leading academic institutions—colleges, medical schools, seminaries, law schools, teaching hospitals, etc.—in the United States and around the world. More than his high intelligence, or his command of his topics, or his excellence as a speaker, he was particularly admired for his humor, humanity, and approachable personality. An unintended consequence of his international exposure was that many academic institutions endeavored to recruit Maynard to lead programs, centers, and departments at their institutions. Consistently, he immediately responded that he was happy with his current position and would not consider changing.

When he was 44 years old, Maynard received a call from his former mentor at Duke, Professor Clarence Foshee.

> **Professor Clarence Foshee:** It is always great to speak and catch up with you, Maynard. However, this conversation will be different. I have an "immodest proposal" to make to you.

Maynard Henden: What did I do to embarrass my alma mater this time?

Professor Foshee: Au contraire, Maynard, we are unequivocally proud of you and your contributions to the world. Your being named several years ago as Duke University's Distinguished Alumnus of the Year is but a small indication of our pride. Your most recent visiting professorship to Duke Medical School caused quite a stir among several of our most influential faculty. They want to bring you back here at a senior level—provost was mentioned repeatedly—preliminary to your someday becoming president of Duke. The problem is that you are still too young. Several senior administrators and key board members at Duke want you to be groomed elsewhere in order to return here as president. They believe that it's best for you to prove your mettle as a president of a smaller university first.

Maynard: As we used to say in my hometown of Beaumont, Texas, "Whoa, partner!" You're moving much too fast for me. I'm happy in my current position. Being a university president has never occurred to me. And by the way, no university is breaking down my doors to ask me to be their president.

Professor Foshee: Funny that you would reference Texas. There is an outstanding university in Texas that wants to recruit a new president to lead them into a new era. They are plenty strong now but want to move up to become a first-tier research university while respecting their history as a religiously based institution. They have asked us to help them identify a candidate. We believe that you would be beyond their highest expectations. Your accomplishments and abilities are a natural fit for them. What we're asking you to do is to go down to Texas and meet with their search committee.

Maynard: Elizabeth, the boys, and I are happy in New York. Once more, I am complimented by everyone's support, but I will have to decline before this goes any further.

Professor Foshee: Where are you right at this moment, Maynard?

Maynard: In my office at Columbia. Why do you ask?

Professor Foshee: Look out your window and tell me *exactly* what you see.

Maynard: You've been to my office many times, Clarence. You *know* what I see. I have a great view of the Columbia Quad: Low Memorial Library, St. Paul's Chapel, Miller Theatre, Dodge Hall, and many wonderful students and professors going to and fro. Again, why do you ask?

Professor Foshee: Now let me tell *you* what *I* would see, Maynard, if I were at the window with you. I would see extraordinary gothic palaces of higher education that *did not build themselves.* I would see students and professors—as you say—going to and fro without giving one thought about who made all these treasures possible for *their* enlightenment. Of course, they are thinking about the moment and entirely about *their* day and *their* responsibilities. They do not think about those who came before them at Columbia who made these resources possible or about the needs of those who will come after them.

You have had the extreme good fortune of being educated and being able to work at Duke, Columbia, and UTS [United Theological Seminary]. These institutions are all blessed with extraordinary resources that people *before* you created for you. *You* have the responsibility to be a builder too—for *others* who need you now and who will come after you. However, Duke, Columbia, and UTS don't need you right now as much as less developed institutions do. You have the rare talents to be both a leader and a builder. I see it as your *obligation.* Please think about it for a week or two, Maynard.

Change and Challenge

Professor Foshee was an experienced and wise mentor for Maynard. He understood his prodigy and his values and structured his argument accordingly. In discussing this event with me in a therapy session many years later, Maynard expressed the following:

> **Maynard Henden:** It was the strangest thing. I was about to leave my office to teach a class when I got Professor Foshee's call. I put it completely out of my mind until he left a message 2 weeks later asking me what I had decided. That night I brought up the subject for the first time with Elizabeth, who I had presumed would tell me, "No way!" I reasoned that I could use her as my excuse to decline.

Maynard was shocked by Elizabeth's response.

> **Elizabeth Henden:** I think we ought to consider the proposition, Maynard.
>
> **Maynard Henden:** You must be kidding, Elizabeth. I thought that you loved living in New York and the life we have here.
>
> **Elizabeth:** You're half right. I love living in New York, but I think that our lives could be much better. With the jobs you have now, you're never home with the family. You have to travel almost every week, and when you are in town, you are always

running back and forth between Columbia College, Columbia-Presbyterian, and UTS. Let's face it, you have three jobs.

Maynard: If I were to get offered the job in Texas—which I don't think is very likely—don't you think that I could get even busier? I have no idea what goes into being a university president, but I could be jumping from the frying pan into the fire.

Elizabeth: It couldn't be any worse than it is right now. At least you won't be running in three different directions, and you would make a lot more money than you do now. Dallas has to be much less expensive to live in than New York. And our condo is worth a fortune these days. We would have much more room for the boys, and they could go outside once in a while.

Maynard: You're sounding a lot like your Dad, Elizabeth.

Elizabeth (*with pique*): He's not exactly, stupid, Maynard. And he always managed to be with his family.

With Elizabeth's strong encouragement, Maynard agreed to permit Professor Foshee to submit his name to the search committee for the university president.

Professor Clarence Foshee: I am pleased that you have decided to throw your hat in the ring, Maynard. The search committee has been constituted for over a year and a half, and they are in the process of inviting back their finalist candidates. Several of the finalists are solid candidates. Six are currently provosts or deans at Ivy League universities.

To his surprise, Maynard was flooded with mixed feelings by what Professor Foshee had just revealed about the search. First, having spent the entirety of his academic career at Duke and Columbia, Maynard had been unwittingly susceptible to academic elitism and provincialism that had surreptitiously percolated and diluted his populist ideals and self-image. He had not anticipated that he would have to compete with so many top-flight candidates to lead a university of lesser prestige…in Texas, no less! Second, his intellectual and athletic gifts had been recognized since he was in middle school. Accustomed to being *pursued* for academic positions, Maynard found himself feeling uncomfortably vulnerable to the possibility of his being *rejected*. To apply for a job would entail "selling himself," which he had never done before. Third, if he got the job, not only would he have to leave positions in which he had been safe and successful but he would also have to prove himself all over again in a new job and in a new environment. What would happen to his career and his family if the move didn't work out? What would happen to *him* if *he* didn't work out?

It also became unsettlingly clear to Maynard that Elizabeth was far more comfortable with change and challenge than was he. He discussed this insight with me in his therapy many years later:

> **Maynard Henden:** I just have to face it: Elizabeth is a much stronger, more secure, and adventurous person than I am. I probably would have never left Duke in the first place if Elizabeth hadn't wanted to work in New York. And certainly, I would have never taken the risk of being rejected by the search committee in Dallas if Elizabeth hadn't encouraged me to do so.
>
> **Stuart Yudofsky:** You have been successful in almost everything you have done, Maynard. We need to discover why you still don't feel secure and confident—despite your proven abilities and accomplishments.
>
> **Maynard:** There are lots of people who were in my graduate school classes at Duke and Columbia who never left those places after they graduated. They found some spot on the faculties and just stayed on forever. Maybe like me, they were afraid to test themselves outside the halo of the powerhouse university. Come to think of it, I'm not alone.
>
> **Stuart:** I have observed the same thing, Maynard. And I have thought long and hard about this phenomenon.

Maynard was invited to Texas to spend 2 days with members of the search committee and with other selected faculty and staff. In spite of the strong competition, his fit with the needs and priorities of the university was exceptional. Similar to Duke, this university, while encouraging secular students, has a strong historical relationship with the Methodist Church. Additionally, the school of divinity is a great source of pride to the university. The university offers master of divinity (M.Div.) and doctor of ministry (D.Min.) degrees as well as a doctor of philosophy (Ph.D.) degree in theology.

The search committee and the Board of Trustees were especially drawn to Maynard's pioneering research and publishing accomplishments in theology, his charisma as a speaker and writer, and his natural leadership potential. His values; his warm, welcoming personality; and his physical attractiveness placed Maynard ahead of the pack by a large margin. Meeting composed, sophisticated, and beautiful Elizabeth on Maynard's second visit to Dallas consolidated

Maynard's appeal to the search committee. Their unanimous first choice, the Board of Trustees allocated significant resources to lure Maynard to Texas. At the end of the day, the Texans got their man.

The Ayes of Texas

Stepping Up

As he began his new role as president of a large urban university, Maynard was deeply concerned that he did not have the administrative experience or the skills to succeed in his new position, which he viewed as vastly different from anything that he had done before.

> **Maynard Henden:** Have you ever seen anyone fall on his face, Stuart?
>
> **Stuart Yudofsky:** Literally, never; metaphorically, many, many times. Which type do you mean?
>
> **Maynard:** Both types. On the very first day on my new job in Dallas, I was walking to my office when I saw a man trip on the curb and fall flat on his face to the sidewalk. He shredded both sides of his face and broke his nose. There was blood everywhere. I must confess that, as disturbing as it was for me to witness the injury of a fellow human being, I was more terrified by what it might portend for my future in Texas. I was pretty sure that it was a sign from Heaven that I was about to fall on my face.

Maynard is a modest man. He had considerably underestimated the broad range of talents that he had brought to his new position. Having flourished in the scholarly crucibles of Durham and New York City, he had learned more than he had recognized from able mentors, peers, collaborators, students, and avid competitors. Also, of a generous and generative nature, President Henden was ever willing to share his vast knowledge and skills with constituents at all levels of his responsibility. These qualities led to his becoming universally beloved by faculty, staff, students, board members, and the Dallas community.

Equally important, Maynard possesses talents as an original thinker, gifted writer, inspiring orator, and transformational teacher. Almost unheard of for modern-day university presidents, he remained the original, productive contributor in the academic foci that made him eligible for the lofty position in the first place. Or as they say in Texas, he continued to "dance with the girl who brung him to the party." In addition to his administrative responsibilities, he was an active educator and researcher in the divinity school; wrote more original papers and best-selling books; preached movingly on special occasions in local churches; and was a spiritual counselor to the families of faculty, staff, board members, and major supporters of the university.

Over time, Maynard's exceptional abilities and hard work paid great dividends for the university. Historically high levels of funding poured in from alumni and community supporters. These funds were invested to establish a profusion of named chairs, to recruit top faculty, to develop new programs, to rebuild and expand the campus, and to provide an unprecedented number of new academic and athletic scholarships.

Duke and other preeminent academic universities took notice:

Professor Clarence Foshee: Well, you did it, Maynard: just like we drew it up 12 years ago. Our current president at Duke is about to step down, and I've been deputized by the search committee to enlist your interest in being a candidate. Although I'm not on the search committee, given your background and what you have done in Texas, I have every confidence that you're a shoo-in. Time to come back home, Maynard.

Maynard: Clarence, do you remember when you called me at Columbia and asked me to look out my window?

Professor Foshee: Of course I do, Maynard.

Maynard: Well, I'm looking out of my office window right now. Like at Columbia, I see many beautiful buildings and profusions of bright students and faculty. Unlike at Columbia, most of these buildings are new. I also see dozens of derricks sprouting out of even newer structures that are presently under construction. It looks like an East Texas oil field. Duke is so strong and prestigious that you will have no trouble recruiting the top talent for the new president. We're not there yet in Dallas. I'm still needed here, and Elizabeth and I are happy in Texas. I want to stay here, Clarence. And I think you'd want me to stay as well to finish what I've started. You are a man of enormous principle.

Professor Foshee: I understand. And Maynard....

Maynard: Yes, Clarence?

Professor Foshee: I'm proud of you.

Dreams of My Father

As Maynard discussed with me many years later in our treatment, Professor Foshee's expression of being proud of him was especially moving and meaningful to him:

> **Maynard Henden:** Right after I hung up from Clarence's call, I broke out into uncontrollable sobs. That's really unlike me. I've never done such a thing before or since. I've thought about that call many times over the years, and I'm still not sure why I broke up like that. I know that I had very mixed feelings about my decision. I truly love Duke, and the presidential position certainly carries far more prestige than I will ever have here. At the same time I love where I am and what I have been doing. Maybe I was upset because I had closed an important chapter in my life. Do you agree, Stuart?
>
> **Stuart Yudofsky:** Did your father ever tell you he was proud of you, Maynard?
>
> **Maynard:** Not in so many words, but I think he was proud of me. Dad showed his care for me by his interest in me—especially in teaching me to play golf.
>
> **Stuart:** You're an educator, Maynard. You know that different teachers have different teaching styles. How did your father teach you?
>
> **Maynard:** Mainly by showing me how to do stuff the "right way." He was a real stickler for proper golfing form, and he would focus on how I could improve my swing.
>
> **Stuart:** What did he say when you got it right?
>
> **Maynard:** Not much, really. Even when I won tournaments, he would tell me what I could I have done better. He called it "constructive criticism." Now that I think of it, Dad wasn't big on compliments.
>
> I just remembered something, Stuart. When I was 12, I had missed two putts on the 18th hole in a state tournament. Even though I was the youngest player in the finals, I could have won the tournament if I had sunk just one of those putts. My father was furious with me. He didn't speak to me on the 2-hour ride back home from Austin.
>
> That very night he went into the hospital for the first time that I knew about. Within 3 months he was dead. Although I saw him several times over those months, no one told me that he was so sick. Even after he died, our family didn't discuss what had happened to him. They just didn't talk about those things like that in those days. At least not in Beaumont. It was many years later that I found out that he had bladder cancer.

Stuart: Right after your father's death, did anybody help you deal with your loss?

Maynard: Like I said, Stuart, we didn't talk about those sorts of things back then. But now that I think about it, I remember being afraid to go to sleep for several years after he died.

Stuart: Do you recall what you were thinking about before falling to sleep? Can you remember any dreams that you had around that time?

Maynard: Both, now that I think about it. Let me tell you about my recurrent dream first.

I was on the green of the 18th hole of the public golf course in Beaumont. As usual Dad was at the edge of the green watching me play. He was staring at me intently to make sure that I kept the proper form and that I read the green correctly. Even before I putted, he was frowning, as if he were cross with me.

Instead of using my putter, I took out my number 1 wood from my golf bag and swung at the ball as hard as I could. The ball hit my father squarely in his mouth—full force. As crazy as this sounds, I hit the ball so hard that it knocked out his front teeth and went down his throat. He began choking violently, as if he were about to suffocate.

I would wake up screaming before my dream ended. I was horrified that he might be dead. That I had accidentally killed him. After I woke up, I would at first be relieved to realize that I was just having a terrible dream. That none of it had really happened. Then I'd remember that Dad was *really* dead, and that he would *never* come back. After that, I would start to cry out of control. So loudly that I had to bury my face in the pillow, in order not to wake up Mom, who was sleeping in the next room of our tiny apartment. I didn't want to go back to sleep because I was afraid that I would have that horrible dream again.

Maynard and I spent many hours analyzing the meaning and implications of his dream. We agreed that the dream symbolized his guilt over feeling responsible for his father's death by his (Maynard's) *choking* on the important putts in the tournament that he had lost—as well as his anger at his father for having abandoned him. A lasting feeling that Maynard harbored was that he had disappointed his father and that, somehow, *that* disappointment led to his death.

Maynard could never recall a time that his father said that he loved him or was proud of him. A most disturbing aspect of the "finality" of the death of his father was that he would never tell Maynard that he was proud of him. The historical and current implications of the dream for Maynard's self-esteem, his key psychological conflicts, and his decision making included the following:

- *Maynard changed his life goal from being a professional golfer to becoming a minister.* Soon after his father died, Maynard decided that he would "dedicate my life to my Creator" and become a small-town minister like his grandfather. Many of his grandfather's sermons centered on "the vanity in mankind's material strivings" and the "wisdom and power of living a spiritual life like Jesus."

- *Maynard no longer enjoyed golf after his father's death.* Golf became Maynard's means to the end of becoming a minister by helping to garner a scholarship at Duke. Although he remained an excellent golfer, Maynard did not find playing golf to be fun or relaxing. It was a job. At the time he began psychotherapy, he played golf mainly in foursomes for fund-raising events in the Dallas community. Because he was still outstanding, technically, in golf, Maynard was often asked to play by business and community leaders.

- *Maynard's principal academic interest became death and dying.* His choice of this field was related to his need to achieve mastery over the unexpected, unexplained, and unexamined traumatic event that had changed his life so dramatically.

- *Maynard became uncomfortable resting, taking vacations, or having fun outside of his working obligations.* This was related to his guilt over believing that he was responsible for his father's death. Additionally, Maynard felt uncomfortable accepting the merits of his true accomplishments, and this left him feeling perennially insecure, anxious, and vulnerable.

- *Maynard's self-esteem became dependent on the approval of male authority figures.* Whether it were Dr. Poole, Professor Foshee, or Mr. Jamison, the chairman of the university Board of Trustees to whom Maynard reported, he was deferential to a fault when interacting with powerful men. He was anxious and insecure if they expressed disapproval of him and felt elated and contingently safe when he was complimented by his so-called "superiors."

- *Maynard denied the implications of his aging.* Maynard lived in the fear that he would die suddenly, which he did his best not to think about. Having a realistic work schedule or entertaining and implementing succession plans for his university presidency or retirement would be to acknowledge his own mortality.

Bullied Pulpit

Maynard was 65 years old when he began treatment with me. His initial concern was the amount of time that his psychotherapy would take away from his work by having to fly back and forth to Houston from Dallas—a trip made more efficient by his use of the university's jet plane. The following discussion took place at our first meeting:

> **Stuart Yudofsky:** If it makes it more convenient for you, I can see you on Saturdays when I also have office hours.
>
> **Maynard Henden:** I work a full day on Saturdays. That might be my busiest day. I have meetings in the mornings with my tenured professors, department chairs, and senior staff on a rotating basis. This allows me to spend at least 1 hour each year with them one on one without having some problem to fix. We can talk about their current job satisfaction and academic aspirations. On Saturday afternoons, I attend university athletic events, and the evenings are prime times for student concerts, theater productions, and going to dinner with new faculty recruits.
>
> Sundays are also pretty busy. Of course I attend church in the mornings, occasionally delivering the sermon. I usually take graduate students to lunch, and then I have research and academic meetings scheduled in the afternoons. On Sunday evenings I clean up the unfinished paperwork from the previous week and prepare for the meetings and lectures of the next week. By 9:00 P.M., if I have the time and energy, I get to do some writing and recreational reading for a couple of hours. I look forward to those 2 hours all week long.

In systematically going over Maynard's calendar with him, I realized that what Elizabeth had said was true: He worked literally all of the time. He almost never took vacations, and he traveled only for business. After Maynard and I spent about 20 minutes in a futile effort to carve out a spot for our weekly psychotherapy, Elizabeth interrupted, impatiently.

> **Elizabeth Henden** (*with exasperation*): Enough already!! This will go on forever, and Maynard will *never* find the time to meet with you, Dr. Y. Trust me; I know that from bitter experience. I suggest you pick a time that fits into *your* schedule, and it will be Maynard's responsibility to be there without excuse or exception. If not, I have my answer: he'll never change, and I can finally stop hoping and waiting.

Stuart Yudofsky: Friday afternoons from 2:00 to 4:00 P.M. Let's meet for 2 hours each time to justify your long trip and, if possible, in order to accelerate the process. It'll take me a few weeks to work you into my schedule on a regular basis, Reverend Henden.

Entertaining Retirement

Over the next year, Maynard "religiously" attended his weekly 2-hour sessions with me. In addition to securing a relevant psychosocial history from his grandparents to the current time, I worked systematically with Maynard on the matter at hand: the prospect of his retirement. Remarkably, he had never considered retiring prior to Elizabeth's recent insistence that he do so.

The Role of Employment and Position in Maynard's Identity, Sense of Self-Worth, and Self-Esteem

Stuart Yudofsky: If, for some reason, you had to leave the university today, what do you think that you would miss the most?

Maynard Henden: As I have said to you so many times, Stuart, I lead a blessed life. I would miss being *relevant* to others, especially having the unique privilege to be a part of their lives during those stressful hours that they need spiritual support. I would miss teaching and mentoring a new generation of theologians— both scholars and ministers. I'd miss helping to build the future of a great university that will touch and better the lives of countless others. In short, I would miss my blessed opportunities to give to others. Does that seem about right to you, Stuart?

Stuart: Not entirely. I'd say you're *half right* about what you'd miss if you leave your position of university president.

Maynard: I'm not surprised that you'd be a tough grader, Stuart. Fifty percent is usually a failing grade. What did I miss?

Stuart: You're clear that your position gives you a powerful platform to *help others*, but what you did not include is how your position *helps you*.

Maynard: You're missing my point, Stuart. By helping others, I feel good about myself.

Stuart: I got *that* point, but here is what I believe that you are leaving out.

What ensued was a long discussion of many of Maynard's other, more selfish, needs, about which he had been oblivious. Over time, it became clear to both of us that had he retired *without* these issues being addressed and accounted for, his retirement years might have been disappointing to him at best. At worst, both he and Elizabeth would have been miserable.

The following is a brief outline of what was missing from Maynard's predictions of what he would have missed most in retirement from his position.

Power

Although Maynard viewed himself as "a humble servant of the Lord," as the president of a great university, he wielded enormous power. Large numbers of people *had to listen* to what he said and *had to do* what he directed. The fact that he delivered his commandments with grace and graciousness did not mean that his commands could be disobeyed.

Like CEOs of large companies, presidents of large universities are like lords of medieval European manors: their word is the law. For example, if a powerful Dallas businessman wanted his granddaughter to be interviewed for admission to the undergraduate college at the university, he would call President Henden, who would then call the Dean of Admissions, who would see to it that the young woman would be interviewed—sooner rather than later. No discussion. The day that Maynard left the position of president of the university, the normal rules and policies would no longer pertain in all of the many domains over which he had presided. A change in Maynard's job status would constitute an enormous loss of power for him.

It was essential for Maynard to understand his attraction to and dependency on that power and be prepared for its loss *before* he relinquished it. Otherwise, there would be hell to pay.

> **Maynard Henden:** I've been so busy over the last 20 years that I never really thought about cutting back. For me, looking long into the future has always been about new projects that we are undertaking at the university, and there has never been any shortage of those. Beyond that I have barely had time to think beyond what I needed to get done that week.

Admiration and Affirmation

In my subspecialty area of psychiatry, neuropsychiatry, I treat the psychiatric aspects of brain illnesses such as stroke, traumatic brain injury, seizures, or Parkinson's disease. Many of my patients (and their caregivers) have significant problems walking and negotiating the traffic and dense maze of buildings in the Texas Medical Center, where my office is located. Consequently, I make frequent house calls to my patients. Invariably on these visits, I gain important information about my patients' environments, family dynamics, and life experience that likely would have remained undiscovered in a traditional doctor's office visit.

> **Stuart Yudofsky:** For a few days next month I will be a visiting professor at the University of Texas Health Sciences Center in Dallas. Would you like to have our session in Dallas on that week?
>
> **Maynard Henden:** Sure. It will save time and jet fuel. Where would you like to meet?
>
> **Stuart:** In your office on campus, if you are comfortable that your confidentiality would not be compromised.
>
> **Maynard:** Totally comfortable. If anyone recognizes you, they will think that I am either trying to recruit you to our faculty or shake you down for a donation to the university—or both. If *you* are comfortable, I would also like to show you around the campus personally to point out all the great things that are going on. You'll get a good idea about why it's so hard for me to retire at this point in the university's history.
>
> **Stuart:** That's one of the prime reasons that I would like to visit you at your home base, Maynard.

In my many years in academics and practice, it has been my privilege to tour several university campuses with their presidents. Unwittingly, I have collected an informal baseline for comparison of how these presidents interact with and are received by the students, faculty, and staff at their respective universities. At a level beyond any prior experience and expectation, I learned that President Henden is beloved by all. His easy, outgoing, open, joyous, friendly, and loving manner was repeatedly and universally reciprocated by those whom we encountered while walking around the university campus. Faculty greeted him with the warmth, high spirits, trust, and confidence of teammates; staff working in offices and in cafeterias or mowing the grass exchanged the personal familiarities of close, trusted friends; and students interrupted what they were doing to run up, bring him the news of their worlds, and hug him. With almost every step of our tour, Maynard received positive *affirmation* of his role, importance, and acceptance.

In a subsequent session in Houston, we discussed my visit to Dallas.

> **Maynard Henden:** OK, Stuart, what did you learn by your visit to the university?
>
> **Stuart Yudofsky:** For one thing, Maynard, if you were running for reelection to the presidency of your university, you would win by a landslide. You're a wonder and a winner in your current role. But as we have discussed, too many blessings can also pose problems.
>
> **Maynard:** What problems in specific?
>
> **Stuart:** Problems with keeping your life in balance. Problems in letting go and moving on to something new and different. Countless times each day you receive both *admiration* and *affirmation* of who you are and how much you have accomplished. Both have enormous psychodynamic significance for you.

Over many ensuing sessions we discussed how losing his father at a critical stage in his development led to Maynard feeling lost, lonely, powerless, and without a strong sense of identity. Although his father prioritized Maynard, he was also critical of him and emotionally cold. Maynard's response was to gain power, love, and self-definition through true accomplishment and with a winning personality. As with many successful people, an unbalanced proportion of Maynard's self-definition was related to his positions and work product. His three professional titles—Reverend Henden, Professor Henden, President Henden—reflect the importance and priority to Maynard of his work role.

But what would become of his sense of self-definition, self-worth, and relevance were he to walk away from the positive reinforcements of his lofty positions? To do so without realistic anticipation of their monumental loss and preparation for such consequences would be foolhardy.

Likes and Dislikes About Current Employment

> **Stuart Yudofsky:** What do you like and what don't you like about what you are doing now, Maynard?
>
> **Maynard Henden:** If you can believe it, Stuart, I never once asked myself that question. It's not about what I *like*, but what I *have to do* that day. And up until now, it's all that I can do to get my daily stuff done. Like a mule dragging a plow, I bend my head and trudge forward.

Stuart: Oh, I believe you, Maynard. But you are now in a place in your career where you have earned the privilege to choose what you do—and what you don't do.

Maynard: I'm not sure that I believe that. In any case, that prospect makes me very anxious.

After deliberate consideration of Maynard's professional demands, we learned that he *enjoyed* many aspects of his work: teaching; spiritual counseling; preaching; writing; doing research; reading; and meeting with students, colleagues, and faculty. He *tolerated*, but no longer liked, fund-raising, long-range planning, recruiting faculty, and the many recurrent administrative and ceremonial obligations associated with being university president. He strongly *disliked* the weekly administrative meetings with his senior faculty and staff, working on budgets, writing annual reports, and preparing for and leading large university-wide administrative meetings.

Current Interests and Enjoyment Outside of Work

Maynard revealed that he has many interests outside his work that he rarely has time to pursue. He loves reading Elizabethan English dramatists and poets, as well as the works of twentieth-century American novelists and poets. He also enjoys attending with Elizabeth live performances of Shakespeare, especially Shakespeare's revenge tragedies, as well as classic American theater—especially plays by Tennessee Williams, Arthur Miller, and Eugene O'Neill and the musical theater of George and Ira Gershwin, Rodgers and Hammerstein, and Stephen Sondheim.

Maynard also loves most sports—both as a spectator and a participant. He is a devoted fan of the Dallas Cowboys, Mavericks, and Rangers but rarely has time to watch even part of a game on television. His favorite participatory sports had become playing tennis with Elizabeth and pick-up basketball with his sons, but he rarely had the opportunity to participate because of his and his sons' busy schedules. Fortunately, Maynard did carve out time to exercise. He ran on a treadmill for about 55 minutes every day in the early hours of the morning and especially enjoyed the unusual occasions that he could run outdoors. Always athletic, when Maynard turned 50, he entered a 5-kilometer run in Dallas. He finished third among many others in his age group. He longed to train for more races and to compete regularly. Finally, since childhood Maynard also loved to be outdoors. He was interested in conservation of all types, especially indigenous birds, fish, and reptiles in the Gulf of Mexico, whose tepid waters slap the coastal plain of his native Beaumont, Texas, 50 miles inland.

Fears About Retirement

Maynard came from a working-class family and lived in a working-class neighborhood in a working-class town. Almost all of the fathers of his neighborhood friends did not attend college and worked in oil refineries or chemical plants, and their wives did not work outside their homes. Because his father had completed college and was a supervisor at his work, Maynard grew up feeling financially secure and socially advantaged. That all changed with his father's sudden death when Maynard was 16 years old. Because his father's death from bladder cancer was not considered to be work related and because Mr. Henden had no life insurance or savings, the family became destitute within less than a year. Not being able to keep up the mortgage payments on their modest home, Maynard's mother was compelled to sell the house, rent a small apartment nearby, and secure a part-time job in the public library. With insufficient funds for food and the other necessities of life, the family went on welfare until Maynard went to college on full scholarship.

> **Maynard Henden:** Being poor and hungry is not an abstract concept for me, Stuart. For most of high school my main meal was the school lunch. I was embarrassed and teased because I had to pay for my lunches with food stamps. I gave to Mom the little money that I made being a caddy at the Beaumont Country Club to spend on rent and food.
> **Stuart Yudofsky:** How do you measure the value of a dollar today, Maynard?
> **Maynard:** I would get about one dollar for carrying two heavy golf bags for 18 holes. If the golfers decided to play an extra 9 holes, I would get another 50 cents. On the occasions that they were generous enough to give me a 50 cent tip, I would earn 2 dollars for about 6 hours of pretty hard work. As you guessed, Stuart, that's what a dollar means to me this very day.
> **Stuart:** Are you afraid you'll become poor again if you retire and lose the steady income from your job?
> **Maynard:** Absolutely. "Terrified" is much closer to the truth.
> **Stuart:** Have you discussed this with Elizabeth?

> **Maynard:** Never. Believe it or not, I'd be embarrassed to. She comes from such a wealthy family, I'm not sure she would really understand. I also worry that she would think less of me.

Many people are much more comfortable talking with their therapists about the intimate details of their sexual lives than they are in discussing their personal finances. As mental health professionals, we are obligated to talk directly about both topics without embarrassment. In doing so with Maynard, I learned that he was well compensated for his work, had no debt, and had accumulated personal assets of more than $7 million—not including Elizabeth's trusts and inherited wealth from her parents' estates. Nevertheless, he felt that he was too poor to relinquish his salary in retirement. He had many associated fears.

> **Maynard Henden:** If I were to retire at age 65, Elizabeth and I could live for another 30 years without any income. Who knows what could happen over those many years living solely off our savings? We, or our children or grandchildren, could have a catastrophic illness that could wipe out our savings. There could be a terrible depression in America that reduces the value of our investments and other assets. With interest rates being so low, we would have to dip into our capital. That would be like burning the planks of a sinking ship for fuel.
>
> **Stuart Yudofsky:** Are you afraid of something happening unexpectedly that would leave you destitute, like what occurred with the death of your father?
>
> **Maynard:** Yes, that's a real fear of mine. And it's hard for others to understand unless you've been dirt poor and hungry at some point in your life.

My patients who have undergone tragic life events such as the loss of a young child through illness or accident have shared with me their distress when well-intentioned friends say something like, "I understand how painful your loss must be." The bereft parents will comment, "We get that they mean well; but comments like this infuriate us. There is no way possible that they can understand what it means to have lost a child without having lost one of their own." Gratuitous comments of understanding by well-intended mental health practitioners are even less favorably received.

> **Stuart Yudofsky:** I won't pretend to understand what you are feeling, Maynard. I have not personally experienced prolonged

hunger or poverty. But let's do our best to examine the implications of your financial assumptions—from both psychological and economic perspectives. Would you consider involving Elizabeth in this discussion as well?

Maynard Henden: Yes. Clearly, I have strong feelings about the differences in our backgrounds. And I bet that she does too.

In subsequent meetings Elizabeth and Maynard discussed financial issues in their marriage and related to retirement. The couple expressed strong feelings and issues that they had never previously broached in their marriage. Maynard disclosed his deep-seated and hurt feelings that Dr. Poole never fully accepted him into the family because of his impoverished background. At first highly defensive and protective of her doting father, Elizabeth ultimately accepted the validity of her husband's feelings and beliefs. She also made the compelling argument that because she, her mother, and her brothers loved, admired, and accepted Maynard fully, his unbalanced focus on her father reflected his own insecurities and prejudices about his background—not theirs. The differences in Maynard's and Elizabeth's socioeconomic backgrounds and experiences also helped explain their divergent attitudes toward retirement and taking risks. Never having been poor and hungry, Elizabeth was less fearful than her husband of that occurring in their futures.

> **Elizabeth Henden:** Maynard is afraid of change. He would've never considered looking into the job in Dallas had I not encouraged him to do so. Now he can't bear to leave it. I'm beginning to understand that he *truly* believes that the sky will fall down on all of us if he makes any changes whatsoever. No wonder he has essentially been doing the same thing for the last 40 years.

On my recommendation, Maynard and Elizabeth sought the advice of a financial planning specialist in Dallas. The advisor concluded that with the inclusion of Elizabeth's assets, the couple had substantially more resources than they had calculated—in excess of what would be required to support long, comfortable lives.

Aspirations for Retirement

Many people have unrealistic expectations for their retirements. They believe that the sources of their stress and anxieties are exclusively related to their work, from which their retirement will be a lifelong solution and reprieve. By anticipating and *expecting* that their retirements will be endless, sun-drenched, fun-filled vacations, they have set themselves up for bitter disappointments. They have neglected to anticipate that their difficult relationships with their spouses and children might intensify with increased contact; that their unhealthful and unsavory habits and personality traits will persist; that their health might decline—gradually or precipitously; that they will feel bored, unstimulated, dispassionate, and irrelevant without the challenges of work; and that they will overdose on the daily pursuit of the pastimes that were enjoyable in smaller servings and when fitted into weekends and holidays.

Having waited her entire marriage for Maynard to prioritize her and their children over his work, Elizabeth looked forward to Maynard's retirement as an opportunity to spend extended time with her husband when he wasn't distracted and exhausted by the demands of his job. She believed that her love and admiration for him and the newfound opportunity to spend more time with their children would be sufficient to sustain him in retirement. Elizabeth did not appreciate that her family experience and, thus, her needs were vastly different from those of Maynard, who had become dependent on a work environment suffused with admiration and affirmation—all in an unconscious attempt to fill the void left by the loss of his father.

> **Maynard Henden:** I had a dream last night that I'd like to share with you, Stuart.
> *I was in our university's new natatorium. It was just completed and is one of the best swimming venues in the country. We are very proud of it. I was at the deep end of the pool with the lead architect on the project. He was wearing a hard hat and white lab coat. We were inspecting the diving well. He asked me to climb up to check out the diving platform with him. The next thing you know I am up there alone standing blindfolded on the edge of the 10-meter diving platform. It's really not a blindfold, but an executioner's mask; you know, the type that covers the entire head. I am somewhat afraid of heights in general, and I am particularly terrified at this point. From the deck of the pool, the architect starts yelling, "Jump, Maynard! Jump down!" But I wasn't sure whether or not the pool had been filled up with water yet. I couldn't remove my blindfold, and there would be no way that I could find the stairs to climb back down to the deck. So I was stuck. The only thing I could do was to jump. I woke up at that point in a state of panic.*

It's one of the weirdest dreams I've ever had, Dr. Y. What do you think it means?

After a succession of questions about the dream and Maynard's associations to it, we agreed that the dream represented his unconscious and conscious fears and conflicts about retirement.

> **Stuart Yudofsky:** At best, your dream reveals that you regard retirement as something you won't be able to deal with—that you would be over your head. At worst, you feel that retirement is a rapid route to death—in the same way that many elderly people view being placed in a nursing home. Certainly, the architect who is wearing the white lab coat represents me, Maynard. Apparently, you experience me as encouraging you to take *a blind leap of faith*—a leap that would lead to sudden disaster and death. A leap that I seemingly don't want to take myself.
> One more thing. For the first time in a long while, Maynard, you just addressed me as "Dr. Y." I am no longer your friend and colleague "Stuart" but now both the architect and executioner of your retirement.

Because Maynard had never seriously thought about or sought retirement prior to Elizabeth's insistence that he do so, his fears far exceeded any aspirations he might have held. He would be moving from his secure, familiar, and reinforcing terrain to a murky destination that was unknown, unexplored, and, by and large, unwanted. For Maynard, retiring was equivalent to taking a blind leap of faith from a high-diving platform into an unfinished pool that may or may not have water.

> **Stuart Yudofsky:** My job is not to tell you what to do, Maynard, but to help you remove the blindfold so that *you* can determine for *yourself* what is in *your* best interest. In arriving at this determination, you should consider as many variables as you can think of related to retirement—including Elizabeth's expectations for your relationship with her and your children. You should also fully explore your retirement options. Only then can you make a decision that won't have a disastrous outcome. That will be an important focus of our work going forward.

Options for Retirement

In considering retirement, Maynard had three basic options from which to choose:

1. To continue in his current position—or *not* to retire
2. To relinquish fully his position—or to retire *entirely*
3. To relinquish selected aspects of his position—or to retire *partially*

Each option had distinct implications for his psychological status, his relationships, and for how and where he would live. Systematically, Maynard and I carefully explored each option and the full range of its respective implications. We paid particularly close attention to the everyday demands of his position as university president.

> **Maynard Henden:** I haven't asked myself what I really want to do since I was 15 years old. That was when I decided that I wanted to be a minister. Once that decision was made, one thing sort of led to the next. And here I am. Also, I never really asked myself if I were *enjoying* doing what I was doing. For the last 50 years, enjoyment has been a distant and abstract concept for me—something that applied to *other people*—but certainly never to me.
>
> **Stuart Yudofsky:** In our discussions, you have been quite clear what you like and what you dislike about your current position. For example, you like the influence and admiration associated with being university president, but you don't enjoy the many administrative headaches, political hassles, and ceremonial responsibilities of the job. Also, Maynard, you don't believe you have the *right* or the *power* to do what you want or enjoy. In actuality, you *do* have the power to decide what you want to do. However, you can't have everything that you want. There are trade-offs inherent in staying in your job—the politics, meetings, and political hassles—as there will be with any decision that you make to change your role at the university—which will involve a loss in your power and influence.

Table 14–1 summarizes retirement considerations that Maynard and I explored in his therapy.

TABLE 14–1. Topics to consider prior to retirement

The role of employment and position in identity, sense of self-worth, and self-esteem

Psychological and symbolic significances of retirement

Likes and dislikes about current employment

Current interests and enjoyment outside of work

Fears about retirement

Aspirations for retirement

Options for retirement

The Case of Reverend Maynard Henden: D2 (Decision) and D3 (Discipline) Components

Key Features of How Maynard Henden Is Stuck in Pause

1. *How Maynard is stuck:* He wants to please his wife and enjoy life but is fearful of transitioning from his full-time work to retirement
2. *Goal for change:* Enjoyment of both his professional and his personal life
3. *Central, unresolved conflicts* (approach-approach): Wants the power and prestige of his position; wants to enjoy life and please his wife and family
4. *Hallmarks of Maynard's being stuck:* Exhaustion, irritability, anxiety, marital problems, confusion, impaired perspective, diminished enjoyment
5. *Binary problem/solution:* Prioritizing work versus prioritizing self and family
6. *Critical decision points:* Retire from university presidency; establish balance between profession and family
7. *Corollary factors required to achieve resolution:* Work on relationships with wife and children; cultivate interests outside of profession; make structural changes in lifestyle in order to travel with wife and spend more time with family; continue with psychotherapy to help him and Elizabeth with transition

8. *Resolution:* Meet with the university's Board of Trustees to relinquish presidency and negotiate part-time position; work with wife to structure a lifestyle that includes more leisure, pleasure, and family time

Taking the Leap

Maynard ultimately determined that the best course for him was to let go of his presidency and to petition the university's Board of Trustees to permit him to work part time. He would ask to move back to the Divinity School, where he would teach, do research, and provide spiritual counseling in hospital settings. He would also agree to be available to the Board of Trustees to assist the university with fund-raising and community relations.

Once Maynard had *decided* to seek part-time retirement, his next task was to exhibit the Power of Go by scheduling a meeting with Mr. Neil Jamison, chairman of the university's Board of Trustees, to relinquish his position as president and to request to work part time. He was apprehensive about doing so.

> **Maynard Henden:** The board is going to be furious with me. I have already indicated to them that I would sign on for 5 more years, and they have made all kinds of plans based on what I have committed to do.
> **Stuart Yudofsky:** Let's assume that you are correct about how the board will *feel* about your decision; what do you think they will *do* about it?
> **Maynard:** I think that their most likely response will be to fire me on the spot. I will have destroyed their trust in me.

The following dialogue was with Mr. Neil Jamison, president of the university's Board of Trustees.

> **Mr. Neil Jamison:** As a board member, Maynard, I've known you for many years. This is the first time that I've ever heard you ask anything for yourself.
> **Maynard Henden:** I apologize for being so brazenly self-advocating. My wife has been encouraging me to spend more time with the family, and I am starting to become more tired and less efficient. I also think that it's responsible for me to make more definitive plans for my succession.
> **Mr. Jamison:** You don't have to apologize, Maynard. Both as your friend and as a successful businessman, let me tell you some-

thing off the record. Like big corporations, large universities are selfish masters. They serve their own purposes by getting what they can out of their employees. They also have very short memories about what people have accomplished in the past. What you will do for the university in the future is about all that counts. Everyone on the board knows that you are a valuable asset. We also know you work your ass off and don't ask anything for yourself. You have done a great job helping me to place our finances in line. You raised a ton of money for the university and have kept expenses way down. Because you never have asked us for any raises, we haven't given you any. You're pretty much working at the same salary we recruited you here with 25 years ago. So you're one of the lowest paid university presidents in America. You've been a real bargain. I'm going to meet with the executive committee and finance committee of the board and recommend that we give you everything that you asked for. I'm also going to recommend that we give you a small raise right now that will continue until we recruit the next president. That is if you assure us that you will stay on until the new person comes aboard.

The executive committee and, thereafter, the full board approved and funded Mr. Jamison's recommendations. In his therapy, Maynard later discussed his meeting with Mr. Jamison.

Maynard Henden: I know that I should be elated by how well Mr. Jamison treated me. But I've been upset since meeting with him, and I'm not sure why. Probably because he hit the ball squarely into my court. I'm most likely nervous because my retirement is now a reality. Don't you agree, Stuart?

Stuart Yudofsky: Not entirely, Maynard. Although Mr. Jamison was complimentary to you, his remarks about universities were cynical and somewhat dismissive of what you have done with your life.

Maynard: That's it, Stuart. I don't agree with him that universities are selfish and thankless places. And I would hate to think that my only accomplishments have been financial. But that's the only part of my job that he talked about. He really didn't say much about our missions and product. Or about our people. What we do can't be measured in profits and losses. I understand that Mr. Jamison doesn't have to give so much of his time and treasure to our university. And I assume that he does so for only good reasons. But why is he so cynical?

Stuart: Let me tell you about "Yudofsky's Law."

Yudofsky's Law
People tend to overvalue what *they* do and to judge others by what *they* do best.

Mr. Jamison is a successful Dallas venture capitalist who has acquired, restructured, and sold many large businesses. During the 6 years that he was chairman of the university's Board of Trustees, he had worked hard to increase the university's operational efficiency and fiscal stability. The university had moved from running a small annual deficit to one with a positive annual operating balance of many millions of dollars. Together with a successful capital campaign and his own generous contributions, Mr. Jamison had doubled the university's endowment in 5 years. This enabled the university to recruit many talented research and teaching faculty and to expand the campus. Mr. Jamison was widely recognized as one of the nation's most successful university board chairmen.

One of Mr. Jamison's favorite sayings was

We're a *not-for-profit* university. But we're also a *not-for-loss* university.

The downside of Mr. Jamison's leadership was that he tended to view and value the university and Maynard's contributions exclusively through the lens of finances. He evaluated Maynard by his success in maintaining financial discipline among the university's faculty and staff, by his ability to inspire philanthropists and to bring in donations, and by the annual increases in dollar totals of federal grants to the university that occurred under his leadership.

Although Mr. Jamison was a consummate manager, he had little interest in the intellectual or social product of the university. What Mr. Jamison did *not* recognize about Maynard was

- His rare intellectual brilliance spanning both the humanities and the sciences that garnered the respect of the faculty and students
- His honest, warm, caring, and compassionate nature that engendered the loyalty, trust, and commitment of faculty, staff, students, and the Dallas community
- His charisma as a tall, model-handsome scholar-athlete whom central casting of a Hollywood movie studio would have selected for the part of a great leader

Without Maynard's leadership, the faculty, staff, and students of the university would have become demoralized by the fiscal harshness and hardships imposed by Mr. Jamison. The most capable faculty, staff, and students would have left the university for greener pastures, and Mr. Jamison would have certainly failed as chairman of the university's Board of Trustees.

Completing the Course

An additional task requiring the Power of Go was for Maynard to engage in regular couples counseling to work out the logistical details of his partial retirement.

> **Elizabeth Henden:** I don't know what "partial retirement" means, Maynard. Just giving up being president and going back to work at the Divinity School probably won't change a thing. When you were "just" a professor at Columbia, you still worked all the time.
>
> **Maynard Henden:** You're right, Elizabeth. I don't trust myself either. I'm vulnerable to working just as hard as ever, even though I will have a part-time job. What do you suggest, Stuart?
>
> **Stuart Yudofsky:** What do you think about limiting the time you spend at the university to 3 days a week? For example, you would go to your office on campus only on Tuesdays, Wednesdays, and Thursdays. That would be 60%, and it would still leave 4 consecutive days a week for you to do things that aren't work related. Alternatively, you could arrange to have several months of vacation time each year so that you and Elizabeth could travel together or do anything else that you might want to do together. How does that sound?
>
> **Maynard:** Sounds absolutely frightening. But I *should* go along with it. No, I *will* do it. Isn't that what you mean by the Power of Go, Stuart?
>
> **Elizabeth:** It sounds like a plan that I can live with too. Anyway, it will have to do for now—until Maynard "sees the light" and retires altogether.

For the first time in his adult life, Maynard did not organize each day of his life with school or work-related classes, meetings, and deadlines. Initially, he found this new state of affairs to be disorienting and anxiety provoking.

> **Maynard Henden:** I wake up on the days that I don't go in to work, and I'm not sure what I am going to do with my time. Nothing

is hanging over my head that I have to get done that day—or feel that I'm going to fail at something. That form of anxiety has been replaced by my overriding dread that something terrible will happen on that day—probably as punishment.

Stuart Yudofsky: Punishment for what?

Maynard: I don't know. Maybe because I'm not earning my right to live another day.

Stuart: If someone were to say that to you in your role as a minister, how would you respond?

Maynard: I would say that it says in the Good Book, "This is the day the Lord hath made; let us be glad and rejoice in it." We are commanded to celebrate each new day as a gift from God. I would add that only God can grant the gift of another day of life to mankind—we don't earn it.

To Maynard's great surprise, he rapidly grew to enjoy the times that he did not have to go in to work. He began to develop a broad range of avocational interests, most of which he shared with Elizabeth. After 3 years of partial retirement, he decided to retire in full. The university took advantage of the occasion to honor Maynard with a record-breaking fund-raising benefit. (Mr. Jamison was not entirely wrong.)

Elizabeth and Maynard sold their home in Dallas and purchased a condominium apartment in New York to be closer to their children and grandchildren and their many friends from the years that they had lived there. Maynard began spending extensive amounts of time with his grandchildren.

> **Maynard Henden:** Elizabeth was so right. I was never "in the moment" when our children were young. My mind was always somewhere else—invariably work related. Now I look forward to and cherish every second that I can be with our sons and grandchildren. Next to being with Elizabeth, it's the most important thing that I do. I should say, "it's the most important thing that I *am*: father and grandfather."

Although Maynard had initially looked forward to writing succeeding editions of his two standard textbooks on spiritual counseling in palliative care, he decided to turn the task over to younger colleagues. "I'm done with deadlines," he reasoned.

Elizabeth reestablished her ties with UNICEF, and she and Maynard spent 3 months each year in the field in Africa to help stem the

AIDS epidemic in young people. Maynard joined the voluntary faculty at Columbia Medical School and taught palliative care to divinity and medical students and to resident physicians of many specialties. Additionally, he volunteered as a spiritual counselor and preacher at the same small church in Greenwich Village where he did his pioneering work 30 years earlier with gay men who had contracted AIDS. "I finally feel like the small-town minister that I set out to become in the first place," he noted.

Although they did extensive volunteer work, Elizabeth and Maynard also took ample time to have fun. They traveled extensively and especially enjoyed attending summer Shakespeare festivals in various cities in the United States, Canada, and England. Maynard began to share Elizabeth's interest in—and, later, passion for—collecting rare furniture that was manufactured in the colonial South. Scholarly by nature, he read extensively on the subject and soon gained expertise in the field that rivaled that of his wife, who is a lifetime collector.

Maynard also began to play golf more frequently.

> **Maynard Henden:** I'd never really *enjoyed* playing golf. I was just good at it. My father put a lot of pressure on me when I played. Certainly, that was never much fun. As you explained, Stuart, I began to believe that his death was associated with my not playing perfectly. Somehow, that all changed after I went into semiretirement. When the head coach of the university golf team became sick, I was asked to fill in for a few months as the assistant coach. After so many years, I got immersed in the game again. To my surprise I began to really enjoy golf—probably for the first time in my life. I think the psychotherapy actually helped.
>
> **Stuart Yudofsky:** Can you imagine that?

Elizabeth and Maynard began to play both golf and tennis together regularly. Additionally, Maynard began to compete with great success in age group amateur golf tournaments. Several years after they moved back to New York, I received a phone call from Elizabeth.

> **Elizabeth Henden:** Maynard is going to be in Houston to compete in the Senior Games National Championships. He noticed that you qualified for quite a few swimming events. Would you mind if he comes by to watch you swim?

Stuart Yudofsky: I have a better idea. Why don't I watch Maynard play? He's the true athlete.

Elizabeth: I'm sure that will be fine with him. I'm sorry that I won't be able to join you both at the golf game. One of our grandchildren is in a soccer tournament, and she expects Grandma to be there.

I went to the golf course to watch Maynard's match. Although Maynard was 70 years old at the time, he was in a foursome of 50-year-old golfers with handicaps equivalent to his. By the final hole, Maynard's score was sufficiently low for him not only to win his age group but also to be in the running to win the entire tournament. This had never before been done by someone of his age. Maynard was left with a difficult 20-foot putt for the win, which he sank. Afterward, Maynard came to the edge of the green where I was standing.

Maynard Henden: Hi, Stuart. Thank you for coming by. I have missed you…. I saw your smiling face right before I took that last putt. I couldn't help but think of my Dad, who was always standing right where you were. Only he would have been frowning.

Stuart Yudofsky: Congratulations on your win, Maynard. I don't know a lot about golf, but I *do* know that your father would have been proud of how you completed the course. I also know that he would have been *very* proud of you.

Maynard: Thanks, Stuart. You know how much that means to me. By the way, what have you been doing these days?

Stuart: Pretty much the same things that I have been doing for a long time. I'm still a department chairman and have ever-increasing administrative demands. I try, often without success, to find time to do what I love most—patient care, teaching, writing, and being with my family.

Maynard: As an ordained minister, I have the right to advise you to practice what you preach, Stuart.

Stuart: Are you saying that I should take my own medicine?

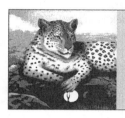

Appendix

Treatment Principles

The treatment principles that appear in in this appendix are from the case examples that appear in chapters throughout the book. These principles highlight special concepts of and approaches to treatment that apply to most patients in psychotherapy.

Treatment Principles

Treatment Principle 1 (*Chapter 4*)
Patients frequently seek psychiatric treatment for symptoms such as anxiety and depression that they do not directly connect to their being stuck in pause. Often they are unaware of being stuck in pause. In the course of assessment and treatment, patients become aware of where they are and how they became stuck. At that point patients have the opportunity to decide to become unstuck and exercise the discipline and behaviors necessary to bring that about.

Treatment Principle 2 (*Chapter 4*)
Effective treatment is a two-step dance: learn and do. Insight and understanding about the problem and its causes are important but insufficient. The application of this knowledge in life to effect change is essential. To do the former without the latter is more an intellectual exercise than anything that is useful, practical, or, at the end of the day, meaningful. To do the latter without the former is to shoot in the dark: one might get lucky with a "ready-fire-aim" approach, but don't count on it.

Treatment Principle 3 (*Chapter 4*)
People rarely become stuck in pause in a single area or for a single reason. Usually, being stuck is the result of the interaction of a multiplicity of biological predispositions, prior and current experiential issues and stresses, and psychosocial dynamics. In addition, patients often have two different but related psychological and medical disorders. Examples include major depressive disorder and alcohol use disorder or antisocial personality disorder and traumatic brain injury. In treatment, the individual contributing issues of each condition must be identified and their sources must be discovered. The role of each causal factor as well as the interplay of the individual factors must be understood and addressed in the process of becoming unstuck.

Treatment Principle 4 (*Chapter 4*)
Psychiatric disorders such as depressive disorders and bipolar disorders distort perceptions and cloud judgment, so major life decisions such as changing jobs, leaving a spouse, quitting school, moving to a different state, and the like must be deferred until the condition is successfully treated. Because these disorders are, in large measure, brain disorders, one cannot count on making rational decisions using a "broken brain."

Treatment Principle 5 (*Chapter 4*)
Educating patients about what is known scientifically and what is unknown about their psychiatric disorder and psychiatric treatment *prior to the initiation of treatment* is respectful and humane and enhances treatment compliance and response.

Treatment Principles *(continued)*

Treatment Principle 6 *(Chapter 4)*

In the initial stages of treatment, beware of entering into patterns and pacts with patients that replicate their central unconscious conflicts and dynamics that perpetuate their symptoms and dysfunctions. Early in treatment, such pacts and patterns appear to enhance the therapeutic alliance, but they will disable your relationship with your patient over time.

Treatment Principle 7 *(Chapter 4)*

People who are stuck in pause are often unaware of precisely where they are stuck. Determining the central conflict and the critical decision points that must be addressed through the Power of Go will clarify this confusion.

Treatment Principle 8 *(Chapter 4)*

"Catching" patients with inconsistencies in their communications to you or using "treatment ploys" (such as sugar pills) creates distance and distrust between you and your patients, and patients will respond by shutting you out.

Treatment Principle 9 *(Chapter 10)*

Mental health professionals should avoid getting into power struggles over weight and diet with their patients with eating disorders. Such interactions, which are about the patient's need for control, reflect therapeutic attention away from the underlying conflicts that have led to the eating disorders and will interfere with the therapeutic alliance between patient and clinician.

Treatment Principle 10 *(Chapter 10)*

Because eating disorders often reflect patients' conflicts between dependence and autonomy, mental health professionals should avoid assuming the roles of *omniscient advisor* or *decision maker* for their patients.

Treatment Principle 11 *(Chapter 11)*

Humor, when not distracting, is an essential component of psychotherapy. It is a gentle way of providing perspective. *Humorless* treatment is *dead* treatment.

Treatment Principle 12 *(Chapter 13)*

The patient's strengths and assets should always be in the forefront of psychiatric care. Not only should these resources form the basis of the alliance between the patient and clinician but also they must be mobilized and directed to effect therapeutic change.

Treatment Principles *(continued)*

Treatment Principle 13 (*Chapter 14*)

The psychodynamics of personality do not change just because a person makes major situational or behavioral alterations in his or her life—such as finding a new job, moving to a different locale, giving up alcohol, or retiring to spend more time with the family. With important change, however, the "steady-state" of interpersonal relationships can be significantly disrupted. These interpersonal stresses are best anticipated and addressed in treatment before retirement in order to obviate shattered expectations and disastrous unintended consequences.

Index

Page numbers printed in **boldface** type refer to tables or boxes.

Opiates
for treatment of alcohol use
disorder, 301
Overmentalization, 399

Panic disorder, 53–95
DSM-IV-TR diagnosis of, 79
medical/psychiatric diagnoses
of, 76
treatment of, 79–86, 80,
84–86
Parasympathetic nervous system,
14
Parents, 498–503
Pastoral counseling, 489–498
Patient
analytical nature of, 186–187
attractive persona of, 187
competitiveness of, 186, 210
confrontation/avoidance of, 323
exploitation of others, 189–190
history, 443–444
inconsistencies in
communication with, 90–
93
insight from treatment, 85–86
oversensitivity, 322
perfectionism, 323
presentation of history, 27–28
psychiatric care of, 227–241
psychiatric history of, 59–75,
255–285
"reading" people, 187
standard psychiatric history and
treatment plan, 26–29, **29**
strengths as a gateway to
treatment and change, 73–
75, 475
transition difficulties of, 323–
324
treatment plan for, 26–29, **B29**
victim mentality of, 323
Pause, ix–x
3-D diet and, 147–177
case example of, 86–87

hallmarks of being stuck in, **26**
key elements of being stuck in,
137, 224, 232, 315–316,
385, 460–461, 532–533, **42**
key principles for getting
unstuck, **43**
Personality disorders, 332. *See also*
Narcissistic personality
disorder
comorbidity with traumatic
brain injury, 233–234
psychiatric treatment of, 235
Pharmacology, for treatment of
alcohol use disorder, 296–297,
301
Pleasing
common features of people who
are stuck in pleasing others,
384
guidelines and techniques to
overcome overpleasing
others and underpleasing
yourself, **396**
how to overcome overpleasing
others and underpleasing
yourself, **395**
need to please, 381, 383–385
stuck in, 380–381
Stuck in Pleasing Scale, **382–
383**D
Pornography, 477–478. *See also*
Internet gaming disorder
Power of No and the Power of Go,
23–52, 533
3-D diet and, 134–136
application of, 51
with autism spectrum disorder,
461–462, 479–480
case example of, 88–94
definitions of, 37
discipline and, 385–386
getting unstuck through, 316–
321
key elements of being stuck in
pause, **42**